AAOS

Symposium on

Sports medicine: the knee

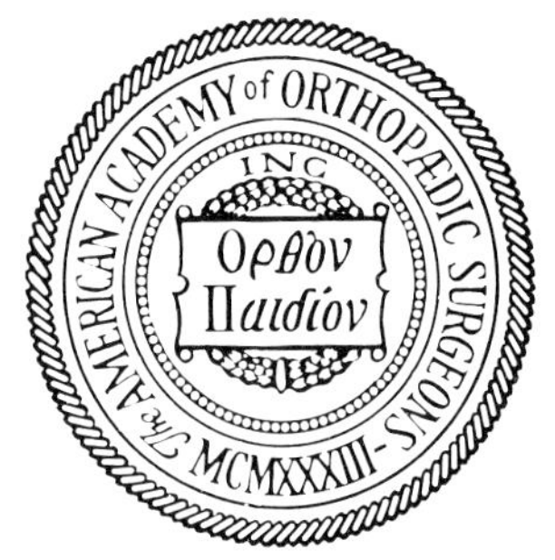

American Academy
of
Orthopaedic Surgeons

Symposium on
Sports medicine: the knee

Denver, Colorado
April, 1982

Edited by

Gerald Finerman, M.D.
Professor of Orthopaedic Surgery,
Department of Orthopaedic Surgery,
School of Medicine, Center for the Health Sciences,
University of California, Los Angeles, Los Angeles, California

with 154 illustrations

The C. V. Mosby Company

ST. LOUIS • TORONTO • PRINCETON   1985

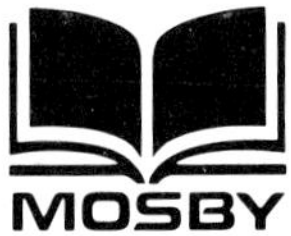

A TRADITION OF PUBLISHING EXCELLENCE

Acquisition editor: Eugenia A. Klein
Assistant editor: Jean F. Carey
Editing supervisor: Elaine Steinborn
Manuscript editor: Carol Sullivan Wiseman
Design: Staff
Production: Gail Morey Hudson, Mary Stueck, Barbara Merritt

The C.V. Mosby Company
11830 Westline Industrial Drive, St. Louis, Missouri 63146

Library of Congress Cataloging in Publication Data

Symposium on Sports Medicine, The Knee (1982: Denver, Colo.)
Symposium on Sports Medicine, The Knee.

Sponsored by American Academy of Orthopaedic Surgeons and National Institutes of Health.
Bibliography: p.
Includes index.
1. Knee—Wounds and injuries—Congresses. 2. Sports—Accidents and injuries—Congresses. 3. Sports medicine—Congresses. I. Finerman, Gerald. II. American Academy of Orthopaedic Surgeons. III. National Institutes of Health (U.S.) IV. Title.
[DNLM: 1. Knee Injuries—Congresses. 2. Athletic Injuries—Congresses. WE 870 S9895s 1982]
RD561.S952   1982   617'.582   84-18955
ISBN   0-8016-0025-1

GW/MV/MV   9 8 7 6 5 4 3 2 1   05/C/608

Contributors

Wayne H. Akeson, M.D.

Acting Chairman, Department of Surgery, Professor and Head, Divison of Orthopaedics and Rehabilitation, Department of Surgery, University of California, San Diego, San Diego, California

David Amiel, M.S., Dip. Ing.

Division of Orthopaedics and Rehabilitation, University of California, San Diego, San Diego, California

Thomas P. Andriacchi, Ph.D.

Associate Professor and Director, Section of Orthopaedic Research, Department of Orthopaedic Surgery, Rush-Presbyterian-St. Luke's Medical Center, Chicago, Illinois

Cecil G. Armstrong, Ph.D.

Department of Mechanical and Industrial Engineering, Ashby Institute, Belfast, Northern Ireland

Steven Paul Arnoczky, D.V.M., Dipl. A.C.V.S.

Associate Professor of Surgery (Orthopedics), Cornell University Medical College; Director, Laboratory of Comparative Orthopedics, The Hospital for Special Surgery, New York, New York

David L. Butler, Ph.D.

Associate Professor, Department of Aerospace Engineering and Applied Mechanics; Research Associate Professor, Department of Orthopaedic Surgery, University of Cincinnati, Cincinnati, Ohio

H. Edward Cabaud, M.D.

Assistant Clinical Professor of Orthopaedics, University of California, San Francisco; Research Orthopaedic Surgeon, Letterman Army Institute of Research, San Francisco, California

William G. Clancy, Jr., M.D.

Associate Professor of Orthopedic Surgery and Head Team Physician and Team Orthopedic Surgeon, University of Wisconsin, Madison, Wisconsin

J. Michael Donohue, M.D.

Resident, Department of Orthopedic Surgery, University of Minnesota, Minneapolis, Minnesota

John A. Feagin, M.D.

Orthopaedic Surgeon, St. John's Hospital, Jackson, Wyoming

Cyril B. Frank, M.D.

Assistant Professor, Department of Surgery, University of Calgary, Calgary, Alberta, Canada

James G. Garrick, M.D.

Director, Center for Sports Medicine, St. Francis Memorial Hospital, San Francisco, California

Philip D. Gollnick, Ph.D.

Professor of Physiology, Department of Comparative Anatomy, Physiology, and Pharmacology, College of Veterinary Medicine, Washington State University, Pullman, Washington

Edward S. Grood, Ph.D.

Associate Professor of Orthopaedic Surgery Research, Department of Orthopaedic Surgery, University of Cincinnati, Cincinnati, Ohio

Wilson C. Hayes, Ph.D.

Associate Professor and Director, Orthopedic Biomechanics Laboratory, Department of Orthopedic Surgery, Beth Israel Hospital and Harvard Medical School, Boston, Massachusetts

James A. Hill, M.D.

Associate, Department of Orthopaedic Surgery, Northwestern University, Chicago, Illinois

Helmut H. Huberti, M.D.

Orthopaedic Surgeon, Department of Orthopaedic Surgery, University of Heidelberg, Heidelberg, West Germany

Murali Jasty, M.D.

Clinical Instructor, Department of Orthopedic Surgery, Harvard Medical School; Assistant in Orthopedics, Massachusetts General Hospital, Boston, Massachusetts

Gary M. Kramer, B.S.

Research Assistant, Department of Orthopaedic Surgery, Rush-Presbyterian-St. Luke's Medical Center, Chicago, Illinois

Glenn C. Landon, M.D.

Assistant Professor, Department of Orthopaedic Surgery, Rush-Presbyterian-St. Luke's Medical Center, Chicago, Illinois

Robert L. Larson, M.D.

Orthopaedic Consultant, Athletic Department, University of Oregon, Eugene, Oregon

William D. Lew, M.S.

Research Engineer, Rehabilitation Engineering Program, Department of Orthopaedic Surgery, Northwestern University, Chicago, Illinois

Jack L. Lewis, Ph.D.

Professor, Department of Civil Engineering and Orthopaedic Surgery, Northwestern University, Chicago, Illinois

Keith L. Markolf, Ph.D.

Adjunct Associate Professor, Department of Orthopaedic Surgery, University of California, Los Angeles, Los Angeles, California

Van C. Mow, Ph.D.

Clark and Crossan Professor of Engineering, Department of Mechanical Engineering, Aeronautical Engineering and Mechanics, Rensselaer Polytechnic Institute, Troy, New York

Elizabeth R. Myers, Ph.D.

NATO Postdoctoral Fellow, Kennedy Institute of Rheumatology, London, England

Frank R. Noyes, M.D.

Clinical Professor, Department of Orthopaedic Surgery, University of Cincinnati Medical Center; Director, Cincinnati Sports Medicine and Orthopaedic Center, Cincinnati, Ohio

Theodore R. Oegema, Jr., Ph.D.

Associate Professor, Department of Orthopedic Surgery and Department of Biochemistry, University of Minnesota, Minneapolis, Minnesota

William G. Rodkey, D.V.M., Dipl. A.C.V.S.

Chief, Operative Services Group, Letterman Army Institute of Research, Presidio of San Francisco, San Francisco, California

George T. Shybut, M.D.

Associate, Department of Orthopaedic Surgery, Northwestern University, Chicago, Illinois

Peter Snell, Ph.D.

Instructor, Pauline and Adolph Weinberger Laboratory for Cardiopulmonary Research, Department of Internal Medicine, University of Texas Health Science Center, Dallas, Texas

Roby C. Thompson, Jr., M.D.

Professor and Chairman, Department of Orthopedic Surgery, University of Minnesota, Minneapolis, Minnesota

Russell F. Warren, M.D.

Associate Professor, Department of Orthopedic Surgery, Cornell Medical School; Director of Sports Medicine, The Hospital for Special Surgery, New York, New York

Carl R. Wirth, M.D.

Professor of Orthopaedic Surgery, Division of Orthopaedic Surgery, The Albany Medical College of Union University, Albany, New York

Savio L.-Y. Woo, Ph.D.

Professor of Surgery and Bioengineering, Division of Orthopaedic Surgery, Department of Surgery, University of California, San Diego, San Diego, California

Preface

The fitness explosion in this country has resulted in the public's increasing involvement in recreational sports. Unfortunately, an estimated 25 million people are injured each year while participating in these recreational activities. Studies indicate that the knee is the most commonly injured area of the body and possibly accounts for over 45% of sports-related injuries.

This course, sponsored jointly by the American Academy of Orthopaedic Surgeons and the National Institutes of Health, was held in Denver, Colorado, April 30-May 2, 1982, in an effort to bring together the most current scientific and clinical sports medicine research relating specifically to knee injuries. The authors' presentations stress meniscal injuries, ligamentous instability, and cartilage damage. Biomechanical information with relevant basic science is included, as well as a discussion of surgical techniques and alternative treatments.

As chairman of this symposium, I wish to thank the authors for their generous efforts in preparing this course and these papers.

Gerald Finerman, M.D.

Contents

PART ONE

Functional principles

1. Physiologic basis for athletic training

Peter Snell

Human physical performance depends on a large number of physical, psychologic, and environmental factors (Fig. 1-1). These factors affect performance to an extent that is largely determined by the nature of the task to be accomplished. Training programs are generally designed for the specific requirements of a particular athletic

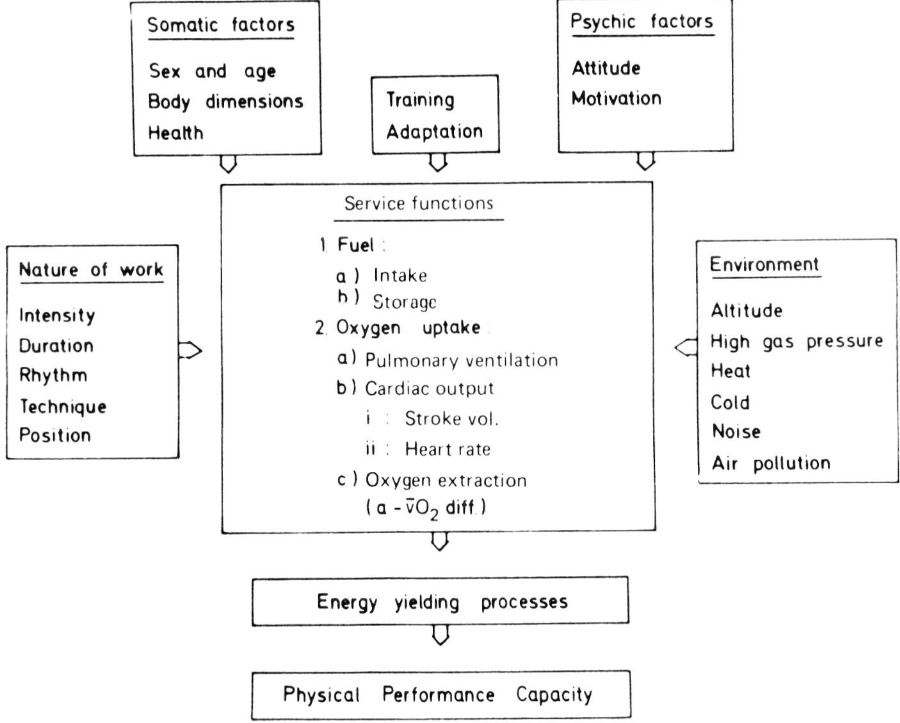

Fig. 1-1. Factors affecting physical performance capacity. (From Astrand, P.O., and Rodahl., K.: Textbook of work physiology, New York, 1970, McGraw-Hill, Inc.)

event. Because athletic performance has multiple determinants, understanding, measuring, and evaluating the relative contribution of each physical component should lead to a more rational approach to training.

Historically, coaches and athletes assess speed, strength, and endurance by using empirically derived criteria. This approach has been successful, since few insights or training innovations originated from physiology laboratories; instead researchers have been active in documenting the physical characteristics of individuals who are successful in various sports. These studies include descriptions of anthropometric features[15,60] and measurement of physiologic function.[11,16,49,52] While these studies have been important in identifying the physical qualities needed for top-level performance, the goal of research now tends toward a better understanding of the nature of the adaptive response, the mechanisms involved in fatigue, and the means by which physiologic function and characteristics may be modified.

Although the development of endurance in running and cycling has been most studied in the laboratory, the principles offered here may be applied to other endurance activities such as swimming, rowing, and cross-country skiing.

METABOLIC COMPONENTS OF PERFORMANCE

Muscular contraction requires energy in the form of adenosine triphosphate (ATP), and performance in any running event may be considered in terms of the amount of ATP that the athlete produces and uses during the race. ATP production involves processes that will ultimately require oxygen. Therefore the ability of the body to use oxygen and to acquire an *oxygen debt* provides a means of assessing the capacity for energy production.

Aerobic metabolism

The relationship between oxygen uptake ($\dot{V}O_2$) and increasing levels of work is linear until reaching a point when increases in the work rate do not result in any increase in $\dot{V}O_2$ (Fig. 1-2). This plateau of $\dot{V}O_2$ indicates the maximal rate of total body use of oxygen, and in healthy persons it is limited by the capacity of the oxygen transport system to deliver oxygen to the working muscles.[44,45,51,58,61] The primary factor in oxygen transport is the cardiac output ($\dot{Q}$), and a high $\dot{Q}$ depends on a high stroke volume. Data from world class middle-distance and long-distance runners.[49,54,62] indicate that values in excess of 70 ml/kg/min are needed for success. This corresponds to a running speed of approximately 350/min or 4½ min/mile. Thus events up to 3000 meters are run at speeds equal to or greater than that necessary to elicit max $\dot{V}O_2$.

Although a high max $\dot{V}O_2$ (also known as maximal aerobic power) is an important factor in endurance performance, the limits will be set by the aerobic capacity. This capacity is the total quantity of oxygen that can be used for the duration of an event. In essence, it depends on the $\dot{V}O_2$ that is maintained without provoking excessive anaerobic metabolism and the rate of rise of $\dot{V}O_2$ to this level.[26] During maximal

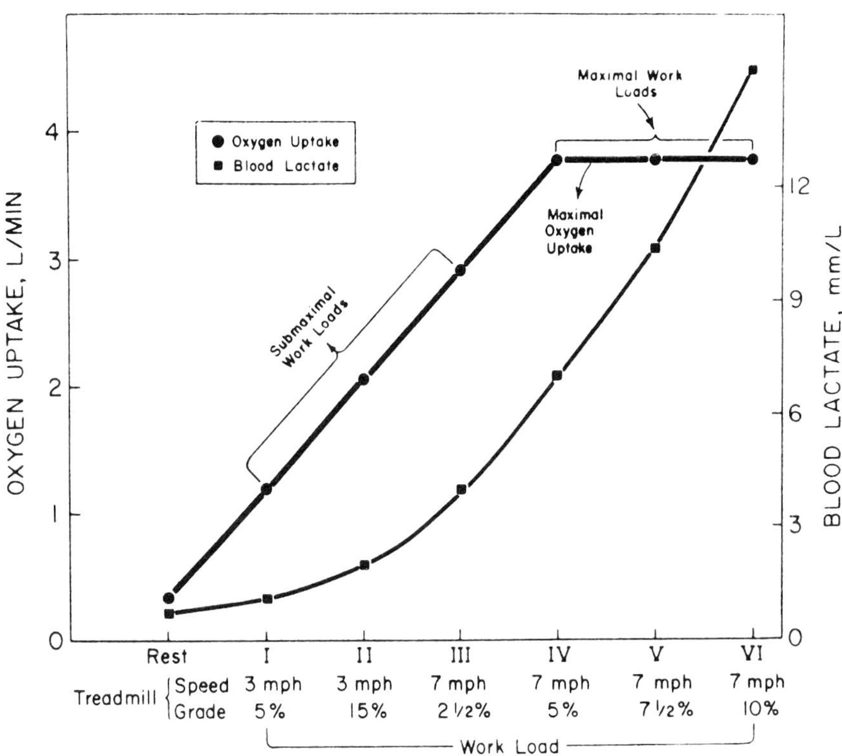

Fig. 1-2. Oxygen uptake and blood lactate response in subject running at increasing speed and grade on treadmill. (From Mitchell, J.H., and Blomqvist, C.G.: N. Engl. J. Med. **284:**1018, 1971.

work, the energy-producing substrate is almost exclusively muscle glycogen,[22] but as work becomes prolonged, plasma free fatty acids (FFA) released from adipose tissue play a major role with an additional contribution of glucose released from the liver.[28] Generally, in well-trained individuals substrates do not limit performance in races up to 1½ hours' duration when depletion of muscle glycogen may become a factor.

For events of shorter duration the time an athlete is able to sustain max $\dot{V}O_2$, or a high percentage of it, depends on the oxidative capacity of the muscle fibers in use.[19,37] Fibers with high oxidative capacity contain a high density of mitochondria and a well-developed capillary supply[14,36] that allows a given submaximal exercise to be performed with less lactate production than when fibers of lower oxidative capacity are recruited. The concept of oxidative capacity is illustrated in Fig. 1-3. In this example max $\dot{V}O_2$ can be sustained for only a brief period, and as the duration of the work is extended the percentage of max $\dot{V}O_2$ that can be used declines. Although this concept has been used to explain variability of performance in distance runners,[8,9]

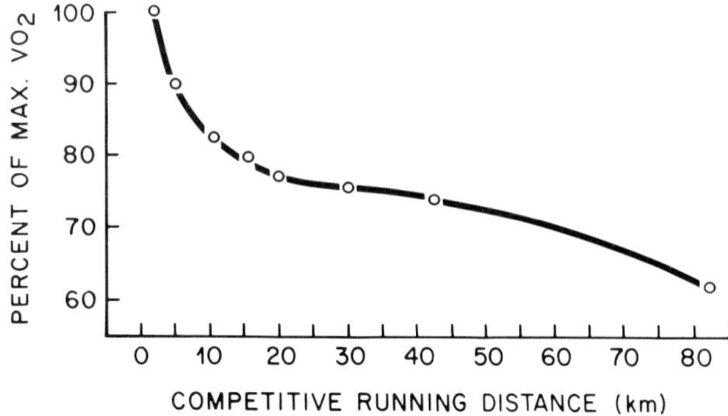

Fig. 1-3. Maximal energy expenditure expressed as percentage of max $\dot{V}O_2$, that may be used by well-trained marathon runners during various distance races. (Modified from Costill, D.L., and Fox, E.L.: Med. Sci. Sports 1:81, 1969.)

it may be relevant for events as brief as 2 to 3 minutes when the oxygen demands are supramaximal.

Anaerobic metabolism

The ability to produce a large amount of energy rapidly and to increase the level of work beyond that which elicits max $\dot{V}O_2$ (Fig. 1-2) is provided by anaerobic pathways. Two systems are important: (1) energy residing in the muscle in the form of ATP and creatine phosphate (CP), which is immediately available for muscle contraction, and (2) energy produced by metabolic pathways that results in the accumulation of an end-product that cannot be readily excreted, such as lactic acid.

Anaerobic power is the rate at which energy can be released over a short period of time. Factors governing the use of ATP are: (1) the number of muscle fibers recruited, (2) the rate of hydrolysis of ATP, and (3) the rate of replenishment of ATP stores. In short bursts of effort, like those in weight lifting, the amount of energy released depends on the cross-sectional area of muscle involved in the task and the ability to recruit a large fraction of the available muscle fibers. In repetitive movements or in single *explosive* movements such as jumping, the rate of ATP hydrolysis will govern the energy release. Individuals who perform well at these activities tend to have muscle comprised of a high percentage of fast-twitch fibers (FT). These fibers have a more rapidly acting enzyme (myofibrillar adenosine triphosphatase [ATPase]) than slow-twitch fibers (ST).

The speed at which ATP can be resynthesized is governed by the rate of glycolysis.[10] Newsholme[47] hypothesizes that individuals who are able to produce energy quickly may have their muscle glycolytic pathways primed for action as a result of *substrate cycles* operating through the rate-limiting step catalyzed by phosphofructokinase in the forward direction and fructose diphosphatase in the reverse direction. Although it is not clear what factors contribute to such a cycle, hormone-induced

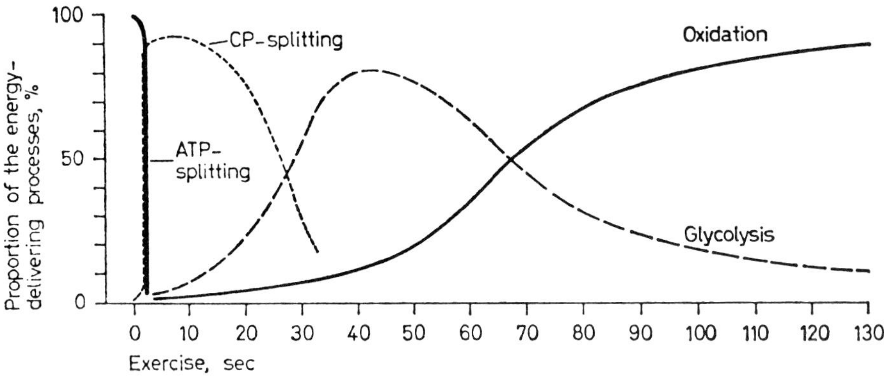

Fig. 1-4. Schematic representation of relative contribution of energy-supply substrates to total energy requirement. (From Keul, J., Doll, E., and Keppler, D.: Energy metabolism of human muscle, Baltimore, 1972, University Park Press.)

increases in the level of cyclic adenosine monophosphate (AMP) in muscle fibers are responsible for the acceleration of glycogenolysis.[10]

Anaerobic capacity also refers to the total amount of energy that may be released in excess of that produced by the complete oxidation of substrates to carbon dioxide and water. Muscle stores of ATP and CP are theoretically capable of providing sufficient energy for approximately 5 seconds of a maximal activity such as sprinting. Glycolysis may sustain maximal energy requirements for another 30 to 40 seconds depending on the state of training. Anaerobic metabolism is probably limited by the lowering of intracellular pH as a consequence of lactic acid production.[32,53]

•   •   •

The relative contribution of aerobic energy and the various sources of anaerobic energy during strenous activity are represented schematically in Fig. 1-4.

DETERMINANTS OF PHYSICAL PERFORMANCE
Heredity

The extent to which athletes are *born* rather than *made* is the subject of long-term debate. It is clear to coaches that there is considerable variability in the adaptation of individuals to similar training programs. Much of our knowledge in this area comes from studies of identical and fraternal twins.[42,43] These studies indicate that performance capacity has a significant genetic component (Fig. 1-5). The possibility does exist, however, that early intervention in the development of an individual may affect the ultimate level of max $\dot{V}O_2$ that may be attained in adulthood.

Age

While it is known that age results in a substantial decline in athletic performance, experience with athletes who maintained good physical condition and remain injury

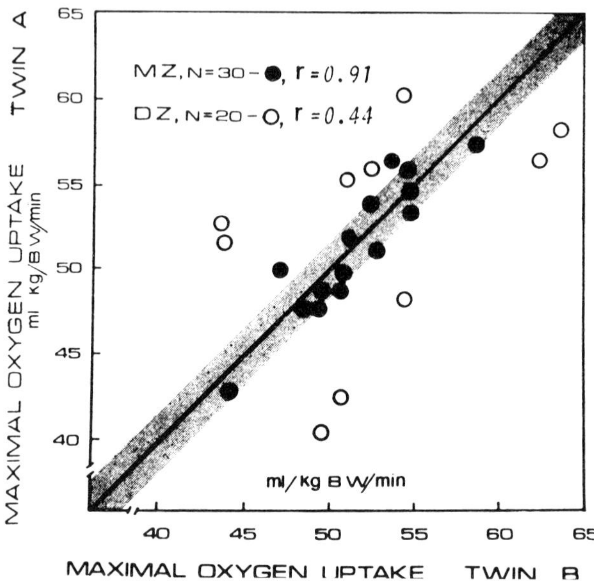

Fig. 1-5. Max $\dot{V}O_2$ in monozygous (filled circles) and dizygous (open circles) twin pairs. (From Klissouras, V.: J. Appl. Physiol. **31**:338, 1971.)

free indicates that a high level of performance can be sustained to a greater age than previously believed. Increasing evidence suggests that a high max $\dot{V}O_2$ may be maintained into the fifth decade.[24,50] Recently Heath and others[29] showed that the differences in max $\dot{V}O_2$ between a group of middle-aged athletes and a group of young athletes could be accounted for by differences in maximal heart rate.

It is interesting that persons over 40 years old are able to compete successfully in international marathon races, yet it is unusual to see an athlete over 30 years old performing well in track events requiring either speed or high levels of oxygen debt.

Environment

Environmental factors exert their effect by altering either the energy requirements of the activity or the amount of energy that the athlete can produce. The major emphasis of studies has been on the effects of temperature and high altitude. With the Olympic Games scheduled for Los Angeles in 1984, concerns have been raised about the effects of air pollution on both health and performance.

Training

The effects of physical training on the cardiovascular system and skeletal muscle are the subject of reviews by Clausen[5], Blomqvist and Saltin[3], and Holloszy and Booth.[34] Generalizations on the degree of adaptation to training are difficult since it depends on the previous history of physical activity and the intensity, frequency, duration, and mode of training.[59] The contribution of physical activity during the developmental years to later physical performance is still unknown. Many of the best athletes do not reach their peak until after several years of training. The nature of long-term physiologic changes has not been resolved, but it is likely that both the peripheral and the central determinants of aerobic capacity are modified.[6,57] A large number of training studies are limited in two important ways: the length of the training period and the intensity of the training.

Efficiency of movement

An important determinant of endurance performance is the energy cost of the task. It is expected that novice runners use more energy at a given running speed. However, a recent study of 12 runners who were highly ranked in a nationally prominent 10-kilometer race found that 65% of the variation in race performance could be explained by a variation in running economy.[7] Little data exist on the energy cost of running at speeds close to maximal, but it appears that at 90% of top speed the oxygen cost of running changes from a linear to an exponential function of speed. This suggests that under certain conditions there is an advantage in training for speed so a smaller percentage of maximal speed is used during the race.

METHODS OF TRAINING

Although a plethora of methods have evolved for the training of competitive runners, there are certain common features that enable these methods to be described as four basic types of training. In this way, complex combinations of intensity, duration, frequency, and recovery period can be reduced to a specific stimulus on body systems[20] and structures that contribute directly or indirectly to improved performance.

Prolonged continuous exercise

Continuous exercise covers a wide variety of running speeds in which the heart rate response (an index of intensity) varies from 130 to 175 beats/min. In young persons exercising in cool conditions, this corresponds to 60% to 85% max $\dot{V}O_2$.

Interval training

Interval running was popularized as a training method in the 1930s by the German 800-meter world-record holder Rudolf Harbig. The method introduced by coach Gerschler and cardiologist Reindell requires periods of effort of 30 to 70 seconds at an intensity that elevates the heart rate to about 180 beats/min. The effort phase is followed by sufficient recovery time to allow the heart rate to return to 120 beats/ min. This method allows the athlete to perform a large volume of work at an intensity similar to that experienced in competition.

Variations on this basic idea have proliferated. In an effort to achieve work that was close to max $\dot{V}O_2$, Saltin and others[56] used a system of 3 minutes of running followed by 3 minutes of rest in the training phase of the Dallas bed rest study. Others used work periods of 10 to 15 seconds and recoveries of 20 to 30 seconds.[18]

Anaerobic training

Anaerobic training is used to describe work that improves anaerobic capacity. This includes all maximal efforts, especially those up to 5 minutes' duration. Interval training with brief recovery periods and repeated sprints with a short recovery are examples of anaerobic training. Since the objective is to develop resistance to the production of metabolic fatigue products particularly lactic acid, this training is very stressful.

Speed and strength training

These types of training are treated together in this chapter because training for strength is done with the goal of improving speed. Training for speed includes two components. One involves quick reactions and rapid movement patterns, while the other is concerned with power and the combination of force and velocity. There is an important difference between sprinting for speed development and sprinting for anaerobic improvements. In speed training, the duration and recovery are adjusted so that fatigue does not interfere with the practice of fast movement patterns.

Alternative modes of training

An important consideration for the injured athlete is the maintenance of fitness levels until normal activity is resumed. In addition, athletes (particularly middle-aged runners) may be able to avoid *overuse* injuries by using other training methods that produce either a cardiovascular conditioning effect or a local conditioning effect. Alternative training methods with cardiovascular conditioning effects are cycling, skating, rowing, swimming, cross-country skiing, and roller skiing. Weight training will not improve max $\dot{V}O_2$ but may extend performance time in some activities limited by muscle strength such as the arms in swimming and the thighs in cycling. Thus weight training can be of indirect benefit by increasing the amount of endurance training that can be accomplished.

In the case of a knee injury, training may be continued with the noninjured leg on a cycle ergometer. Even more effective is the combination of arm cranking with one-leg cycling, which uses muscle mass equivalent to that used in running.

EFFECTS OF TRAINING
Oxidative potential

The observation that endurance performance improves without an increase in max $\dot{V}O_2$[12] and the levels of oxidative enzymes continue to rise after max $\dot{V}O_2$ has plateaued[2,23,31] suggests that changes at the fiber level are important. Thus it would seem reasonable to expect that the more times a given fiber is required to contract per day, the greater the oxidative adaptation. However, to ensure that all fibers in a muscle receive a training effect there must be a balance between exercise intensity and duration. For example, the ultra-marathon runner who runs 3 to 4 hours/day does so at an intensity that allows the conservation of glycogen stores with the consequence that not all muscle fibers receive a training effect. Davies and Thompson[13] estimated in studies of 12 highly trained individuals that they were able to complete a 50-mile race at 67% of their max $\dot{V}O_2$. The average running time for this distance was 5 hours and 54 minutes, which corresponds to 14.34 km/hr or 6 min 44 sec/mile. The max $\dot{V}O_2$ of these runners was a high 72.5 ml/kg/min, yet their performance at 5 kilometers was not outstanding. Data from Gollnick and others[23] provide some insight into the paradox surrounding the effects of continuous exercise. Their study shows that it requires 2 hours of exercise at 64% of max $\dot{V}O_2$ to achieve any appreciable depletion of glycogen in the FT fibers. Since the glycogen in the ST fibers was almost totally depleted in the biopsy sample, it appears that sufficient exercise time is required before FT fibers are recruited. At a much higher exercise intensity (84% of max $\dot{V}O_2$), significant reduction of glycogen remains in almost all of the ST fibers. This suggests that FT fibers are recruited at an early stage of the higher intensity exercise and before depletion of the ST fibers.

On a practical level, athletes who spend many months on long, slow distance running probably develop highly oxidative ST fibers that are able to produce a large proportion of energy-using fat metabolism[30,35]. On the other hand, the athletes' FT fibers may not be receiving any training effect[23] with the consequence that these fibers fatigue rapidly when running speed is sufficient to require their participation. Some Olympic athletes who compete in the 10,000-meter race have trained almost exclusively using long-distance running. It is important, however, that their runs have been at a high intensity and not surprisingly accompanied by a high incidence of structural injury.

Interval running seems to have effects similar to those of continuous running.[18,21] Theoretically, this method is appealing because a greater intensity of training is possible, and consequently, FT fiber training effects can be achieved with shorter training sessions. However, the total amount of work that can be accomplished during interval training is less than that which may be achieved at a lower intensity of continuous effort. Glycogen depletion of FT fibers during high-intensity interval training may result and thus limit performance time. For muscle-fiber training, interval training, limited to 10 to 15 seconds[18] may be preferable, since blood lactates levels are lower at the same intensity than when longer work periods are used (Fig. 1-6).

There is evidence that anaerobic training does not increase oxidative capacity.[35] The reason for this is not clear, since a large amount of muscle fiber activity can be achieved in a motivated individual. Ibara and others[35] report a decrease in the oxidative marker enzyme succinated dehydrogenase after 6 weeks of anaerobic training. Another factor, which may limit improvements in oxidative capacity, is the increase in the diffusion distance of oxygen that results from fiber hypertrophy that accompanies intensive training.[58]

Oxygen transport

Improvement in oxygen transport mainly occurs from an increased maximal stroke volume of the heart,[17] which results in a greater maximal cardiac output, and consequently, a higher max $\dot{V}O_2$. The increased stroke volume may result from an improvement in cardiac dimensions and contractility,[41,46] from an increase in blood

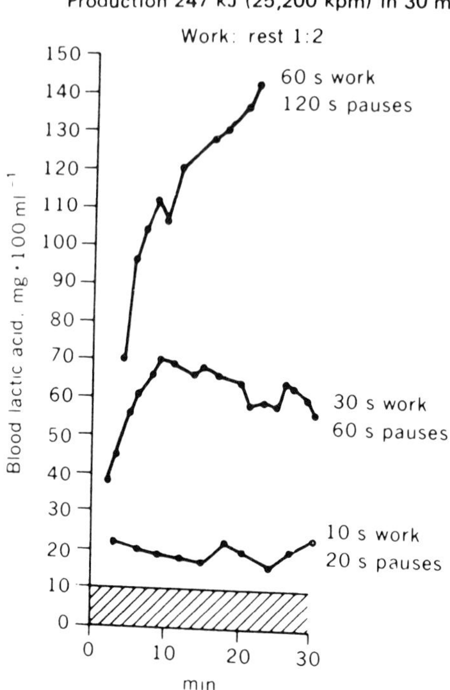

Fig. 1-6. Blood lactate response to same level of work (412 watts) for 10, 30, or 60 sec, followed by recovery period of 20, 60 and 120 sec, respectively. (From Astrand, P.O., and Rodahl, K.: Textbook of work physiology, New York, 1970, McGraw-Hill, Inc.)

volume and total hemoglobin,[39,48] or from an increase in systemic conductance.[3,5] Studies indicate that continuous training and interval training are about equal in their effects on max $\dot{V}O_2$ provided the intensity of the continuous work increases in proportion to the increase in max $\dot{V}O_2$. The intensity of training should be kept at a constant level relative to max $\dot{V}O_2$. However, specific central or peripheral adaptations resulting from these different training methods are not entirely clear. Gains of 50% in max $\dot{V}O_2$ have been reported in programs using a combination of intermittent and continuous activity.[33] Studies on athletes[49,54] indicate that the highest values for max $\dot{V}O_2$ are achieved by cross-country skiers. These athletes are able to sustain a higher percentage of their max $\dot{V}O_2$ during training because of the greater muscle mass involved in the exercise. A higher $\dot{V}O_2$ during training would be matched by a higher cardiac output and consequently a higher volume overload on the heart. This volume overload may be the critical stimulus to improving end-diastolic dimensions and thus stroke volume.[3]

SUMMARY

Improved endurance performance may be attained by increasing energy production or by improving the efficiency of energy use. Although the limits of performance may be set by max $\dot{V}O_2$, which has a strong genetic component, the capacity of the muscles to use a high fraction of max $\dot{V}O_2$ is important. Both high and moderate intensity training have similar effects on the oxidative capacity of muscle provided the moderate work is of sufficient duration. During rehabilitation from injury, alternative forms of endurance activity may help in maintaining cardiac performance. Increases in the pumping capacity of the heart appear to result from sustained activity using a large muscle mass that induces a large systemic blood flow.

REFERENCES

1. Astrand, P.-O., and Rodahl, K.: Textbook of work physiology, New York, 1970, McGraw-Hill, Inc.
2. Benzi, G.: Endurance training and enzymatic activities. In DiPrampero, P.E., and Poortsmans, J.R., editors: Physiological chemistry of exercise and training, Basel, 1981, S. Karger, AG, Medical and Scientific Publishers.
3. Blomqvist, C.G., and Saltin, B.: Cardiovascular adaptation to physical training, Annu. Rev. Physiol. **45:**169, 1982.
4. Reference deleted in proofs.
5. Clausen, J.P.: Effect of physical training on cardiovascular adjustment to exercise in man, Physiol. Rev. **57:**779, 1977.
6. Clausen, J.P., and others: Central and peripheral circulatory changes after training of the arms or legs, Am. J. Physiol. **225:**675, 1973.
7. Conley, D.L., and Krahenbuhl, G.S.: Running economy and distance running performance of highly trained athletes, Med. Sci. Sports Exerc. **12:**357, 1980.
8. Costill, D.L., and Fox, E.L.: Energetics of marathon running, Med. Sci. Sports Exerc. **1:**81, 1969.
9. Costill, D.L., Thomason, H., and Roberts, E.: Fractional utilization of the aerobic capacity during distance running, Med. Sci. Sports Exerc. **5:**248, 1973.
10. Danforth, W.H.: Activation of glycolytic pathway in muscle. In Chance, B., and Estabrook, R.W., editors: Control of energy metabolism, New York, 1965, Academic Press, Inc.
11. Daniels, J., and others: Aerobic responses of female distance runners to submaximal and maximal exercise, Ann. NY Acad. Sci. **301:**726, 1977.
12. Daniels, J.T., Yarbrough, A., and Foster, C.: Changes in $\dot{V}O_2$ max and running performance with training, Eur. J. Applied Physiol. **39:**249, 1978.
13. Davies, C.T.M., and Thompson, M.W.: Aerobic performance of female marathon and ultra marathon athletes, Eur. J. Applied Physiol. **41:**233, 1979.
14. Davies, K.J.A., Packer, L., and Brooks, G.A.: Biochemical adaptation of mitochondria, muscle, and whole-animal respiration to endurance training, Arch. Biochem. Biophys. **209:**539, 1981.
15. DeGaray, A.L., Levine, L., and Carter, J.E.L.: Genetic and anthropological studies of olympic athletes, New York, 1974, Academic Press, Inc.
16. DiPrampero, P.E., Pinera Limas, F., and Sassi, G.: Maximal muscular power, aerobic and anaerobic, in 116 athletes performing at the XIXth Olympic Games in Mexico, Ergonomics **13:**665, 1970.
17. Ekblom, B., and others: Effect of training on circulatory response to exercise, J. Appl. Physiol. **24:**518, 1968.
18. Essen, B., Hagenfeldt, L., and Kaijser, L.: Utilization of blood-borne and intramuscular substrates during continuous and intermittent exercise in man, J. Physiol. **265:**489, 1977.
19. Farrell, P.A., and others: Plasma lactate accumulation and distance running performance, Med. Sci. Sports Exerc. **11:**338, 1979.
20. Faulkner, J.A.: New perspectives in training for maximum performance, JAMA **205:**117, 1968.
21. Fox, E.L., and others: Intensity and distance of interval training programs and changes in aerobic power, Med. Sci. Sports Exerc. **5:**18, 1973.
22. Gollnick, P.D., Piehl, K., and Saltin, B.: Selective glycogen depletion pattern in human muscle fibres after exercise in varying intensity and at varying pedal rates, J. Physiol. **241:**45, 1974.
23. Gollnick, P.D., and Saltin, B.: Significance of skeletal muscle oxidative enzyme enhancement with endurance training, Clin. Physiol. **2:**1, 1982.
24. Grimby, G., and Saltin, B.: Physiological analysis of physically well trained middle-aged and old athletes, Acta Med. Scand. **179:**513, 1966.

25. Reference deleted in proofs.
26. Hagberg, J.M., and others: Faster adjustment to and recovery from submaximal exercise in the trained state, J. Appl. Physiol. **48**:218, 1980.
27. Reference deleted in proofs.
28. Havel, R.J.: Influence of intensity and duration of exercise on supply and use of fuels. In Pernow, B., and Saltin, B., editors: Muscle metabolism during exercise, Karolinska Institute symposium, vol. II, New York, 1971, Plenum Press.
29. Heath, G.W., and others: A physiological comparison of young and older endurance athletes, J. Appl. Physiol. **51**:634, 1981.
30. Henriksson, J.: Training induced adaptation of skeletal muscle and metabolism during submaximal exercise, J. Physiol. **270**:661, 1977.
31. Henriksson, J., and Reitman, J.S.: Time course of changes in human skeletal muscle succinate dehydrogenase and cytochrome oxidase activities and maximal oxygen uptake with physical activity and inactivity, Acta Physiol. Scand. **99**:91, 1977.
32. Hermansen, L.: Effect of acidosis on skeletal muscle performance during maximal exercise in man, Bull. Eur. Physiopathol. Respir. **15**:229, 1979.
33. Hickson, R.C., Bomze, H.A., and Holloszy, J.O.: Linear increase in aerobic power induced by a strenuous program of endurance exercise, J. Appl. Physiol. **42**:372, 1977.
34. Holloszy, J.O., and Booth, F.W.: Biochemical adaptation to endurance exercise in muscle, Annu. Rev. Physiol. **38**:273, 1976.
35. Ibarra, G., Fisher, A.G., and Conlee, R.K.: Effects of anaerobic training on selected aerobic factors in well-trained endurance runners, Med. Sci. Sports Exerc. **13**:109, 1981.
36. Ingjer, F.: Effects of endurance training on muscle fibre ATP-ase activity, capillary supply and mitochondrial content in man, J. Physiol. **294**:419, 1979.
37. Ivy, J.L., and others: Muscle respiratory capacity and fiber type as determinants of the lactate threshold, J. Appl. Physiol. **48**:523, 1980.
38. Jones, N.L., and others: Fat metabolism in heavy exercise, Clin. Sci. **59**:469, 1980.
39. Kanstrup, I.-L., and Ekblom, B.: Acute hypervolemia, cardiac performance and aerobic power during exercise, J. Appl. Physiol. **52**:1186, 1982.
40. Keul, J., Doll, E., and Keppler, D.: Energy metabolism of human muscle, Baltimore, 1972, University Park Press.
41. Keul, J., and others: Effect of static and dynamic exercise on heart volume, contractility and left ventricular dimensions, Circ. Res. **48**:1162, 1981.
42. Klissouras, V.: Heritability of adaptive variation, J. Appl. Physiol. **31**:338, 1971.
43. Komi, P.V., and others: Skeletal muscle fibers and muscle enzyme activities in monozygous and dizygous twins of both sexes, Acta Physiol. Scand. **100**:385, 1977.
44. Mitchell, J.H., and Blomqvist, C.G.: Maximal oxygen uptake, N. Engl. J. Med. **284**:1018, 1971.
45. Mitchell, J.H., Sproule, B.J., and Chapman, C.B.: The physiological meaning of the maximal oxygen intake test, J. Clin. Invest. **37**:538, 1958.
46. Morganroth, J., and others: Comparative left ventricular dimensions in trained athletes, Ann. Intern. Med. **82**:521, 1975.
47. Newsholme, E.A.: Control of carbohydrate utilization in muscle in relation to energy demand and its involvement in fatigue. In DiPrampero, P.E., and Poortsmans, J.R., editors: Physiological chemistry of exercise and training, Basel, 1981, S. Karger, AG, Medical and Scientific Publishers.
48. Oscai, L.B., Williams, B.T., and Hertig, B.A.: Effect of exercise on blood volume, J. Appl. Physiol. **24**:622, 1968.
49. Pollock, M.L.: Submaximal and maximal working capacity of elite distance runners. I. Cardiorespiratory aspects, Ann. NY Acad. Sci. **301**:310, 1977.
50. Pollock, M.L., Miller, H.S., and Wilmore, J.H.: Physiological characteristics of champion American track athletes 40 to 70 years of age, J. Gerontol. **29**:645, 1974.
51. Rowell, L.B.: Human cardiovascular adjustments to exercise and thermal stress, Physiol. Rev. **54**:75, 1974.
52. Rusko, H., Havu, M., and Karvinen, E.: Aerobic performance capacity in athletes, Eur. J. Applied Physiol. **38**:151, 1978.
53. Sahlin, K., and others: Effects of lactic acid accumulation and ATP decrease on muscle tension and relaxation, J. Appl. Physiol. **23**:353, 1967.

54. Saltin, B., and Åstrand, P.-O: Maximal oxygen uptake in athletes, J. Appl. Physiol. **23**:353, 1967.
55. Saltin, B., and others: Fiber types and metabolic potentials of skeletal muscles in sedentary man and endurance runners, Ann. NY Acad. Sci. **301**:3, 1977.
56. Saltin, B., and others: Response to exercise after bed rest and after training, Circulation (suppl. 7)**38**:1, 1968.
57. Saltin, B., and others: The nature of the training response: peripheral and central adaptations to one-legged exercise, Acta Physiol. Scand. **96**:289, 1976.
58. Saltin, B., and Rowell, L.B.: Functional adaptations to physical activity and inactivity, Fed. Proc. **39**:1506, 1980.
59. Shephard, R.J.: Intensity, duration, and frequency as determinants of the response to a training regime, Int. Z. Angew. Physiol. **26**:272, 1968.
60. Tanner, J.M.: The physique of the Olympic athlete, London, 1964, George Allen & Unwin (Publishers), Ltd.
61. Taylor, H.L., Buskirk, E., and Henschel, A.: Maximal oxygen intake as an objective measure of cardiorespiratory performance, J. Appl. Physiol. **8**:73, 1955.
62. Wyndham, C.H., and others: Physiological requirements for world-class performances in endurance running, S. Afr. Med. J. **43**:996, 1969.

2. The epidemiology of knee injuries in sports

James G. Garrick

Injuries involving the knee receive more attention than any other injuries associated with athletics. The impact of injuries in sports can be appreciated by looking at the table of contents of O'Donoghue's book.[5] Nearly one fifth of the entire volume is devoted to the knee, which is 50% more space than is allocated to either the shoulder or the ankle and spine combined.

The knee offers a variety of structures available for injury unparalleled in the muscuoloskeletal system. Sprains, strains, dislocations/subluxations, and a variety of overuse problems occur in and around only the knee with such frequency to merit serious attention.

The number of structures commonly injured is exceeded only by the variety of mechanisms causing those injuries. No body part is associated with more sport-designated syndromes or injuries. Such problems include *swimmer's knee, jumper's knee, runner's knee, football knee,* and *skier's knee.* All with different pathologic entities.

The variety of demands placed on the knee in various athletic activities further complicates the task of assessing knee injuries. For example, *breaststroker's knee,* which is devastating to the swimmer, would be of little consequence to the offensive tackle in football. Similarly, patellofemoral overuse syndromes are among the most common time-loss injuries in distance runners, but even if present they would be a mere annoyance to the wrestler. Thus knee injuries are present as true problems only in the context of the specific athletic event in which one participates.

From an epidemiologic standpoint this wide array of variables surrounding the injuries presents almost insurmountable problems. The first problem is defining what constitutes a knee injury. Because so few of the knee problems result in either direct visualization of the pathology by surgical intervention or visualization of abnormalities on X-ray, one is almost totally dependent on the history and physical examination. Normally these are sufficient for evaluating musculoskeletal problems, but lacking in knee injuries as evidenced by the variety of evalution methods used in knee instability and patellofemoral overuse syndromes.

The changing character of diagnostic tests also complicates any study of knee injuries. The frequent use of arthroscopy may reveal that the patient who previously was diagnosed as having chondromalacia by history and physical examination may in fact have a normal appearing articular cartilage and now requires a new pathologic description. Arthroscopy has also permitted a critical look at the fallibility of portions of the physical examination, such as the drawer test, and the efficacy of the Lachman test, which reveals that the anterior cruciate ligament may be among the most frequently injured structures in and around the knee.

Even considering these problems, an epidemiologic approach to knee injuries is valuable. This approach allows the establishment of the relative risk of injury as it pertains to specific activities. This is an important factor when advising the patient who has been previously injured. It allows us to marshall our forces to be prepared to provide care for specific athletic events. For example, crutches and a knee immobilizer are more important at a football game or ski area than at a marathon. Finally, the epidemiologic approach allows medical professionals to compare experiences. This may reveal the efficacy of a safeguard (e.g., use of prophylactic knee braces in football) or the danger in an item of equipment (long, conical cleats on grass fields).

An epidemiologic study of athletic injuries was carried out in four Seattle area high schools over 2 years. It was unique, because it involved all school-sponsored sports for males and females, employed a common and rigidly adhered to definition of injury, and most important was conducted by four specially trained athletic trainers. Their sole responsibility was to gather data and deal with athletic injuries. Although the data were gathered nearly a decade ago, before the use of some current diagnostic tests, the data provide a level of precise and uniform information that would be financially impossible to gather today.

In this study an injury was defined as a sport-related medical problem causing a participant to be removed from or miss a practice or competitive event. Among the 3049 participants in 19 sports, 1197 were injured according to this definition.

Although 42% of the injured athletes required an examination by a physician, the majority of the injuries would not be considered severe since 73.4% returned to full athletic participation in less than a week. Of the 1142 injuries allowing specific pathologic and anatomic classification, 166 (14.5%) involved the knee. Among the sports studied (Table 2-1), knee injuries contributed as many as 33% of the total problems in female cross-country to none of the problems in male gymnastics, swimming, and tennis and female swimming and badminton.*

More meaningful than the percentage of injuries involving the knee is the rate at which these injuries occur in the various sporting activities. This takes into account the number of individuals actually exposed and is expressed in the number of knee injuries per 100 participants per season of sports activity (Table 2-1).

---

* While conventional knowledge reveals that knee injuries are a problem in all of these events, one must bear in mind that the high level athletes usually studied in these sports are not represented here, since those high levels of competition usually occur in the extra-scholastic or club environment.

Table 2-1. Knee injuries in high school sports

Sport	Sex	Knee injuries %	Knee injury rate* per 100 players
Badminton	F	0	—
Baseball	M	13.0	2.0
Basketball	M	9.6	2.9
Basketball	F	24.1	6.1
Cross-country	M	27.5	7.8
Cross-country	F	33.0	11.5
Football	M	15.2	12.3
Gymnastics	M	0	—
Gymnastics	F	5.1	2.0
Softball	F	14.3	6.2
Soccer	M	19.0	5.7
Swimming	M	0	—
Swimming	F	0	—
Tennis	M	0	—
Tennis	F	30.0	2.2
Track and field	M	13.0	4.2
Track and field	F	12.3	7.2
Volleyball	F	11.8	1.1
Wrestling	M	15.5	14.1
All males		14.9	6.9
All females		14.1	3.1

* Knee injury rate $= \dfrac{\text{No. of knee injuries}}{\text{No. of participants}} \times 100.$

The contact sports of football and wrestling showed the highest rate of knee injuries. The character of these activities reflected the fact tht 63% of the football knee injuries and 73% of those seen in wrestling were fractures, sprains, and contusions. The two sports with the next highest rate of knee injuries were male and female cross-country. While the knee injury rates in cross-country approach those in contact sports, the type of injuries were predominantly caused by overuse.

Although there is a high knee injury rate in distance running, there is the tendency to dismiss these overuse injuries as less severe than the sprains seen in contact sports. The knee sprain requiring surgery is important to the sports physician. Thus the *football knee* seems more consequential than the *runner's knee*. However, the facts are that the vast majority of knee sprains do not require surgery and allow return to participation in a matter of weeks.[1,2] The average overuse injury may be more severe when viewed in terms of the time lost from sports participation, since a higher proportion of cross-country injuries (especially those in females) resulted in more than a week of time lost than those seen in football.

The types of knee injuries (Table 2-2) reflect the demands of the various sports.

Table 2-2. Knee injuries (N = 166)

Injury	Total (%)	Males (%)	Females (%)
Fracture	4.2	4.9	—
Sprain	42.2	43.3	34.8
Laceration	1.2	1.4	—
Contusion	17.5	18.9	8.7
Strain	7.2	6.3	13.0
Inflammation	10.2	7.7	26.1
Other	17.5	17.5	17.4
TOTALS	100%	100%	100%

The greater incidence of male knee sprains is caused primarily by the large number of injuries resulting from football and wrestling. These two activities account for 66% of all knee injuries reported. Similarly, the high proportion of knee inflammations in females (mostly extensor mechanism overuse problems) is partially a result of both the absence of contact sports like football and wrestling and the popularity of sports in which running and jumping are the major activities, such as basketball, track, cross-country, and volleyball. These sports involved some 60% of the total number of female participants.

Although there was a difference of injury types seen in males and females, there is nothing in these data to suggest that this was anything more than a reflection of the activities in which these young people participated. Thus the most important predictive variable is a specific athletic activity in which one participates.

Comparing the type and frequency of knee injuries in various sports is often less meaningful in an epidemiologic sense. An example of this is the attempt to draw far-reaching conclusions regarding the cause of injuries from anecdotal medical information. Orthopaedists dealing with athletic injuries often see an inordinate number of patients with a specific diagnosis participating in a single sport.

Gymnastic knee injuries

A recent report[1] studied 12 injuries involving the anterior cruciate ligament. All occurred in female gymnasts, and seven of the maneuvers resulting in the injury involved a "twist." Although this group of patients was homogeneous from a medical standpoint (all had sprains of the anterior cruciate ligament), it was heterogeneous in nearly every other sense: (1) injuries occurred in each of the four gymnastic events; (2) two injuries occurred as a result of unintentional falls; (3) seven injuries occured in practice, which raised the issue of proficiency rather than a specific movement being involved; and (4) the gymnasts were competing at various levels. Any of these factors could play an important role in the production of the injuries.

A torn anterior cruciate ligament presents a real problem to the gymnast sustaining

Table 2-3. Knee injury rates in gymnastics

Level	No. of participants	No. of knee injuries	Knee injury rate*
High school (4)	98	2	2.0
High school (12)	221	5	2.3
Club (3)	72	3	4.2
College (2)	24	3	12.5

From Garrick, J.G., and Requa, R.K.: Am. J. Sports Med. 8:261, 1980.
*Injuries per 100 gymnasts per season.

the injury. Whether this represents a real problem to the sport of gymnastics remains to be seen. As pointed out by Dr. Douglas Jackson[4] in his discussion of the paper, one must know the number of gymnasts from which this group was drawn as well as their level of both proficiency and activity.

To emphasize the potential influence on injuries by the level of competition, a comparison of knee injury rates was made among participants at three levels (Table 2-3).[3] This comparison revealed a six-fold variation in the probability of sustaining a knee injury. Yet without knowing at least the actual time at risk (i.e., time actually spent working out), these data only suggest a greater incidence at the college level.

Football knee injuries

Football serves as an example of a sport producing a high frequency of knee injuries, and the causes may be appreciably different than they appear on the surface. During five seasons of play (1978 to 1982) in the National Football League, 324 film clips depicting surgically treated injuries were analyzed.* The circumstances surrounding the injuries were divided into three groups. The first group was called *football* and included blocking, tackling, being blocked, and being tackled; it resulted in 53.4% of the injuries. The second group (25.18%) was termed *accidental* and included such mechanisms as being fallen on by another player. The third group or *noncontact* (21.4%) included injuries sustained as a result of cutting or decelerating and did not involve contact with another player.

The knee was involved in 73.1% of the injuries. The medial collateral ligament was the most frequently injured structure (46.1% of all knee injuries), and the anterior cruciate ligament was the next most frequently injured (33.8%). A detailed review of the 77 knee injuries sustained during the final 2 years of the study revealed that the isolated medial collateral ligament injuires (N = 18) and the isolated anterior cruciate ligament injuries (N = 16) occurred under appreciably different circumstances (Table 2-4).

---

* Study sponsored by the National Football League Joint Safety Committee: National Football League Players Association and National Football Management Council.

Table 2-4. Isolated ligament injuries of the knee, National Football League 1981-1982 (N = 34)

Circumstances	Medial collateral ligament	Anterior cruciate ligament
Football	10	5
Accidental	8	3
Noncontact	—	8

Half of the isolated anterior cruciate ligaments were not football injuries, but injuries resulting from running, stopping, and turning corners. These circumstances occur in a multitude of sports including soccer and basketball. The epidemiologic question this raises is whether this injury occurs more frequently in football and if so why.

• • •

The knee injuries discussed thus far seem to occur in situations in which an external force is applied (football and wrestling), a high degree of shoe/playing surface cohesion exists (football and gymnastics), and repeated *pounding* foot strikes occur (track and cross-country). What could be expected of a sport in which these circumstances are not present?

Figure skating knee injuries

In 1981, 70 national level figure skaters responded to a survey regarding their previous injuries. These skaters with a combined competitive experience of 464 years reported 150 injuries, each resulting in more than a week of time lost from skating. The injury types were almost equally divided between acute (N = 78) and overuse (N = 72). The knee was involved in 15.3% of the acute and 23.6% of the overuse injuries. No anatomic region was involved more frequently. Thus even in an activity involving no running, little body contact and less than secure foot fixation to the *playing surface* there still exists an inordinate proportion of knee injuries.

SUMMARY

Because sports are voluntary activities, there is a tendency to view athletic injuries in a simplistic fashion. In the past few years it has been suggested that knee injuries in sports can be prevented by prohibiting blocking and tackling below the waist in football, eliminating twisting dismounts in gymnastics, and using orthotics to prevent pronation in runners. While these and other practices may prevent some injuries, they do not provide the answer to the problem of knee injuries in sports. There is no single answer because there is no single problem.

On the optimistic side, athletic activities should be the greatest source of enlightenment regarding the causes of injuries involving the knee. The relative homogeneity of the participants (all come to the activities relatively fit), the high degree of supervision by coaches and trainers, the documentation of the circumstances surrounding the injuries (often on film or videotape), and the sophistication of medical care should all provide laboratorylike setting. It seems that the only missing element is a cooperative multidisciplinary approach to studying the problem.

REFERENCES

1. Derschied, G.L., and Garrick, J.G.: Medial collateral ligament injuries in football, Am. J. Sports Med. **9:**365, 1981.
2. Ellsasser, J.C., Reynolds, F.C., and Omghundro, J.R.: The nonoperative treatment of collateral ligament injuries of the knee in professional football players, J. Bone Joint Surg. **56A:**1185, 1974.
3. Garrick, J.G., and Requa, R.K.: Epidemiology of women's gymnastics injuries, Am. J. Sports. Med. **8:**261, 1980.
4. Hunter, L.Y., and Torgan, C.: Dismounts in gymnastics: should scoring be re-evaluated? Am. J. Sports Med. **11:**208, 1983.
5. O'Donoghue, D.H.: Treatment of injuries to athletes, ed. 3, Philadelphia, 1976, W. B. Saunders Co.

3. The biomechanics of running and knee injuries

Thomas P. Andriacchi
Gary M. Kramer
Glenn C. Landon

The number of people running for recreation, sport, or health has increased from 100,000 in 1968 to current estimates as high as 25,000,000.[10] Concurrently, the number of injuries associated with running has increased substantially. The knee is the most frequently injured joint in runners.[8,10,11] In addition, the knee joint is often traumatically injured during other athletic activities.

Little is known of the relationship between extrinsic loading at the knee during activities such as running or cutting maneuvers and frequently occurring injuries to the knee joint. This is a result of the small number of biomechanical studies of running in comparison to the number of studies of walking. In general, running has been studied from an athletic viewpoint[3,4,6,7,9] with the goal of improving performance. Consequently, there is little information that can be used to study the injury mechanisms associated with running. This chapter examines the biomechanics of normal running associated with commonly occurring injuries to the knee joint. In addition, the biomechanics of running and side-step cutting are examined in the normal knee and the anterior cruciate ligament–deficient knee.

MATERIALS AND METHODS

The forces and moments acting at the knee joint were calculated from kinematic and ground reaction force measurements during running and side-step cutting. Flexion-extension and abduction-adduction motion at the hip, knee, and ankle measured as well as foot contact patterns. The instruments include a 10-meter walkway, force platform, optoelectronic system for motion analysis, and foot contact area transducer; these are described elsewhere.[1,2] Light emitting diodes (LEDs) were placed at the anterior-superior iliac crest, greater trochanter, lateral joint line of the knee, lateral malleolus, base of the calcaneus, and base of the fifth metatarsal head to aid observation. The actual location of the joint center for the hip, knee, and ankle were located relative to the LED placed at the greater trochanter, lateral joint line of the knee, and lateral malleolus. Motion was sampled at a rate of 150 Hz. Inertia properties for the limb segments of the thigh, shank, and foot were derived from data described in the literature.

Local anatomic coordinate axes were placed in the thigh, shank, and foot to locate the anatomic axes of flexion-extension, abduction-adduction, and internal-external rotation. The coordinate systems for the hip, knee, and ankle were fixed in the thigh, shank, and foot, respectively. The three-dimensional limb kinetics were calculated using an idealized three-dimensional model of the lower extremity. This approach assumes the axial rotation of each limb segment is small with respect to the adjacent segment.

A foot contact area transducer[5] was used to measure instantaneous foot contact relative to the pathway of the center of pressure during running. The transducer was placed on the force plate, and the measurements of the ground reaction force and the center of pressure were combined with a computer-generated footprint.

The measurement protocol required each subject to run and walk the length of a 10-meter walkway in a range of speeds. The side-step cut was performed by each subject running to a specific point and cutting at 90 degrees to the direction of progression. Ten normal subjects and three patients with anterior cruciate ligament (ACL) deficiencies were observed. Force measurements were normalized to body weights, and moment measurements were normalized to the product of body weight times height (bw × ht) for comparison.

RESULTS
Running: a comparison of extrinsic joint loading and common injury patterns

A computer-generated stick figure of a single leg going through the support and swing phase of running at a 3 m/sec pace was used for qualitative evaluation of running styles (Fig. 3-1). Three portions from this computer-generated image were selected for detailed analysis of body configuration and extrinsic loading at the knee joint. The three portions include the foot strike, midsupport, and preswing configuration of the limbs and torso (Fig. 3-2).

As the foot strikes, the hip and knee are slightly flexed, and the foot contacts the ground dorsiflexed. During running, the body has a more vertical posture at heel strike with slightly more hip and knee flexion than normally occurs during level walking. Landing in this flexed position provides a potential for absorbing the higher impact that occurs during running. An analysis of the extrinsic loading at the knee at foot strike indicates compressive and posteriorly directed force components and a moment that tends to flex the joint. As the body moves forward to the midsupport phase, the axial force reaches a maximal of 200% body weight compressive load, the posterior shear reaches 100% body weight, and the moment tending to flex the knee approaches 15% body weight times height. The maximal knee flexion moment is greater than 5 times the moment that normally occurs during level walking.

The hip and knee joints extend and the ankle plantar flexes as the body moves

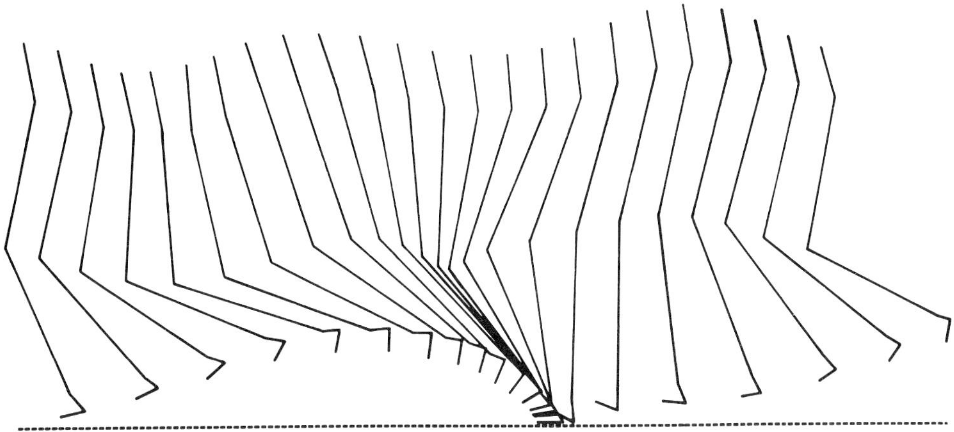

Fig. 3-1. Computer-generated stick figure representation of leg going through support and swing phases of running.

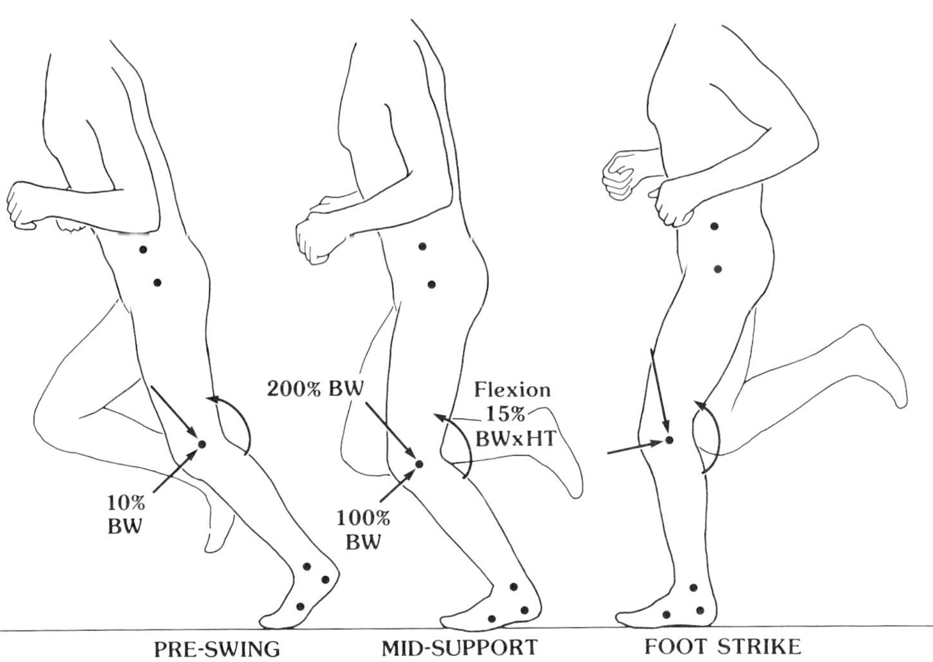

Fig. 3-2. Sagittal plane view of limb configuration and knee joint loading during foot strike, mid-support, and preswing portions of support phase of running. Numbered values indicate occurrence of maxima.

SUPPORT PHASE KNEE JOINT EXTERNAL LOADING
RUNNING 3M/sec

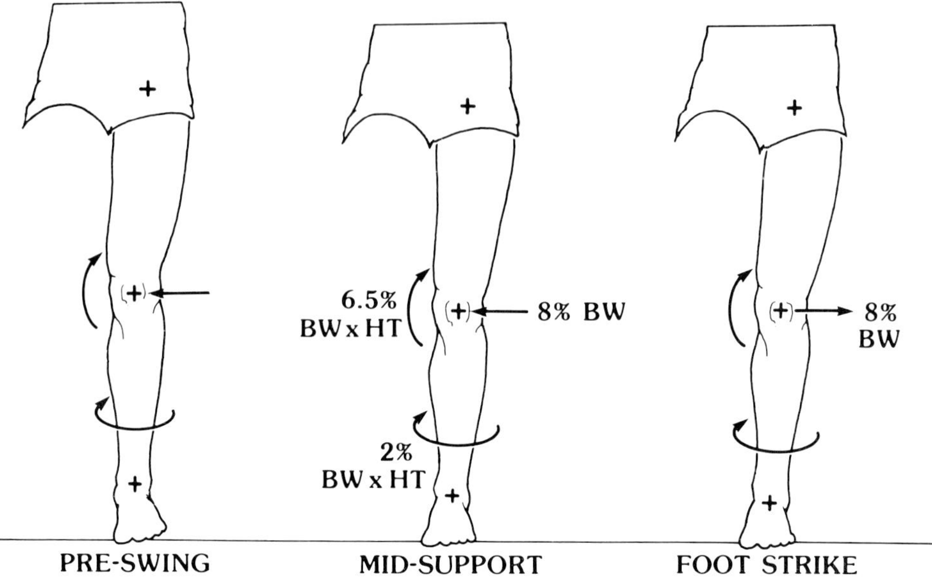

Fig. 3-3. Frontal plane view of leg during foot strike, mid-support, and preswing portions of running with loading at the knee joint. Numbered values indicate occurrence of maxima.

to the preswing phase. The loading decreases and the only significant change is the shear at the knee joint that switches to an anteriorly directed shear of 10% body weight.

Shown in Fig. 3-3 is the configuration of the limb in the frontal plane during three phases of the support phase of running. At foot strike, there is a medially directed shear of 8% body weight as well as a moment tending to abduct the knee and internally rotate the joint. At midsupport, the shear reverses direction to a maximum of 8% body weight directed laterally, the internal rotation moment reaches a maximum of 2% body weight times height, and the moment tending to adduct the knee reaches a maximum of 6.5% body weight times height. As the body moves toward preswing, the internal rotation moment, the abduction-adduction, and the medially directed force continue in the same direction, but reduce in magnitude before the foot leaves the ground.

A comparison of the largest moment components between level walking and running suggests a relationship between extrinsic loading and common injury patterns in runners. For example, the moment tending to flex the knee increases from 2.3% body weight times height during level walking to 13.4% body weight times height when running at 3 m/sec (Table 3-1). Simlarly, the moment tending to adduct the

Table 3-1. Largest moment magnitudes increase over level walking

External moment	Level walking (1.2 m/sec)	Running (3 m/sec)	Factor of increase
Knee flexion	2.29	13.38	5.8×
Hip adduction	5.07	10.15	2.0×
Hip flexion	6.22	12.25	1.9×
Ankle dorsal flexion	9.13	16.81	1.8×

hip joint, the moment tending to flex the hip joint, and the moment tending to dorsiflex the ankle increase by nearly a factor of two over level walking. These results are consistent with reports of injury patterns common to runners, since these moment magnitudes show the largest increase in areas where common running injuries occur. For example, the large increase in the knee flexion moment must be balanced primarily by the quadriceps mechanism and potentially generates stress in the patellofemoral joint, which is a common site of running injuries. Also, the large adduction moment at the hip and knee stresses the iliotibial band. The knee and the patellofemoral joint experience the greatest stress increase over level walking.

Running styles, variations, and effects of shoe design

The pattern of moments about the flexion-extension axes and abduction-adduction axes were reproducible and consistent among different test subjects, with one exception: the ankle inversion-eversion moment. The inversion-eversion moment at the ankle joint depends on the style of running (Fig. 3-4). Curve A in Fig. 3-4 was a heel-toe runner, Curve B is a forefoot runner, and Curve C was a runner who tends to excessively pronate the foot. These three running styles were also demonstrated by the outline of the footprint of each runner, with the pathway of the center of pressure indicated by the solid and dash lines (Fig. 3-5). The tendency to overpronate was associated with a more medial pathway of the center of pressure through the foot. The overpronation of the foot has been associated with patellofemoral problems. In the action of the subtalar joint, as the foot pronates, the tibia rotates and potentially increases the lateral subluxing force on the patella.

The tendency of the foot to overpronate was related to the inversion-eversion moment at the ankle. The maximal magnitude of the eversion moment at the ankle was used as an index for overpronation, and the influence of running shoes on controlling overpronation was studied. Illustrated in Fig. 3-6 is the mean and standard deviation for the maximal eversion moment for 10 trials of barefoot running and 5 trials running with each of five styles of running shoes. Several shoe styles significantly reduce the magnitude of moment when compared to the barefoot trials. If the magnitude of this eversion moment is used as an index for overpronation, these results indicate that some designs of running shoes have a strong influence on controlling the excessive pronation tendency.

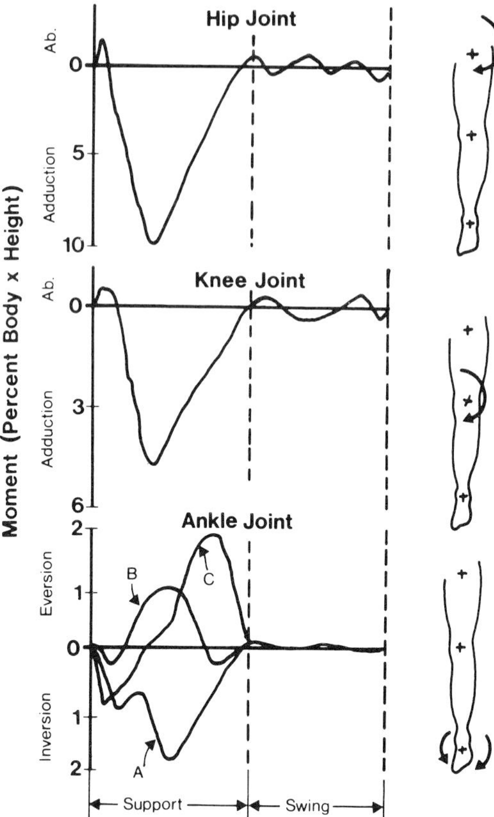

Fig. 3-4. Typical patterns of abduction-adduction moments at hip and knee and inversion-eversion moments at ankle. At ankle, three patterns of moments were observed. Curve *A*, Heel-toe runner; curve *B*, forefoot runner; curve *C*, runner who tended to excessively pronate foot.

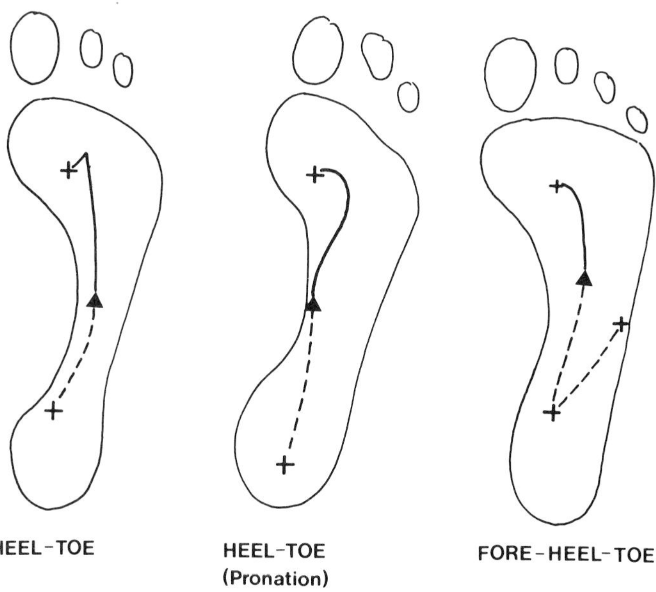

Fig. 3-5. Pathway of center of pressure through foot in three running styles.

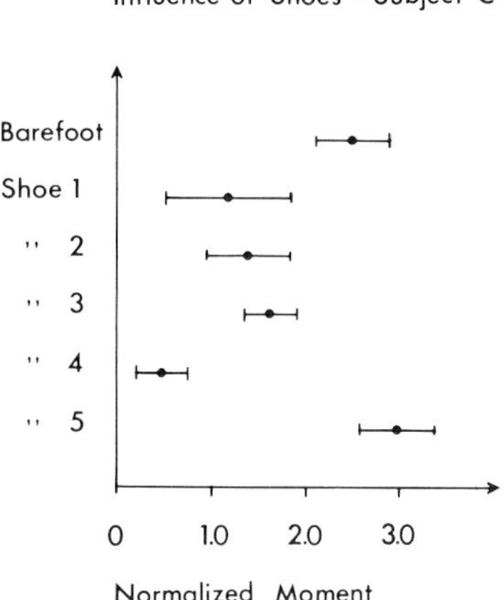

Fig. 3-6. Averages and standard deviations of magnitude of eversion moment at ankle during barefoot running and running with five different sytles of running shoes. Results tended to indicate influence of running shoe while controlling tendency for overpronation.

Side-step cutting

The biomechanics of side-step cutting were measured by the subjects running to a spot and then cutting at 90 degrees to the direction of progression. Illustrated in Fig. 3-7 is a sagittal plane view of three phases of the support phase of the cutting cycle: the foot strike, the midsupport phase, and the preswing phase. At foot strike, the external compressive force at the knee reaches a peak of 250% body weight. This compressive force rises more rapidly than during normal running. The external moments in this plane tend to extend the knee, and there is also an anterior shear reaching a maximal of 10% body weight. In the ACL-deficient knee, this phase would be the most troublesome.

As the subjects go into midsupport phase, the compressive force declines while the shear force reverses to a posterior direction and reaches a maximum of 100% body weight. The external moment at the knee tends to flex the joint and reaches a maximum of 7% body weight times height. The body configuration and the limb configuration are considerably different during the cutting maneuver than during straight running.

When the leg is viewed in the frontal plane during the cutting maneuver (Fig. 3-8), an internal rotation moment of 2% body weight times height and an abduction moment moment of 1.5% body weight times height can be seen. At midsupport, the axial moment reverses to an external direction, and the medial lateral shear reaches a maximum of 70%. As the limb moves toward push-off, the loading reduces in magnitude and the only change is a reversal to an internal rotation moment.

The major differences between loading during running and loading during cutting were the presence of the external rotation moments during midsupport phase, the

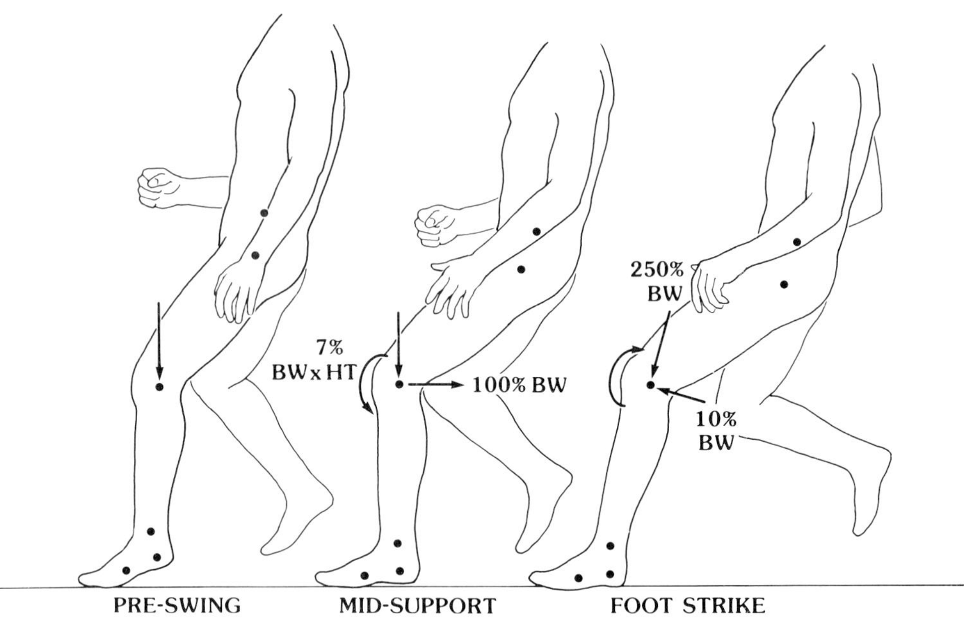

Fig. 3-7. Sagittal plane view of leg during foot strike, mid-support, and preswing phases of 90-degree side-step cut. Numbered values indicate occurrence of maxima.

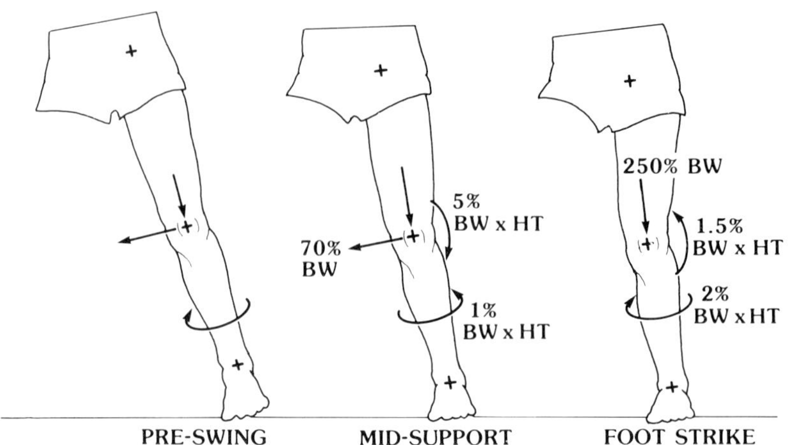

Fig. 3-8. Frontal plane view of the leg during 90-degree side-step cut. Numbered values indicate occurrence of maxima.

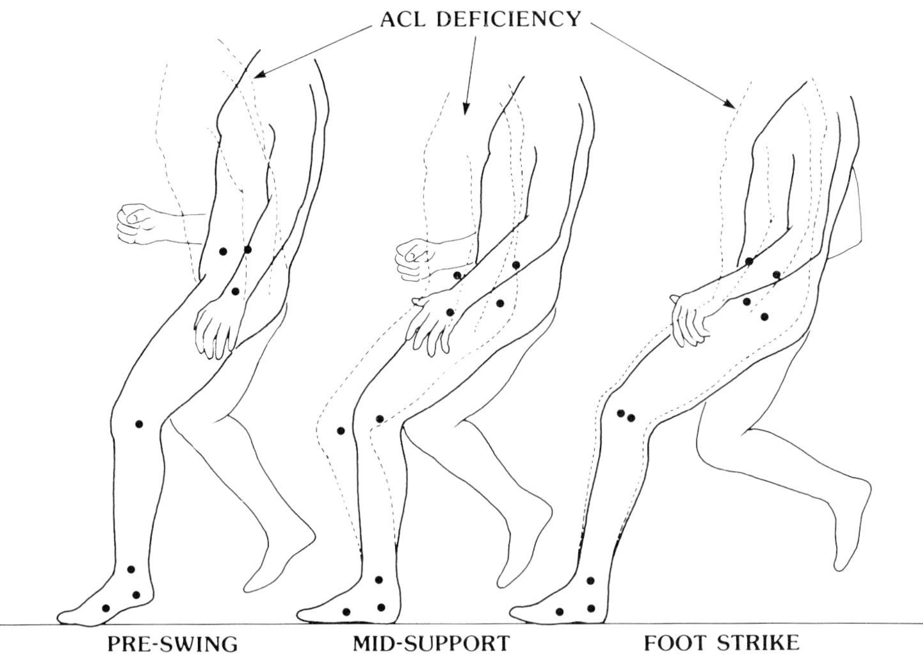

Fig. 3-9. Different mechanisms used during cutting maneuver by patients with ACL insufficiency compared to normal. Patients with ACL insufficiency tended to cut with knee and hip more flexed.

large increase in the medial shear, and the large increase in the loading at the foot strike position.

ACL deficiencies in side-step cutting

The 90 degree side-step cutting maneuver was also observed on three patients with a grade 2 ACL insufficiency. These patients performed the cutting maneuver in a manner considerably different from normal. They performed the cut with the body more flexed at the hip and knee and maintained the torso in a more erect position (Fig. 3-9). Using this body posture, the patients with ACL insufficiency have a larger than normal hip and knee flexion moment during the cut. These patients were also studied during running and stair climbing and were found to perform these activities with the knee and hip in a more flexed position. This flexed limb posture may possibly be associated with the role of the hamstring muscles. By maneuvering with the knee in a more flexed position, the hamstrings are in a better positon to stablize the tibia and prevent abnormal anterior translation and internal-external rotation. These subjects may be using this mechanism as compensation for the ACL insufficiency.

DISCUSSION

These results indicate a relationship between extrinsic loading at the knee joint and common overuse injury patterns. When changing from walking to running there is a large increase in external loading at the knee, which may explain the preponderance of knee injuries in runners. Slight perturbations in body mechanics associated with the mechanisms of running could cause injury. For example, changes in running styles caused by fatigue, shoe design, or running surface, and changes in distance combined with the high loading taking place at the knee may induce injuries. Little is known about these factors at this time. Understanding the compensatory patterns of movement in patients with ligament injuries may provide insight into surgical treatment and rehabilitation methods as well as improve our understanding of the actual nature of the functional knee instability.

REFERENCES

1. Andriacchi, T.P., and others: Three dimensional coordinate data processing in human motion analysis, J. Biomech, Eng. **101:**279, 1979.
2. Andriacchi, T.P., and others: Moments exerted on the lower extremities during running, Trans. Orthop. Res. Soc., Las Vegas, **6:**52, 1981.
3. Cavanaugh, P.R., Pollock, M.L., and Landa, J.: A biomechanical comparison of elite and good distance runners, Ann. NY Acad. Sci. **301:**328, 1977.
4. Dillman, C.J.: Kinematic analyses of running, Exerc. Sport Sci. Rev. **3:**193, 1975.
5. Draganich, L.F., and others: Electronic measurement of instantaneous foot-floor contact patterns during gait, J. Biomech. **13:**875, 1980.
6. Elftman, H.: The work done by muscles in running, Am. J. Phys. **139:**672, 1940.
7. Fenn, W.O.: Frictional and kinetic factors in the work of spring running, Am. J. Phys. **93:**443, 1930.
8. James, S.L., Bates, B.T., and Osternig, L.R.: Injuries to runners, Am. J. Sports Med. **6:**40, 1978.
9. James, S.L., and Brubaker, C.E.: Biomechanical and neuromuscular aspects of running, Exerc. Sport Sci. Rev. **1:**189, 1973.
10. Krissoff, W.B., Ferris, W.D.: Runner's injuries, Physician Sports Med. **7:**12, 1979.
11. Slocum, D.B., and James, S.L.: Biomechanics of running, JAMA **205:**721, 1968.

4. Skeletal muscle: adaptability to altered patterns of physical activity

Philip D. Gollnick

Skeletal muscle comprises approximately 40% of the total body weight of humans. This tissue constitutes the largest single mass of the body devoted to a single function, that is, locomotion. It may also be the most plastic tissue considering the magnitude and rapidity with which it adapts to changes in its pattern of physical activity. The concept of adaptation to altered patterns of use in this chapter encompasses the spectrum of changes occurring in the skeletal muscle of humans and other animals in response to complete inactivity to the most intense physical activity.

This chapter provides a general overview of the characteristics of skeletal muscle, with the emphasis on human skeletal muscle, and briefly describes the adaptive processes that can occur in the tissue in response to altered states of physical activity. A more complete exposition of this subject is contained in recent reviews by Buchthal and Schmalbruch[4] and Saltin and Gollnick.[24]

GENERAL CHARACTERISTICS OF SKELETAL MUSCLE

Most skeletal (striated) muscles have their origins and insertions on the skeletal system. An example of an exception is the diaphragm where the insertion is the central tendon. Although skeletal muscles share many features, such as their general appearance, the skeletal muscle's role in maintaining body posture without conscious control, in the generation of the locomotor activities associated with daily tasks, or in the high power and endurance activities practiced by the elite athlete varies widely. The characteristics of a muscle at any time are the combined effects of heredity and environment.

The class of tissue labeled skeletal muscle consists of the individual muscle cells or fibers that are under the control of the motor nerve and all support tissue. The combination of the motor nerve and the fibers it innervates is the motor unit or functional unit of muscle. Each motoneuron in the motor unit branches as it enters the muscle and innervates a number of fibers. There are a number of important considerations regarding a muscle, how it functions, and its relationship to these motoneurons.

It is observed that there are a variety of muscles, that they possess different contractile and fatigue properties, and that they are used in innumerable ways. Moreover, the same muscle is capable of a wide variety of responses ranging from activities requiring great precision but little force to those requiring high tension development with little regard for overall control. Motor patterns accomplished by the human hand illustrate this diversity of response by single muscles and muscle groups. The first question to be approached is how the diversity of contractile patterns is produced.

Contractile properties of motor units

Foremost in an understanding of muscular adaptability is the realization that most muscles are collections of motor units that possess different contractile properties.[4,5,24] These fundamental properties are used to identify muscle fiber types or motor units. The contractile properties are distinguished from the time to peak tension development following activation and the time of one-half relaxation once attaining the peak tension following the initiation of a single contractile cycle.

In the skeletal muscle of humans and most animals, the contractile properties can be divided into motor units that attain peak tension rapidly and those that peak rather slowly. Fast contracting motor units in the intact human biceps muscle attain maximal tension in about 35 msec whereas 90 msec is the average of slow contracting units.

Differences do exist for different muscles of different species. The fast contracting motor units of the medial gastrocnemius of the cat reach peak tension in times ranging from 32 to 43 msec, whereas in the rat it may be as low as 13 msec. Conversely, the times for slow contracting units are about 85 and 40 msec for the cat and rat, respectively. In these species there are considerable differences between motor units of the same muscle and between muscles. This is similar to humans. These differences in contractile speeds of the motor units can be identified as fast twitch (FT) or slow twitch (ST).

Molecular basis for contractile properties of motor units

The molecular basis for the difference in contractile speeds of motor units is in the myofibrillar complex or the total of the proteins that are assembled into myofibrils. The myofibrillar complex exists in isozyme form that results in differential rates at which they release adenosine triphosphatase (ATPase). This property was first identified in myosin, which, on a molecular weight basis, is the major protein of the contractile complex. Early studies of Bárány[1] reveal that for a variety of species there is a linear relationship between actin-activated ATPase activity and the contractile speed of muscle when expressed as muscle lengths per second. Subsequent studies verify this relationship and also reveal isozymes of the other proteins that comprise the entire contractile element of muscle. Thus it is best to refer to the ATPase activity of the muscle as a myofibrillar ATPase rather than a myosin ATPase, since it is modulated by a number of elements comprising the entire contractile complex. The isozyme exists in the myofibrillar complex, because 8 of the 22 genes involved in the myofibril assembly must be expressed to form a single type of myofibril.[19] Thus a variety of expressions of these genes is possible.

The existence of different myofibrillar ATPases can be identified in muscles by numerous methods. The easiest is the visualization of ATPase in the individual fibers by histochemical methods. This is done with fresh-frozen cross sections of muscle that are pretreated with buffers at selected pHs to take advantage of the fact that different isozymes of proteins in the contractile complex have different sensitivities to either acid or alkali.[3] This method is based on the general finding that exists for all mammalian species: the myofibrillar complex in muscle with fast contractile properties is alkali stable but acid labile. Conversely, those fibers that have slow contractile properties are acid stable, may be acid activated, and are alkali labile. By simply preincubating cryostat-cut fresh sections at a pH of 10.4 before placing them into a reactive mixture at pH 9.4 results in a loss of ATPase staining from the ST fibers, whereas staining in the FT fibers is retained. When the preincubation is carried out at pH 4.35 there is a loss of ATPase staining from the FT fibers, whereas the ST fibers possess an intense staining. This situation is complicated somewhat because there are fibers that respond differently when the ATPase staining is conducted by varying the pH or by changing the ionic composition of the preincubation medium. The most widely used method is to include a third preincubation at pH 4.60. With this preincubation, a portion of the FT fibers retain a moderate staining intensity, whereas others lose the histochemically demonstrable ATPase, that is, they become ATPase negative. There is another class of FT fibers that retain an ATPase staining after all preincubations. On this basis at least three subtypes of FT fibers can be identified in most mammalian muscle, especially humans. These FT fibers have been identified as FTa, FTb, and FTc for those that are labile at pH 4.6, pH 4.35, and acid and alkali stable, respectively.

There are probably more subclassifications of fibers, and the ability to identify them at present is a function of the methodology. The convention of identifying fibers here is to use the designation of FT and ST to identify twitch properties.[24] An alternate method is the system introduced by Brooke and Kaiser[3] in which the ST fibers are identified simply as type I and the FT as type II. The type II are subclassified as IIa, IIb, and IIc. The FT and ST designation as used here is an attempt to include a physiological connotation in the indentification system.

There are other ways to identify motor unit subtypes in skeletal muscle in addition to the acid-alkali preincubation method. Gaining increasing acceptance is the immunocytological method. In this procedure specific antibodies are prepared for the different isozymes that comprise the contractile complex. Fresh-frozen cross sections of the muscle are incubated with the antibodies that react with the proteins and identify the specific subtypes of fibers. The major limitation to this method is that it requires the preparation of an absolutely pure native protein to prepare an antibody that will react with only one species of the polymorphic protein. Failure to do so will result in a reaction with more than one species and confuse rather than clarify the issue. This method is more expensive than the more traditional histochemical methods. Refinements in the acid-alkali preincubation method may increase its sensitivity and make it as useful and less expensive than the immunocytological method.

Individual fibers can also be isolated from muscle and the protein composition determined by a variety of electrophoretic methods. These methods do not hold immediate promise for wide application in routine use.

Metabolic properties of motor unit subtypes

ST fibers generally possess higher concentrations of enzymes associated with the citric acid cycle and the electron transport system than FT fibers.[13,24] The ST fibers are richly endowed with mitchondria and have a high capacity for oxygen uptake. Conversely, they have low concentrations of the enzymes used in the anaerobic degradation of carbohydrates, either muscle glycogen or blood glucose, to lactate. FT fibers can be separated into those that have a reasonably high potential for oxygen consumption, that is, a fairly high complement of mitochondria (FTa), and those that are motochondria poor (FTb). Both of these subtypes have a high glycolytic potential. It is imperative to point out that the metabolic property of muscle is variable[21] and influenced by the state of physical activity,[13,24] and that it is essentially unusable as a consistent criterion for identifying different types of motor units.

Homogeneity of motor units

An important characteristic of motor units of all species is that they are homogeneous with regard to all properties.[4,18] This is the case whether some of these have undergone a mutation as a result of naturally occurring phenomena or experimentally induced perturbations.

ADAPTATIONS WITH ACTIVITY PATTERNS
Muscle size

Skeletal muscles dramatically respond to altered states of physical activity in their size and strength. The changes in size in response to inactivity and heavy resistance exercise are well known. In orthopaedics, one of the most frequently encountered problems is inactivity associated with the surgical repair of deformities or broken bones. Under these conditions there is a rapid loss in total muscle mass and strength.

Knowledge of muscle atrophy in humans comes primarily from investigations made in patients following the application of cast after injury. Reductions in muscle volume were estimated either from anthropometric methods[26] or more recently by the use of computerized tomography.[15] The influence of inactivity on the muscle fibers was assessed from measurements made on biopsy samples taken with the needle method. With immobilization there is a major loss of muscle weight. At the fiber level this loss is characterized by reductions in the cross-sectional areas of individual fibers that correspond closely to the overall loss in cross-sectional areas of muscle. Haggmark[15] demonstrated that this loss occurred intially or preferentially in the ST fibers. However, with up to 213 days' immobilization, Sargeant, and others[26] observed almost equal reductions in cross-sectional areas in all types of human muscle fibers. These data suggest that if there is an initial loss of volume from the ST fibers, this will be matched some time later in the process of atrophy by a similar loss in FT fibers. With a return to normal activity and the institution of exercise programs, growth occurs to reconstitute the original cross-sectional area of the muscle fibers.[15] In these studies, there was also a loss in maximal metabolic capacity as indicated by the one-leg maximal oxygen uptake. Recovery following removal of the cast was not reported.

Hypertrophy versus hyperplasia

Of some interest regarding the growth of muscle is whether skeletal muscle retains the potential for proliferation of the fibers following differentiation. This problem is of some clinical importance in the return of muscle mass and function in instances where losses have occurred as a result of nerve damage, disease, or the physical destruction of muscle tissue because of injury. Minor damage to muscle fibers apparently can be repaired.[28] The genesis of the question regarding hyperplasia arises from studies suggesting that the total number of fibers in skeletal muscle can increase in the muscles of animals during early growth[6] and in response to the accelerated growth associated with heavy resistance exercise.[9,10,22,29] In some cases this suggestion has been extended to humans.[8] This is contrary to early studies that suggest fiber number is established either immediately before or shortly after birth.[24]

The suggestion that there can be an increase in total fiber number in skeletal muscle during exercise training comes from studies where fibers with branch points have been identified or isolated in histologic or teased preparations.[9,10,22,30] The assumption has been made that these branch points represent fibers that are in the process of dividing to produce daughter cells. Clusters of small fibers can also be observed in muscle.[29] These are interpreted as being a single muscle fiber dividing into several new or daughter fibers. It has been reported that the flexor carpi radialis muscles of cats trained with a weight lifting program contain 20% more fibers than found in the muscles of control animals.[9,10] The proliferation of fibers in these studies was attributed to a longitudinal division of preexisting fibers. The validity of these findings is compromised by the fact that the increase in total muscle weight (6% to 16%) is insufficient to accomodate the reported increase in total number (20%) and the average cross-sectional area (20% [estimated from the fiber diameter]) of the fibers. Moreover, with the total number of fibers reported in the muscle and the average weight of the muscle the calculated length of the fibers needed to accommodate the entire muscle weight would have exceeded the total length of the forelimb of the cat.

Gollnick and others[12,14] approached this problem by developing methods in which fibers could be individually dissected from muscle, counted, and examined over their entirety to determine the total number and the frequency of fiber branching. These methods were applied to the study of muscle enlargement where growth is produced by functional overloads. These overloads were produced in the rat[12] by surgical ablation of synergistic muscle with and without exercise and in the chicken[14] by hanging weights on one wing. Studies of control groups of rats demonstrated that although there was a close correspondence between the number of fibers contained in a muscle from the right and left hindlimb of the same animal, interanimal variation was so great that it precluded the possibility of making comparisons between animals. Thus the possibility of a fiber proliferation was evaluated only from comparisons made between normal and enlarged muscles from the same animal.

The general finding from these studies was that the total number of fibers in skeletal muscle was unchanged under conditions where the total weight of the muscle had doubled. Moreover, fibers with points of branching can be found in all muscles including those in young animals, but the frequency is too small to account for a change in the total fiber number of a muscle. In experiments where the weight that could be attributed to the fibers was calculated from their length, cross-sectional area, total number, and density, it was possible to account for approximately 85% of the total weight of the muscle. Since it is generally assumed that 15% of a muscle is extra-fiber material, this accounting is a good indication that the method of evaluating the individual components of the fibers was reasonable. Application of the direct counting method to the cat flexor carpi radialis muscle[12] revealed that the total fiber number, reported in studies where hyperplasia was claimed, was only one-third of the actual total number of fibers contained in the muscle. This large discrepancy appears to have resulted from taking transverse sections cut from the muscle at its point of greatest diameter. Unfortunately, the fiber arrangement of the muscle was multipenniform, and as a result only a small percentage of the fibers traversed the point where the cut was made. These data clearly illustrated the problems of determining the total number of fibers from histologic methods where the fiber arrangement is not parallel to the long axis of the muscle and extends to a point where they are included in the cross section. The increase in the number of fibers contained in a cross-sectional cut of muscles with penniform fiber arrangment appears to be the result of change in the angle of the fibers as they lie in the muscle as a function of changes in their size.[12]

Another problem is that the points of branching on the fibers can occur anywhere along the length of the fiber, and there are instances of multiple branches and instances where cleavages exist in the center of the muscle but fuse into a single fiber. All of these make it unlikely that it will be possible to evaluate the importance of the longitudinal division of fibers, if it does occur, in the overall process of muscle enlargement.

The reports of increases of fiber number in human skeletal muscle in response to exercise programs come from estimates of the total number of fibers in muscle based on the total cross-sectional area of the muscle measured with ultrasonic or computerized tomographic methods and the average cross-sectional area of the fibers in the muscle.[27] In most cases there has not been a clear demonstration that all of the fibers contained in the muscle contributed to the cross-sectional area as it was measured. An alternate method is to measure the cross-sectional area of large muscles, since the fibers contained in these muscles are not particularly large enough to make the assumption that there must have been a proliferation of fibers so that all could retain a constant size. Recent studies suggest that a similar range in the total number of fibers for a given muscle, such as the biceps brachii, is large. This is similar to other animal species. The enlargement of the existing fibers in a muscle can adequately account for the total enlargement that has been induced in humans during controlled experiments.[24]

The findings of Gollnick and others[11,14] support the older concept that the number of fibers in skeletal muscle is established early in life and that the expected enlargement that occurs during normal growth and development and high intensity exercise is the result of hypertrophy and not hyperplasia. The possibility of hyperplasia of muscle fibers as a response to prolonged overuse associated with high intensity exercise cannot be completely discounted. However, definitive proof in support of this possibility is lacking in both humans and other animal species.

Metabolic properties

Changes associated with the oxidative potential are second in magnitude to alterations in muscle size in response to altered patterns of physical activity. If the normal human state is sedentary, training for endurance can increase the concentration of enzymes for the terminal oxidation of fuels by twofold to threefold depending on the time and duration of the training.[13,17,24] This increase in oxidative potential can occur in all fiber types. The response to high resistance exercise, such as weight lifting, is an augmentation contractile element with no change in the total amount of mitochondria. Under these conditions there is a dilution of the total mitochondrial concentration that results in a lower enzyme concentration per unit protein. With short, heavy bouts of exercise, such as sprinting, there is little if any increase in the concentration of aerobic enzymes.[13,24] However, there is no reduction as occurs in weight lifting. With inactivity, whether it be from immobilization of a limb or the voluntary termination of high level training, there is a rapid loss in the activity per unit tissue of the enzymes associated with the use of oxygen by the muscle. Neither training nor inactivity appears to alter the basic kinetic properties of the enzymes in the Embden-Meyerhof pathway or the mitochondria involved in adenosine triphosphate (ATP) production. An alteration of the total amount of enzyme per unit of tissue is the only effect.

The influence of training on the anaerobic capacity of skeletal muscle is not as clear as the aerobic potential.[13,24] There are conflicting reports of the effect of endurance and sprint training on the activities of key enzymes in the Embden-Meyerhof metabolic pathway. At present it would be safe to conclude that if there is an effect of training on the glycolytic pathway it is relatively small. With inactivity there also is little or no overall change in the anaerobic capacity of skeletal muscle. Maintenance of the enzymes of this metabolic pathway at rather constant levels may be an indication that their level is independent of activity patterns. This may be a protective device resulting from a constant endowment of muscle with the potential for short bursts of high intensity activity, such as an extension of the fright and flight mechanism.

Of some interest is the interplay between the increase in oxidative potential in skeletal muscle and the improved work capacity as a result of training. It should be established that the increases in the oxidative potential of skeletal muscle that occur with training outstrip the changes in total body oxygen uptake (the maximal oxygen uptake [max $\dot{V}O_2$]).[24,25] Moreover, it has been demonstrated that increases in max $\dot{V}O_2$ can occur without any change in the concentration of oxidative enzymes in the muscle. In addition, following the termination of training the fall in the concentration of mitochondrial enzymes in the muscles exceeds that of the total body max $\dot{V}O_2$. On this basis it may be best to look for the influence of endurance training on metabolic events during submaximal exercise to discover a possible role for the adaptation that occurs with exercise. This is not an unrealistic proposal, since little exercise is done at maximal or supramaximal levels, particularly by those who train with endurance methods, and the training that produces these changes is mostly of the prolonged submaximal type.

The major effects of endurance training during prolonged submaximal exercise are an increased use of fat with a concomitant sparing of muscle glycogen, a reduced production of lactate as reflected by the concentrations in both the working muscle and the blood, and a prolongation of work capacity.[12,24] These changes occur although the oxygen uptake, the cardiac output, the availability of fat in the form of plasma free fatty acids, and the blood flow through the muscle are the same at a given exercise intensity before and after training. The most important of these changes appears to be a greater reliance on fat as a fuel during exercise and the conservation of the carbohydrate stores of the muscle.

There is a close relationship between the depletion of the skeletal muscle glycogen stores and exhaustion. How does an increase in the concentration of oxidative enzymes result in a greater use of fat when the oxygen consumption of the muscle is the same?[25] It is not the result of a change in the availability or extraction of oxygen from the blood or from a higher concentration of fatty acids in the blood. Gollnick and Saltin[12] postulate that this effect is one of regulation at the enzyme level in a manner that an elevation in oxidative enzyme concentrations retards the rate that glycogen is degraded. The hypothesis set forth is that higher mitochondrial concentrations will result in a more effective transport of adenosine diphosphate (ADP) produced from the breakdown of ATP into the mitochondria. If this rate is elevated and there are elevated concentrations of other oxidative enzymes within the muscle, it will enhance the rate that oxygen uptake occurs. Thus there will be a smaller fall in the cystolic [ATP]/[ADP][Pi] ratio. This ratio is important in controlling a number of metabolic processes including regulating the flux of substrate through the Embden-Meyerhof pathway at the level of phosphofructokinase. Inhibition of glycogenolysis will result in a reduced production of pyruvate that will in effect reduce the competition between acetylcoenzyme A units derived from beta oxidation of fatty acids. Moreover, with the reduced pyruvate production a greater percentage of that formed will be shunted to the citric acid cycle and less will spill over to the formation of lactate. This entire process can be compared to a localized Pasteur effect with the maintenance of a high cystolic [ATP]/[ADP][Pi] ratio being the key to suppressing glycolysis and promoting the use of fat. This entire scheme of an altered control can take place without any alteration in the availability or consumption of oxygen.

FIBER TYPE CONVERSION

The property that endows the muscle with the capacity for a wide variety of contractile patterns used in daily life makes some motor units more suitable for certain types of activity than others. For example, the higher oxidative potential of the ST and FTa motor units than that of the FTb fibers makes them more suitable for prolonged activity where the fuel reserves could be used to the greatest advantage. Conversely, the FTb fibers appear to be well suited for short, intense contractile patterns where the production of lactate could be tolerated. This is how the different motor units are used.

The control over these patterns of motor unit use is based on the general principle of the difference in the size of the motoneurons that innervate the fibers. The smaller the diameter of the motoneurons the easier it is to activate them.[16] ST fibers are innervated by the smallest motoneurons and are always the first to be activated.[7] A continuum exists by which motor units are added in a sytematic manner to provide an orderly increase in the force-developing capacity of the muscle.

Studies in humans revealed that there is a systematic recruitment of motor units during a variety of physical activities.[7,13,24] In prolonged submaximal exercise this recruitment occurs whereby, at the point of exhaustion, all of the motor units, regardless of type, may have been used. This occurs despite the fact that during the course of the exercise the force developed and the power produced remain essentially unchanged. This suggests that during prolonged submaximal exercise some motor units become exhausted and drop out of the contractile process as others are added.

Studies in humans also demonstrated that wide variation exists in the fiber composition of the same muscle in different persons.[13,24] In the general population this variation can be described by the normal bell-shaped curve with the bulk of the population having about equal percentages of ST and FT fibers. However, there are individuals who possess high percentages of either of the two major fiber types. Studies of elite athletes demonstrated that endurance and sprint athletes generally have high percentages of ST and FT fibers, respectively.

Of some interest is whether these unusual fiber compositions are the result of genetic endowment or are produced by the specific training programs in which athletes engage. It is imperative to realize that the identification of a fiber type is based exclusively on its composition of myofibrillar proteins. Earlier reports of changes in fiber types that were based on alteration in oxidative capacity, that is, a change from a *white* to a *red* fiber, are considered erroneous and are discounted except on the basis that they are only reflections of changes in the concentration of mitochondrial enzymes which occur in response to endurance exercise. Existing data demonstrate with cross reinnervation[2] and alterations in the pattern of stimulation, such as that produced with electrical stimulation via the motor nerves,[20,23] changes occur in the contractile proteins that constitute a real conversion of one type of fiber to another. Thus fibers possess the genetic machinery for the production of all of the isozymes of the proteins associated with the various fiber subtypes.

There are only a few longitudinal studies of physical training that have attempted to determine whether these alternate modes of genetic expression can be produced by normal patterns of physical activity. The general conclusion from these studies is that there is little or no interconversion of FT and ST fibers.[13,24] There is an indication that the subtypes of FT fibers may be mutable as a result of normal physical activity. A more complete summary of studies dealing with the effect of training programs on fiber composition of skeletal muscle is contained in Saltin and Gollnick.[24]

SUMMARY

A general overview of the contractile and metabolic properties of human skeletal muscle is presented. Two broad classes of fibers, those with slow twitch and those with fast twitch properties, are described. The fast twitch fibers can be subtyped depending on the sensitivity of the myofibrillar ATPase to acid inactivation. There are differences in metabolic properties of these fiber types, but these differences vary and are influenced to such an extent by physical activity that they are essentially useless in identifying the motor units by standard histochemical methods.

The response of muscle to altered patterns of physical activity is discussed. The major increases or decreases in total muscle strength are the result of changes in the total cross-sectional area of the muscle. These changes are the result of either an atrophy or a hypertrophy of the individual fibers and not a result of alterations in the total fiber number. The metabolic properties of muscle are easily altered by use or disuse of the muscle. The most dramatic alteration is the large increase in the concentration of mitochondria and, concomitantly, an alteration of the enzymes used in the production of ATP via the use of oxygen as a result of endurance training. Heavy resistance training (weight lifting) and sprint activity have essentially no effect on the metabolic properties of muscle, whereas inactivity caused by immobilization results in a rapid loss of mitochondrial enzymes.

The anaerobic potential of muscle is relatively unchanged by modification in physical activity. The bulk of the data suggests that the major division of fiber types found in muscle is a genetic endowment and relatively unchanged by training. There may be, however, some shifts in the subtypes of the fibers with training. This latter situation is an area that needs additional attention. Alterations in fiber composition and metabolic adaptations caused by activity and inactivity are important areas of study in the care and treatment of athletic injuries.

REFERENCES

1. Bárány, M.: ATPase activity of myosin correlated with speed of muscle shortening, J. Gen. Physiol. **50**(suppl. 21):197, 1967.
2. Bŕńy, M., and Close, R.I.: The transformation of myosin in cross-innervated rat muscles, J. Physiol. **213**:455, 1971.
3. Brooke, M.H., and Kaiser, K.K.: The use and abuse of muscle histochemistry, Ann. NY Acad. Sci. **228**:121, 1974.
4. Buchthal, F., and Schmalbruch, H.: Motor unit of mammalian muscle, Physiol. Rev. **60**:90, 1980.
5. Burke, R.E., and Edgerton, V.R.: Motor unit properties and selective involvement in movement, Exerc. Sport Sci. Rev. **3**:31, 1975.
6. Chiakulus, J.J., and Pauly, J.E.: A study of postnatal growth of skeletal muscle in the rat, Anat. Rec. **152**:55, 1965.
7. Desmedt, J.E., and Godaux, E.: Ballistic contractions in man: characteristic recruitment pattern of single motor units of the tibialis anterior muscle, J. Physiol. **264**:673, 1977.
8. Fugl-Meyer, A.R., and others: Is muscle structure influenced by genetical or functional factors? Acta Physiol. Scand. **114**:277, 1982.
9. Gonyea, W., Ericksson, G.C., and Bonde-Petersen, F.: Skeletal muscle fiber splitting induced by weight-lifting in cats, Acta Physiol. Scand. **99**:105, 1977.
10. Gonyea, W.J.: Role of exercise in inducing increases in skeletal muscle fiber number, J. Appl. Physiol. **48**:421, 1980.
11. Gollnick, P.D., and others: Fiber number and size in overloaded chicken anterior latissimus dorsi muscle, J. Appl. Physiol. **54**:1292, 1983.
12. Gollnick, P.D., and Saltin, B.: Significance of skeletal muscle oxidative enzyme enhancement with endurance training, Clin. Physiol. **2**:1, 1982.
13. Gollnick, P.D., and Sembrowich, W.L.: Adaptations in human skeletal muscle as a result of training. In Amsterdam, E.A., Wilmore, J.H., and DeMaria, A.M., editors: Exercise in cardiovascular health and disease, New York, 1977, Yorke Medical Books.
14. Gollnick, P.D., and others: Muscular enlargement and number of fibers in skeletal muscle of rats, J. Appl. Physiol. **50**:936, 1981.
15. Haggmark, T.: A study of morphologic and enzymatic properties of the skeletal muscles after injuries and immobilization in man, thesis, Stockholm, 1978, Karolinska Institute.
16. Henneman, E., and Olson, C.B.: Relations between structure and function in the design of skeletal muscle, J. Neurophysiol. **28**:581, 1965.
17. Holloszy, J.O., and Booth, F.W.: Biochemical adaptations to endurance exercise in muscle, Annu. Rev. Physiol. **38**:273, 1976.
18. Kugelberg, E., and Lindegren, B.: Transmission and contraction fatigue of rat motor units in relations to succinate dehydrogenase activity of motor unit fibres, J. Physiol. **288**:285, 1979.
19. Perry, V.S.: In Milhorat, A.T., editor: Exploratory concepts in muscular dystrophy II, Amsterdam, 1974, Excerpta Medica, Inc.
20. Pette, D., et al.: Time dependent effects on contractile properties, fibre population, myosin light chains and enzymes of energy metabolism in intermittently and continuously stimulated fast twitch muscles of the rabbit, Pflugers Arch. **364**:103, 1976.
21. Reichmann, H., and Pette, D.: A comparative microphotometric study of succinate dehydrogenase activity levels in type I, IIA, and IIB fibres of mammalian and human muscles, Histochemistry **74**:27, 1982.
22. Reitsma, W.: Skeletal muscle hypertrophy after heavy exercise in rats with surgically reduced muscle function, Am. J. Phys. Med. **48**:237, 1968.
23. Salmons, S., and Stréter, F.A.: Significance of impulse activity in the transformation of skeletal muscle types, Nature **263**:30, 1976.
24. Saltin, B., and Gollnick, P.D.: Skeletal muscle adaptability: significance for metabolism and performance. In Peachy, L.D., Adrian, R.H., and Geiger, S.R., editors: Handbook of physiology, Baltimore, 1983, The Williams & Wilkins Co.
25. Saltin, B., and Rowell, L.B.: Functional adaptations to physical activity and inactivity, Fed. Proc. **39**:1506, 1980.

26. Sargeant, A.J., and others: Functional and structural changes after disuse of human muscle, Clin. Sci. Mol. Med. **52:**337, 1977.
27. Schantz, P., and others: The relationship between the mean muscle fibre area and the muscle cross-sectional area of the thigh in subjects with large differences in thigh girth, Acta Physiol. Scand. **113:**537, 1981.
28. Schmalbruch, H.: The morphology of regeneration of skeletal muscles in the rat, Tissue Cell **8:**673, 1976.
29. Sola, O.M., Christensen, D.L., and Martin, A.W.: Hypertrophy and hyperplasia of adult chicken anterior latissimus dorsi muscles following stretch with and without denervation, Exp. Neurol. **41:**76, 1973.
30. Von Eulenberg, A., and Cohnheim, R.: Ergebnisse der anatomischen Untersuchung eines Falles von sogenannter Muskelhypertrophie. Verh. Ber. Med. Ges. **1:**191, 1866.

5. Determination of patellofemoral contact pressures

Helmut H. Huberti
Wilson C. Hayes

Many surgical reconstructive procedures are available for the treatment of chondromalacia and osteoarthritis of the patellofemoral joint. For recurrent subluxation and dislocation of the patella (thought to be one major cause of chondromalacia), there are more than 140 different procedures available.[7] Most of the surgical procedures are based on hypotheses that suggest the disease state is related to abnormally high patellofemoral contact pressures caused by kinematic or loading abnormalities. However, few experimental data are available on patellofemoral contact pressures or on how these surgical procedures influence the contact pressures.

Several researchers[1,15] measured patellofemoral contact areas using a number of different techniques. To measure contact pressures, Burke and Ahmed[6] and Ahmed and others[2,3] interposed a plastic foil in the joint space and determined pressures by evaluating plastic deformations of the foil. Henche and others[9] built an air cushion that contained several electrical contacts and used it to measure contact areas at different pressures. These methods required sophisticated equipment and did not allow sytematic investigation of many of the important mechanical variables influencing patellofemoral contact.

Special features of the patellofemoral joint are the asymmetric and geometric complexities of the patella and its interaction with the femoral groove and the femoral condyles. In addition, at flexion angles less than 90 degrees, the patellofemoral contact force is transferred solely to the patella. At higher flexion angles, an additional tendofemoral contact force occurs between the quadriceps tendon and the femoral groove (Fig. 5-1).

The resultant patellofemoral contact force vector is a function of the knee flexion angle. For given tensile forces F_Q and F_L, acting at the upper and lower pole of the patella, respectively, the contact force increases with the flexion angle. The patello-

☐ Supported by NIH RCDA AM 00749, AM 26740, and by an Orthopaedic Research Fellowship from the Deutsche Forschungsgemeinschaft (Federal Republic of Germany).

femoral force resultant is also a function of the Q angle in the frontal plane (Fig. 5-2). The Q angle is defined by the patellar ligament and the resultant quadriceps vector that is aligned with a line from the center of the patella to the anterior-superior iliac crest.[5] This adds a laterally directed component to the resultant force. Clinically, it is thought that abnormally large Q angles are associated with a high incidence of chondromalacia.[8,11] Thus several surgical procedures are aimed at restoring a normal Q angle (about 15 degrees in full extension).

The objectives of this chapter are to use a new pressure-sensitive film and knee-

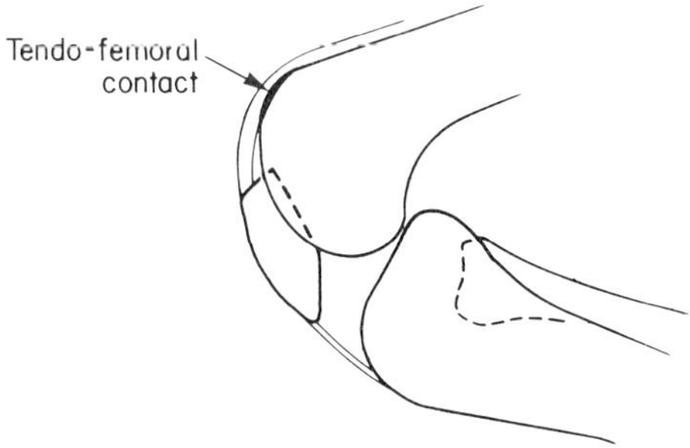

Fig. 5-1. Tendofemoral contact between quadriceps tendon and femoral groove occurring at large flexion angles.

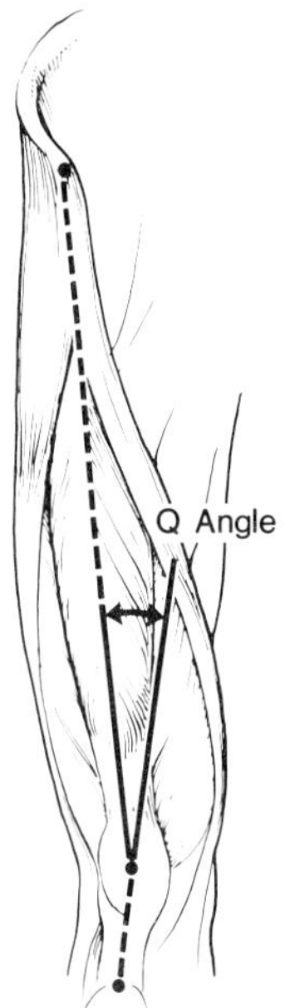

Fig. 5-2. Clinical definition of Q angle. Q angle is angle formed by ligamentum patellae and line from center of patella to anterior-superior iliac spine.

joint loading fixture to conduct parametric studies of patellofemoral contact pressures as functions of joint flexion angle and Q angle. The measured contact pressures serve as baseline data to evaluate surgical reconstructive procedures and to provide more refined estimates of patellofemoral contact stresses for finite element studies of normal and resurfaced patellas.

MATERIALS AND METHODS

Twelve fresh-frozen human knee joints were tested (age 56 to 75, six male and six female). All had macroscopically intact articular cartilage and were tested with intact capsule and patellar retinacula. To apply controlled patellofemoral contact forces, the joints were mounted into an INSTRON 1331 Materials Testing System using a special loading fixture (Fig. 5-3). For mounting, tibia and femur were each sectioned transversely at 25 cm from the joint space. The quadriceps tendon was clamped and attached through a load cell to a metal plate at the proximal end of the femur, which allowed adjustment of the Q angle in the frontal plane. The apparatus was loaded through low-friction spherical bearings at locations representing the hip and ankle by moving the hydraulic actuator under automatic control. This resulted in tension in the quadriceps loop and loaded the patella against the femoral groove. The knee flexion angle was adjusted by varying the length of the extensor tendon.

Contact pressures and contact areas were measured with Fuji PRESCALE pressure sensitive film. The film is 200×10^{-6} mm thick and consists of two paperlike sheets: (1) an A sheet coated with a microencapsulated dye and (2) a C sheet coated with a developing substance that produces a color density proportional to the applied

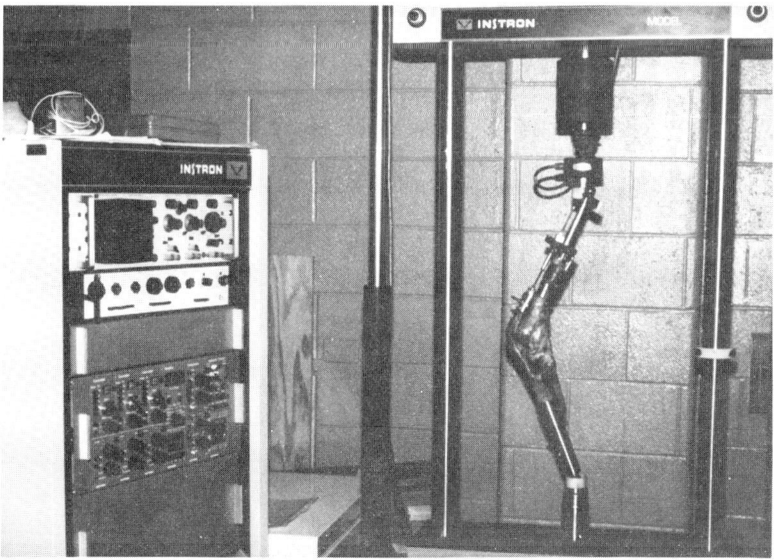

Fig. 5-3. Loading fixture for in vitro testing of patellofemoral joint mounted in INSTRON Materials Test System.

pressure. To allow use of the film in fully lubricated synovial joints and to protect the film against the synovial fluid, we enclosed it between two thin polyethylene sheets each 0.05 mm thick. The layered sheets were inserted through an incision in the superior synovial pouch leaving the capsular apparatus intact. Transducer calibration was accomplished using plane-ended cylinders of cartilage and subchondral bone compressed together to known pressures. Data reduction for the contact pressures was accomplished by visual comparison with the calibration standards. Contact areas were measured by tracing the pressure pattern boundary on a TALOS RP-622 digitizer.

Contact pressures and contact areas were determined in each knee joint at four different flexion angles (20, 30, 60, and 90 degrees) and at three different Q angles: (1) physiologic, (2) 10 degrees increased (more lateral pull of the quadriceps), and (3) 10 degrees decreased (more medial pull). The applied patellofemoral forces were controlled by consistently applying one third of the maximal in vivo isometric quadriceps moments measured in human volunteers.[10,14,18] These previous studies all demonstrated similar variations with flexion angle in the maximal isometric quadriceps moments. Based on these data, we applied 23.6 N-m at 20 degrees, 30.7 N-m at 30 degrees, 47.2 N-m at 60 degrees, and 35 N-m at 90 degrees of flexion.

In a second experiment that tested eight additional knees, pressures were measured at 120 degrees of flexion with an additional tendofemoral contact occurring. At this high flexion angle (and at physiologic Q angles) patellofemoral and tendofemoral pressures were measured simultaneously. In this experiment the joints were loaded with 47.2 N-m resultant bending moment, equivalent to two thirds of the maximum in vivo quadriceps moments. In some cases a problem occurred with use of the film to measure tendofemoral pressures. Because of the dual curvature of the film caused by contact with the tendon at this flexion angle, a wrinkling of the film occurred. In these cases the pressure distribution was remeasured with several small strips of film.

RESULTS

The first experiment was designed to test the influence of knee flexion on patellofemoral contact pressures at both physiologic and altered values of Q angle. Fig. 5-4 shows the pressure patterns at physiologic Q angle and at 20 degrees of flexion, the smallest flexion angle tested in the first experiment. The film was cut to the contact area (after the experiment) and placed in its original position on the patella. For normal Q angles, the pressures were remarkably uniform over the contact area with approximately the same contact pressures on both medial and lateral patellar facets (± 0.25 MPa). At physiologic Q angles, the average contact areas increased more than 60% over the range of flexion angles tested, reaching 4.1 cm^2 (± 1.8, 95% Confidence Interval [C.I.]) at 90 degrees (Table 5-1). The average pressures more than doubled from 20 degrees to 90 degrees. Assuming a uniform pressure distribution and multiplying the contact area by the average pressure, we also calculated

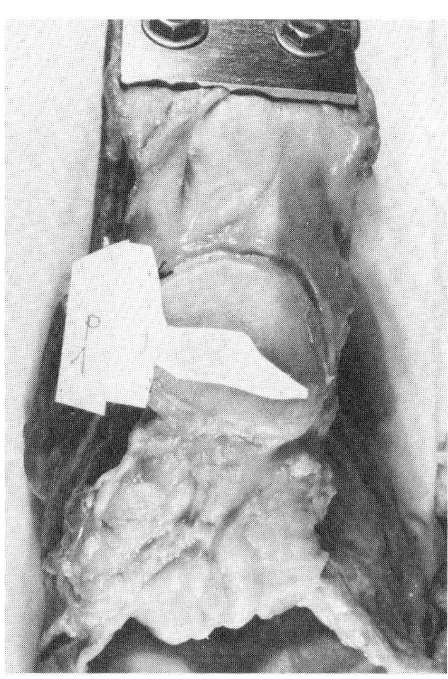

Fig. 5-4. Patellofemoral contact pressure at 20 degrees of flexion and physiologic Q angle. Pressure-sensitive film cut to contact area and placed in its original position on patella cartilage.

Table 5-1. Patellofemoral contact at physiologic Q angle*

Knee flex-ion angle (degrees)	Contact area		Average contact pressure (MPa)	Resultant contact force (N)
	(cm²)	Total articular area (%)		
20	2.6 ± 0.4	20.5	2.0 ± 0.4	497 + 90
30	3.1 ± 0.3	24.9	2.4 ± 0.6	573 ± 125
60	3.9 ± 0.5	30.4	4.1 ± 1.4	1411 ± 331
90	4.1 ± 1.1	32.2	4.4 ± 1.0	1555 ± 419

*Mean values for n = 12 knees (±95% C.I.)

the resultant patello-femoral contact force for each knee. The average contact force varied from approximately 500 N (±150) at 20 degrees to 1550 N (±665) at 90 degrees (Table 5-1). Extrapolation to full maximal in vivo moments amounts to a total contact force of approximately 4500 N or 6.5 times a standard body weight of approximately 687 N (70 kg).

Variations in Q angle resulted in significant changes in the pressure distribution at all four flexion angles. In about half the knees, with both an increase and a decrease in Q angle, a similar pressure distribution consisting of increased peripheral loading of both the medial and lateral facets (Fig. 5-5) was found. The contact area separated nearly completely into two distinct regions. In the remaining knees, a more medially directed quadriceps force resulted in a transfer of the contact area entirely to the medial facet. A more laterally directed force caused a transfer of the load completely to the lateral facet in half of the knees tested.

Despite these changes in the shape of the pressure pattern, the magnitudes of the contact area were only slightly affected by Q angle (Table 5-2) with no statistically significant variations from the values at physiological Q angle. The maximum contact pressures, however, clearly increased both for an increased and a decreased Q angle. Surprisingly, a decreased Q angle resulted in even higher pressures than those obtained with an increased Q angle. Compared with the results at physiologic Q angle, there was a 50% increase in the average peak pressure at 20 degrees of flexion and a 25% increase at 90 degrees of flexion (Table 5-2).

In the second experiment, we measured both patellofemoral and tendofemoral contact pressures at 120 degrees of flexion and physiologic Q angle (Fig. 5-6). In most knees tested at this high flexion angle, the pressure on the patella was uniformly distributed over the medial and lateral facets. However, in two cases at 120 degrees higher pressure was found on the medial facet, which in one case was twice as high on the medial facet as on the lateral facet. The tendofemoral pressure in all cases

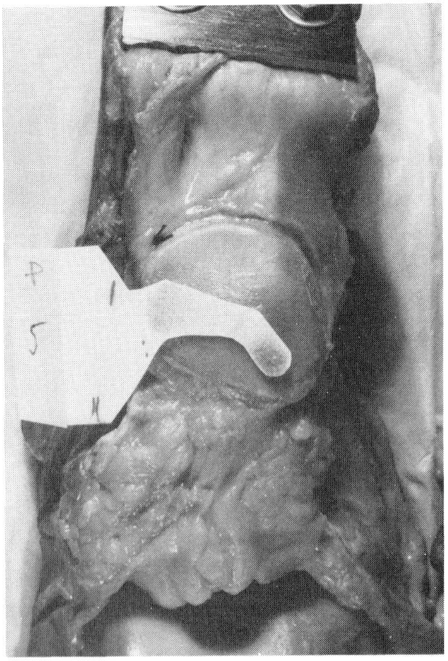

Fig. 5-5. Patellofemoral contact pressure with 10 degrees decreased Q angle in the same joint and same flexion angle as in Fig. 5-4. It shows peripheral loading on both lateral and medial patellar facets with complete unloading of vertical crest region. Identical pattern was found in half the knees after both increased and decreased Q angle.

Table 5-2. Patellofemoral contact for increased and decreased Q angle*

Knee flex- ion angle (degrees)	Contact ±area (cm²)		Maximum pressure (MPa)	
	Decreased Q angle (10°)	Increased Q angle (10°)	Decreased Q angle (10°)	Increased Q angle (10°)
20	2.7 (±0.5)	2.2 (±0.3)	3.1 (±0.6)	2.9 (±0.5)
30	2.8 (±0.6)	2.8 (±0.6)	3.1 (±0.6)	2.8 (±0.5)
60	3.6 (±0.7)	3.0 (±0.7)	5.8 (±1.3)	4.7 (±1.2)
90	3.7 (±0.8)	3.6 (±0.7)	5.4 (±0.8)	5.0 (±1.5)

*Mean values for n = 12 knees (±95% C.I.)

Table 5-3. Patellofemoral and tendofemoral contact at 120 degrees flexion angle*

Contact	Contact area (cm²)	Average contact pressure (MPa)	Resultant contact force (N)
Patellofemoral	4.6 ± 0.7	3.4 ± 0.5	1591
Tendofemoral	3.4 ± 0.5	1.6 ± 0.2	557

*Mean values for n = 8 knees (±95% C.I.)

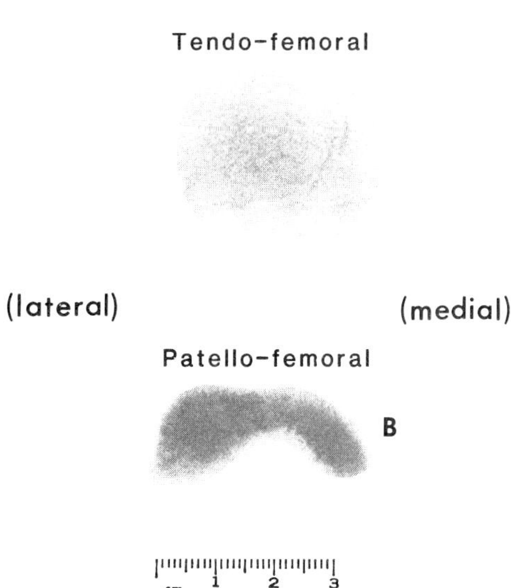

Fig. 5-6. Tendofemoral and patellofemoral contact pressure at 120 degrees of flexion. Two measurements were performed simultaneously. Contact pressure distribution was uniform (±0.25 MPa). Pressure at tendofemoral contact reached approximately 45% of pressures on patella at this flexion angle.

was uniformly distributed and significantly less than the patellofemoral pressure.

Average tendofemoral pressures at 120 degrees flexion reached about 45% of the patellofemoral pressures (Table 5-3). Average tendofemoral contact area at 120 degrees was 3.4 cm² (± 0.5) compared with 4.6 cm² (± 0.7) at the patellofemoral contact. Again assuming uniform pressure distributions and multiplying average pressure by the contact area, we calculated an average patellofemoral contact force of approximately 1600 N (± 232 N) and a tendofemoral contact force of 550 N (± 133) at 90 degrees flexion. This represents a 3:1 ratio between the patellofemoral and tendofemoral contact forces. Adding these two nonparallel vectors by assuming that they form an angle of 45 degrees resulted in a total contact force of about 2000 N. Extrapolation to full in vivo moment amounts to a total contact force of 3000 N at 120 degrees, or about four times standard body weight.

DISCUSSION

At physiologic Q angles, patellofemoral contact pressures were remarkably uniform over the contact area and were unaffected by differences in patellar geometry as classified by Wiberg.[19] In fact, three patellae were Wiberg type I, three were type II, and six were type III. In all cases the patellofemoral contact pressures were uniformly distributed (± 0.25 MPa). This suggests that the radiologically based morphologic classification system of Wiberg cannot be used as a direct indicator of the patellofemoral contact pressures. In our series, Wiberg type III patellae were not associated with abnormally high contact pressures.

For controlled loads, corresponding to one third of maximal in vivo voluntary moments, the resultant contact force more than tripled from about 500 N at 20 degrees to 1550 N at 90 degrees. Extrapolation to full in vivo moments resulted in a total maximum patella contact force of about 4500 N or six times body weight. This finding agrees with the predictions of Bandi and Brennwald[4] but is about twice as high as the values reported by Reilly and Martens.[17]

Altering the Q angle had little influence on the magnitude of the patellofemoral contact area. However, both a decreased and an increased Q angle resulted in higher peak contact pressures. The greatest increase in average maximum pressure (53%) was obtained at 20 degrees and at a decreased Q angle. This indicates that in a chondromalacic but otherwise normal joint, a surgical reduction of the Q angle may not be an appropriate procedure to reduce the contact pressures in the patellofemoral joint. In addition, overcorrection of an enlarged Q angle should be carefully avoided. These results also suggest the possibility of higher patellofemoral contact pressures not only with increased values of Q angle but also with decreased values of Q angle.

At 120 degrees of knee flexion, the tendofemoral pressure reached approximately 50% of the patellofemoral contact pressure. This indicates that tendofemoral contact may indeed play an important role in reducing patellofemoral contact pressures. This could also help explain the higher incidence of chondromalacia observed in patella alta.[11-13,16] In high-riding patellae, tendofemoral contact probably occurs rarely, and this may result in increased patellofemoral contact pressures, which in turn may contribute to accelerated degenerative change.

The results provide baseline data, which eventually may be used to guide surgical reconstruction of the unstable or chondromalacic patellofemoral joint. The measured pressures also provide input data on patellofemoral contact necessary to model normal, arthritic, and prosthetically replaced patellae by the finite element method. The pressure-sensitive film and the knee-jont loading fixture provide a simple and accurate method for determining patellofemoral and tendofemoral contact pressures. The methodology may also be useful in applications to other joints and other compartments of the knee.

ACKNOWLEDGMENTS

The authors wish to acknowledge the help and suggestions of John Granholm, Clement Sledge, and Peter Walker, Brigham and Women's Hospital, Boston, and of John Bodine and John Stone, Beth Israel Hospital, Boston.

REFERENCES

1. Aglietti, P., and others: A new patella prosthesis: design and application, Clin. Orthop. **107**:175, 1975.
2. Ahmed, A.M. and Burke, D.L.: In vitro measurement of static pressure distribution in synovial joints. I. Tibial surface of the knee, J. Biomech. Eng. **105**:216, 1983.
3. Ahmed, A.M., Burke, D.L., and Yu, A.: In vitro measurement of static pressure distribution in synovial joints. II. Retropatellar surface, J. Biomech. Eng. **105**:226, 1983.
4. Bandi, W., and Brennwald, J.: Degenerative joint disease: the significance of femoropatellar pressure in the pathogenesis and treatment of chondromalacia patellae and femoropatellar arthrosis. In The knee joint, Amsterdam, 1974, Excerpta Medica, Inc.
5. Brattstrom, H.: Shape of the intercondylar groove normally and in recurrent dislocation of patella: a clinical and x-ray anatomical investigation, Acta Orthop. Scand. Suppl. **68**:51, 1964.
6. Burke, D.L. and Ahmed, A.M.: The effect of tibial tubercle elevation on patellofemoral loading, Trans. Orthop. Res. Soc., Atlanta, **5**:162, 1980.
7. Cotta, H.: Zur Therapie der habituellen Patellarluxation. Arch Orthop. Unfall-Chir. **51**:265, 1959.
8. Ficat, R.P. and Hungerford, D.S.: Disorders of the patellofemoral joint, Baltimore, 1977, The Williams & Wilkins Co.
9. Henche, H.R., Kunzi, H.U., and Morscher, E.: The areas of contact pressure in the patellofemoral joint, Int. Orthop. **4**:279, 1981.
10. Inman, V.T., Ralston, H.J., and Todd, F.: Human walking, Baltimore, 1981, The Williams & Wilkins Co.
11. Insall, J., Falvo, K.A., and Wise, D.W.: Chondromalacia patellae: a prospective study, J. Bone Joint Surg. **58A**:1, 1976.
12. Insall, J., Goldberg, V., and Salvati, E.: Recurrent dislocation and the high-riding patella, Clin. Orthop. **88**:67, 1972.
13. Lancourt, J.E. and Cristini, J.A.: Patella alta and patella infera: their etiological role in patellar dislocation, chondromalacia, and apophysitis of the tibial tubercle, J. Bone Joint Surg. **57A**:1112, 1975.
14. Lindahl, O., Movin, A., and Ringqvist, I.: Knee extension: measurement of the isometric force in different positions of the knee joint, Acta Orthop. Scand. **40**:79, 1969.
15. Matthews, L.S., Sonstegard, D.A., and Henke, J.A.: Load-bearing characteristics of the patellofemoral joint, Acta Orthop. Scand. **48**:511, 1977.
16. McKeever, D.C.: Transplantation of the tibial tubercle, J. Bone Joint Surg. **33A**:478, 1951.
17. Reilly, D.T. and Martens, M.: Experimental analysis of the quadriceps muscle force and patellofemoral joint reaction force for various activities, Acta Orthop. Scand. **43**:126, 1972.
18. Smidt, G.L.: Biomechanical analysis of knee flexion and extension, J. Biomech. **6**:79, 1973.
19. Wiberg, G.: Roentgenographic and anatomic studies on the femoropatellar joint, with special reference to chondromalacia patellae, Acta Orthop. Scand. **12**:319, 1941.

6. Composition, structure, material properties, and function of articular cartilage: a review

Van C. Mow
Elizabeth R. Myers
Carl R. Wirth

Physical conditioning has become an important part of the life-style of a large segment of the American population. Backed by encouraging data from cardiologists, exercise physiologists, and others, many people are participating in sports. This participation has become a source of enjoyment to many, a challenge to others, and even a social necessity to some. According to Powers,[47] more men of all ages are participating in sports, and there are also an unprecedented number of athletes among women and children. The sports vary from heavy contact sports to cyclic loading activities, such as walking, running, and cycling. Therefore it is anticipated that the number of knee injuries is likely to increase dramatically with this increased athletic participation.

Symptoms relating to problems in the patellar extensor complex of the knee compel many athletes to consult an orthopaedist. Overuse, malalignment, facet syndromes, chondromalacia, and secondary synovitis may disrupt the enjoyment of sports. Patellofemoral joint disease is a major cause of disability in athletes and in extreme cases may contribute to the termination of an athlete's career.

The patellofemoral joint is an integral part of the extensor mechanism of the knee. The patella is a sesamoid bone in the quadriceps complex that is covered on the interior surface by articular cartilage. The patella is tethered to the tibia by the patellar ligament, which permits only a fixed arc of medial-lateral motion. The relationship of the patella to the articular surface of the femur is determined by (1) the angular relationship of the quadriceps mechanism relative to the tibia; (2) the collagenous stabilizing ligaments fixing the patella to the femur, tibia, and meniscus;

□ Research projects supported by the National Institute of Arthritis, Diabetes, and Digestive and Kidney Diseases grants No. AM26440 and No. AM19094.

and (3) the geometry of the articular surfaces of the patella and the patellar groove on the femur.[13,31] The complex stresses and strains experienced by the patella must be sustained by the extensor mechanism, the surrounding structures, and the articulating cartilage surfaces.[12,19]

Articular cartilage serves three primary purposes: (1) it carries the load generated by joint use, (2) it dissipates the energy associated with the load, and (3) it permits smooth, almost frictionless, relative motion to occur between the articulating surfaces of the joint.[1,49] To understand how articular cartilage performs these functions in the knee, it is necessary to understand the relationship of composition and structure to the mechanical behavior of articular cartilage.

COMPOSITION AND STRUCTURE

Patellar articular cartilage normally appears as a white glistening pad firmly attached to the underlying bone. From the material science point of view, articular cartilage is a biphasic material. This material consists of 60% to 80% water, 20% to 40% collagen fibrils (50% to 70% dry weight), 10% to 25% proteoglycan, and 5% to 40% chondrocytes, glycoproteins, and lipids.[46]

Collagen

Type II collagen is the most abundant component of the organic solid matrix in articular cartilage. The basic structural form of collagen in cartilage is the fibril, which is an organized collection of helical protein molecules visible by transmission electron microscopy.[11,46] Of all the soft connective tissues, such as tendons, ligaments, and fibrocartilage, the ultrastructural arrangement of the collagen fibrils in articular cartilage is the most complex and unique. The superficial fibrils are densely packed and arranged in planes parallel to the articular surface and, perhaps, randomly oriented in the plane of the surface.[8,16,44] The fibrils of the middle zone are dispersed in the tissue in a three-dimensional arrangement with wide spaces between them. Benninghoff,[5] using observations from light microscopy techniques, postulated the existence of a columnar fibril arrangement throughout the middle zone. His observations lead to the development of an *arcade* concept to describe the arrangement as the straight columnar fibrils turn and merge into the superficial zone (Fig. 6-1, *A*). However, in recent studies under the scanning electron microscope, the general appearance of the fibrils suggests a random orientation in the midzone.[8,16,24,44] In the deeper third of the cartilage thickness, the collagen fibrils appear perpendicular to the bone as they pass through the tidemark and calcified cartilage and enter the subchondral cortex.[50] This is how articular cartilage is anchored to the ends of the bone. Fig. 6-1, *B* shows a schematic representation of the collagen architecture depicting the three salient ultrastructural zones of normal articular cartilage as interpreted from scanning electron microscopy.[8,16,24,44,50]

Fixation of cartilage to bone is important because if a sharp transition existed between the relatively soft articular cartilage and stiff bone, it could be a source of difficulty under certain loading conditions during joint use.[4,19,50] High shear stresses

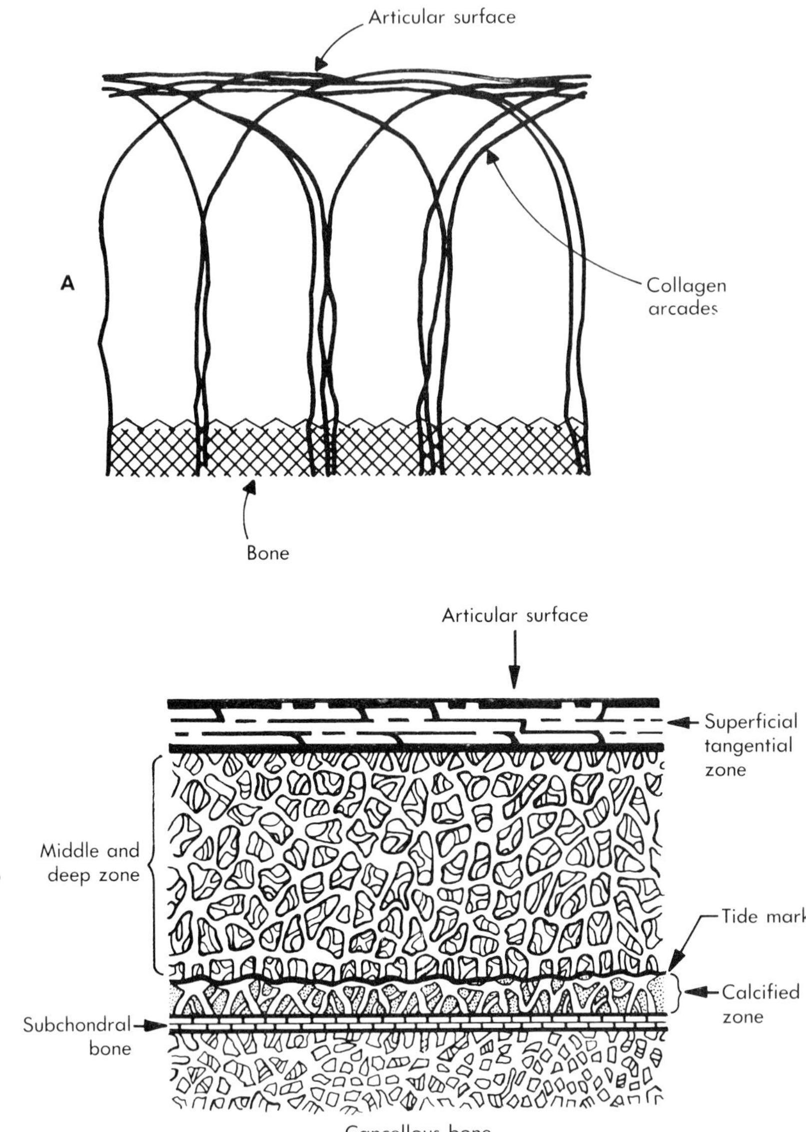

Fig. 6-1. A, Schematic depiction of collagen fibrils forming arcades throughout depth of articular cartilage as proposed by Benninghoff.[5] **B,** Schematic representation of collagen fibril ultrastructure, as seen from the scanning electron microscope, depicting the three salient zones of articular cartilage. (From Mow, V.C., and Lai, W.M., SIAM Rev. **22:**275, 1980.)

could develop at this interface when the joint is subjected to impulsive high loadings during athletic activities.[4,48,49] Thus the increasing density of calcium with depth from the tidemark through the calcified cartilage to the subchondral cortex appears important in creating a region of gradually increasing mechanical stiffness.[50] This transition zone between cartilage and bone allows a smooth transfer of stress from the

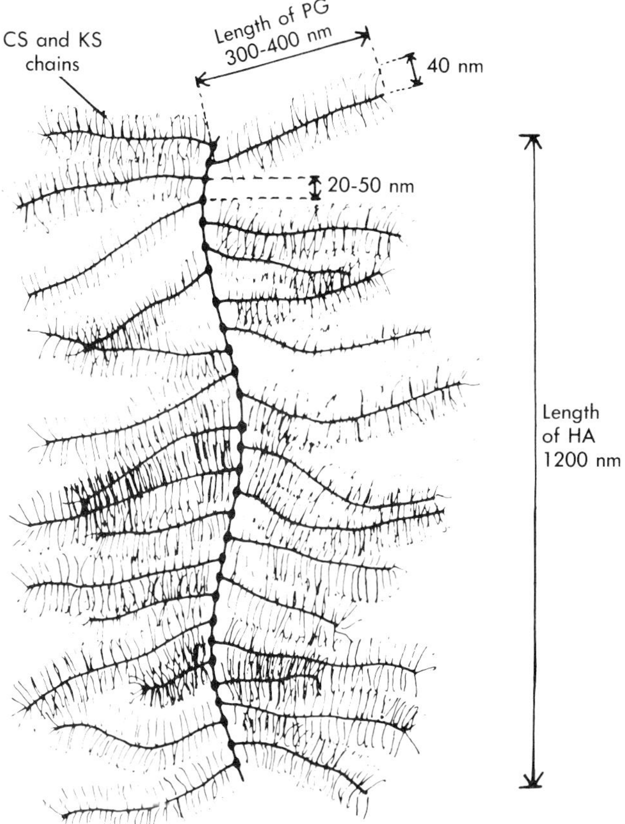

Fig. 6-2. Schematic depiction of proteoglycan aggregate showing subunits attached to HA molecule approximately 1.2 μm in length. (From Muir, H.: Biochemistry. In Freeman, M.A.R., editor: Adult articular cartilage, Kent, England, 1979, Pitman Medical Publishing Co., Ltd.)

cartilage to the bone and may be the biomechanical purpose for the layer of calcified cartilage.

Proteoglycans

The gel portion of the organic solid matrix of articular cartilage consists mostly of proteoglycans. Proteoglycans are complex, serpentine molecules with a central core of hyaluronic acid (HA). Attached to HA by link proteins are proteoglycan subunits, that is, molecules composed of a protein core with laterally attached glycosaminoglycans of chondroitin sulfate and keratan sulfate side chains.[46] Fig. 6-2 illustrates the conformation of this biomacromolecule. The glycosaminoglycans of the proteoglycans are negatively charged, and their proximity to each other, approximately 5 to 15 Å, results in a strong tendency for intramolecular and intermolecular charge repulsion. The proteoglycans of cartilage are stiffly extended molecules that are densely packed into the collagen network of the solid matrix. Thus significant charge repulsion exists in situ.[33,34] Maroudas[32,35] has calculated the charge density of this molecular packing. This densely charged population of proteoglycans causes cartilage to swell to the maximum volume permitted by the surrounding tensed collagen fibrillar network;[33,43] this swelling pressure influences the tensile behavior of articular cartilage.[17]

The degree of swelling in normal tissues depends on the ultrastructure of the surrounding collagen network. Recent results of experiments on swelling obtained by Mow and co-workers[42,43] show that swelling is anisotropic, that is, greater for specimen strips obtained perpendicular to the Hultkrantz split lines[21] than for those obtained parallel to the split lines, and inhomogeneous, that is, greater for specimen strips obtained from the middle and deep zones than for those obtained from the superficial zone.[43] These findings are consistent with known cartilage composition and tensile properties, which show that swelling is greater in regions where the proteoglycan/collagen ratio is higher[46] or where the tensile stiffness is lower.[23,52,62] Although the exact details of collagen-proteoglycan interactions are unknown,[46] most researchers believe that these interactions make the collagen-proteoglycan matrix into a cohesive solid substance with a definite, measurable set of material constants. A stable biomechanical state for articular cartilage is maintained only if the integrity of the collagen fibrillar network at the ultrastructural level, the proteoglycan aggregate at the molecular level, and their mutual physical interactions and entanglements are all normal.[40,46]

MECHANICAL BEHAVIOR
Tensile properties

It has been postulated that the main mechanical function of collagen is to resist tension.[9,58] This postulation is based on collagen fibril morphology, anatomic position, and mechanical tests on tissues primarily composed of the protein, such as tendon and ligament tissue. Therefore to study the mechanical behavior of collagen in cartilage, uniaxial tension tests are often performed on thin microtomed sections. These specimens are mounted in the jaws of a universal testing machine and pulled at a constant, slow rate until the piece fractures. The initial *toe* region of the resulting stress-strain curve (Fig. 6-3) is usually attributed to the straightening of the native coiled fibril configuration. The force required in this region of the stress-strain curve is attributed to the viscous drag of the fibrils sliding through the ground substance.[23] The relatively straight portion of the stress-strain curve (Fig. 6-3) is attributed to the stretching of the collagen fibrils or network, and the ratio of stress to strain is generally used to define Young's modulus of the tissue.[23,62] The fracture point of the specimen is a measure of strength, since the more stress required to break the cartilage, the greater the failure strength of the tissue.

Bovine articular cartilage from immature animals appears not only to have high

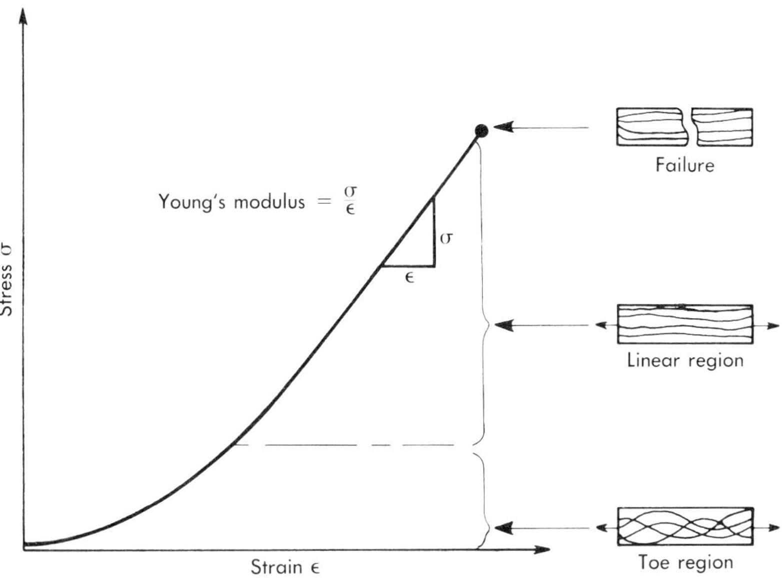

Fig. 6-3. Schematic diagram of typical stress-strain curve and representation of change of collagen fibril orientation during tensile experiment on cartilage.

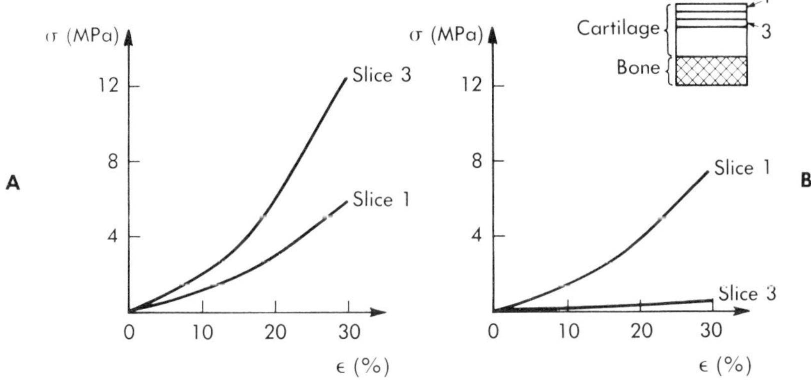

Fig. 6-4. Stress-strain curves for bovine articular cartilage samples pulled in uniaxial tension. Slice numbers correspond to position of samples with depth from articular surface, as illustrated in inserted depiction of cartilage and bone. **A,** Stress-strain curves for samples taken from immature joints. **B,** Stress-strain curves for samples taken from mature joints.

tensile stiffness and strength in the superficial tangential zone (STZ), but also increasing strength and stiffness with increasing depth (Fig. 6-4, *A*).[52] When the physis closes, however, the mature articular cartilage exhibits progressively less tensile stiffness and strength with increasing depth (Fig. 6-4, *B*). These results suggest that the STZ acts as a tough, wear-resistant skin covering the weaker, deeper layers of articular cartilage in mature and aging animals.[25,52] In a similar study using human patellar articular cartilage, Wirth and others[61] showed that the tensile properties are greatest in the teenage years and gradually diminish with age. The failure stress of each of the zones of human articular cartilage also appears to diminish with age. Kempson and others,[23] Woo and others,[62] and Roth and Mow[52] have all shown that the strength and stiffness of articular cartilage samples vary with orientation to the Hultkrantz split lines.[21] These studies show that, similar to swelling properties, articular cartilage test specimens taken parallel to split lines demonstrate greater stiffness and strength than those specimens taken perpendicular to the split lines for all depths and all age groups.

Compressive properties

In contrast to the role of collagen in providing tensile stiffness and strength for cartilage, proteoglycans may be thought of as enabling cartilage to resist compression. Before establishing a relationship between compressive properties and cartilage composition, the response of cartilage when compressed must be understood. Hirsch[20] used an indentation test to show that the articular cartilage of the human patella is not a purely elastic material. He found that indentation of the cartilage results in an instantaneous compressive deformation followed by further compression, which is characterized by a slow creeping process. Because the biphasic nature of cartilage precludes a simple explanation for this observed behavior, it took 40 years of intensive research to develop an understanding of the role of fluid movement in the compressive *viscoelastic* creep process.[3,20,40,42,55]

Patellar articular cartilage is an inhomogeneous layered structure in which the superficial region (approximately 20%) contains mostly collagen and water, and the deeper regions contain less closely packed collagen and more proteoglycans. Movement of fluid in and out of the tissue depends on the porosity and permeability of the collagen network at the STZ.[40,42,45] Movement of fluid in the deeper zones requires movement through the molecular pores of the collagen-proteoglycan matrix.[3,34,42] Fluid flow through the tissue is impeded by a large frictional drag developed between these molecular pores and the flowing interstitial fluid.[10,40,42] Movement of fluid through the articular cartilage matrix can be caused by a direct compression of the tissue or by creating a pressure gradient across the tissue.[41] Mow and co-workers[40,42] developed a two-phase model of articular cartilage (solid and fluid) that accounts for both the mechanical properties of the solid matrix and the flow of the interstitial fluid during compression. For example, when patellar cartilage suddenly receives an applied load via a porous filter, water is rapidly driven out causing a rapid loss of tissue volume. This water loss creates additional *space* into which the matrix can flow. This exchange of space between the fluid phase and the solid phase occurs slowly and simultaneously, that is, no physical void is actually created during the compressive creep deformation. This whole deformational process continues until a compressive equilibrium state is achieved, then fluid flow stops and the applied load is borne by the solid matrix.

Table 6-1. Mean values of intrinsic mechanical properties of articular cartilage from lateral facet of 103 human patellas as measured from biphasic confined compression creep experiment

Variable	N	Minimum	Maximum	Mean	Standard deviation
Age (yr)	103	16	85	56.40	19.13
Permeability $\times\ 10^{14}$ (m^4/N $\cdot$ s)	103	0.05	1.95	0.47	0.36
Modulus (MPa)*	103	0.13	1.91	0.79	0.36
Thickness (mm)	103	1.69	5.17	3.12	0.72
Water content (%)	58	72.80	88.40	78.63	3.86

From Armstrong, C.G., and Mow, V.C.: J. Bone Joint Surg. **64A**:88, 1982.
*1 MPa = 145 psi.

Realizing that these biphasic properties of articular cartilage affect the deformational response under a compressive load, Armstrong and Mow[3] performed a study using human patellar cartilage to determine the variation of compressive properties in composition and structure. One hundred three human patellar specimens were prepared in the form of cylindrical plugs and placed in a chamber that confined the cartilage laterally and permitted only uniaxial compression. The articular cartilage adjacent to the plug was studied using the histologic-histochemical grading system of Mankin and others.[30] The morphologic changes associated with aging and osteoarthritis showed little correlation with the mechanical properties of articular cartilage in confined compression. Despite the known biochemical alterations that occur with aging, the matrix compressive modulus (ratio of the compressive stress to the compressive strain after the loaded specimen has reached equilibrium) did not change as a function of age. However, there was a direct linear relationship between the matrix compressive modulus and uronic acid content, and an inverse linear relationship between the modulus and water content.[2,3] In the same studies, Armstrong and Mow found that the permeability is porportional to the inverse of the frictional resistance offered by the microporous collagen-proteoglycan solid matrix against the flow of the interstitial fluid (Table 6-1).

Shear properties

The mechanical properties of cartilage in shear may be determined in small shear-strain experiments. Hayes and Bodine[18] were the first to directly assess the shear modulus of cartilage. To avoid fluid flow, small shear-strain amplitudes (approximately 30×10^{-6}) were applied to a thin strip of the tissue between two oscillating planar piezoelectric plates. Since this technique is believed to not induce fluid flow, internal frictional flow resistance is not generated and therefore only the shear stiffness of the proteoglycan-collagen solid matrix is measured. The application of shear strain permits determination of the elastic energy stored (G_1) in the matrix (storage modulus) and the viscous energy dissipated (G_2) by the matrix (loss modulus). The complex

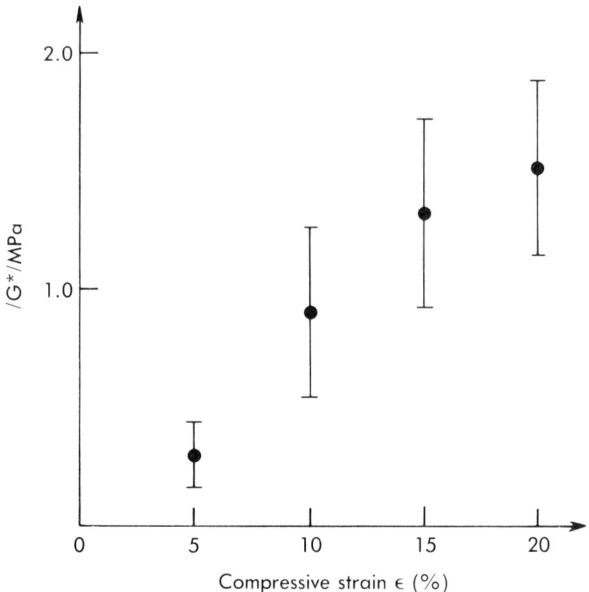

Fig. 6-5. Variation of magnitude of complex shear modulus $|G^*|$ with applied compressive clamping strain ϵ. The torsional test was performed at frequency of 1.0 Hz and shear strain of 0.1%. Linear regression analysis yields $|G^*| = 0.081\ \epsilon$ (%) for 18 plugs tested in torsion. The low value of $|G^*|$ at $\epsilon = 5\%$ is believed a result of sample-platen slippage.[53]

shear modulus (G^*) quantifies these two moduli (G_1, G_2), and the magnitude of the complex shear modulus $(|G^*| = [(G_1^2 + G_2^2)^{1/2}])$ can be thought of as a measure of the total external energy required to deform the solid matrix in shear.

To perform these tests, a compressive strain had to be applied normally to the cartilage strip to create enough frictional force to prevent slippage between the grips and the test specimen. It was later found that during this process the magnitude of the complex shear modulus increased when more compressive strain was applied.[6] It was also found that the compressive stiffening of the cartilage under load disappeared when articular cartilage was depleted of proteoglycans. This effect of compressive strain on the magnitude of the shear modulus was recently confirmed by Roth and others.[53] Thin circular disks of cartilage specimens were sheared in torsional oscillation with 0.1% shear strain at the sample periphery (Fig. 6-5).

The findings of both Hayes and Bodine[18] and Roth and co-workers[53] suggest a positive correlation between collagen content and the magnitude of the complex shear modulus and a negative correlation between collagen content and viscous energy dissipation. It appears that the collagen network plays an active biomechanical role in contributing to the shear properties of articular cartilage. This may be understood by visualizing the stretching of the randomly distributed network in the middle zone during shear; this stretching is a mechanism for elastic energy storage within the tissue. The complex shear modulus measurements reported by Mak and others[28] on proteoglycan solutions at 50 mg/ml (a concentration similar to those found in cartilage) show that proteoglycans contribute a minute amount toward the shear stiffness of cartilage. It must be stressed, however, that these shear results are tentative and more work needs to be done before any firm conclusions are established.

FUNCTION
Load carriage within cartilage

Load transmission across a joint, in particular the patellofemoral joint, means that loads are applied from one articular surface to the opposing articular surface. Loads several times body weight are applied across the patellofemoral joint and are sustained over an area usually not more than several square centimeters.[12,13,31] Consequently, the articular cartilage of the patella in daily use regularly experiences a compressive stress of 5 to 10 MPa (725 to 1450 psi) applied to its surface. Moreover, this load is not constantly fixed in relation to the surface, but moves about as the joint is being used. This leads to a complex mechanical situation within the cartilage: the microstructure must be able to sustain the stresses developed within the tissue, and an effective lubrication mechanism must exist at the surface.

Askew and Mow[4] showed that the relatively stiff collagen-rich layer at the surface protects the interior of cartilage by lowering the level of stress experienced by the tissue at these locations. Significant tensile stresses and strains exist at the surface. These are sustained by the tough collagen-rich superficial zone. Also, significant shear stress is predicted at the tidemark. In normal cartilage, the compression stiffening effect against shear will protect the lower zone of cartilage from shear scission at the tidemark.[4,51]

Under pathologic conditions when the collagen network is weakened, proteoglycans are lost and water content is increased.[2,3,33,35,40] These compositional changes and structural damages result in an increase of tissue permeability and a decrease of matrix stiffness.[2,3] Using computer models, Askew and Mow[4] and Roth and Mow[51] simulated the biomechanical consequences following these pathologic changes. Local loss of proteoglycans can lead to local soft spots and a significant increase of tensile stresses and strains experienced by the superficial collagen-rich zone, which can cause additional collagen network disruptions.[60,61] Loss of proteoglycans defeats the compression stiffening effect[6] and its protective role at the tidemark. Finally, the increase in tissue water content and permeability will defeat the role of the interstitial fluid in contributing toward load support through a hydrostatic mechanism and the ability of cartilage to lubricate itself.[1,40] The detailed mechanisms relating the cause and effect between changes of cartilage biochemistry, biomechanics, and function are now actively being pursued.

The role of articular cartilage in joint lubrication

According to Gardner and co-workers,[14,15] the articular cartilage surfaces are rough, not smooth. Using a size scale relevant to lubrication mechanisms, they described a set of secondary irregularities, approximately 0.5 mm in diameter, tertiary hollows and mounds approximately 20 to 45 μm in diameter, and quaternary ridges approximately 1 to 4 μm in length.[1] These irregularities are accentuated in aging joints, where microcracks and fibrillar tufts are seen in the frayed areas on the articular surface. These surface flaws are precursors to gross cartilage loss through wear. Wear rates of the cartilage surface have recently been reported,[27] and for normal cartilage they are minuscule. Since 1934, the coefficient of friction has been repeatedly measured. These measurements range from 0.005 to 0.03.* These values for the frictional coefficient compare favorably to artificial bearing systems.

The dual characteristics of low wear rates and low frictional coefficients have made biologic bearings, such as the knee or hip, the envy of lubrication engineers. Under abnormal conditions, however, breakdowns of bearings occur, and in biologic situations, osteoarthritis results. Thus it is important to know how the properties of articular cartilage contribute to the lubrication efficiency of diarthrodial joints.

Basically, boundary and fluid film are the two types of lubrication.[1] Boundary lubrication depends on adsorption of a monolayer of lubricant molecule to the articular surface. The characteristics of this adsorbed molecule were first identified by Swann and Radin.[56] This molecule, known as the lubricating glycoprotein fraction (LGF), is found in the synovial fluid. It is a single polypeptide chain containing oligosaccharides or single sugar molecules distributed along the length of the protein core. The molecular weight is about 250,000. This molecule has a tremendous affinity for articular cartilage and is not easily rubbed off. However, if a molecule is lost through attrition, another molecule of the LGF easily replaces it.

In fluid film lubrication, a thicker film of lubricant exists between the two bearing surfaces. There are two sources for this lubricant. First, under normal conditions, there is a minuscule amount of synovial fluid (typically for normal joints no more than 2 ml exists within the entire joint cavity). The synovial fluid contains nutrients for the cartilage, hyaluronic acid, LGF, and other electrolytes. Under lightly loaded and fast-moving conditions, synovial fluid serves as the lubricant for the joint. Under heavier loads and slower conditions, which is the predominant condition, the interstitial fluid in the articular cartilage becomes the major source of lubricant. It is instructive to assess the amounts of fluid available to the joint as a lubricant. Generally, a fluid film of 10 to 20 μm is required for effective function as a lubricant. Since synovial fluid probably acts as a fluid film lubricant under lightly loaded conditions, there are approximately 10 to 20 μm of synovial fluid covering the articulating surfaces. However, articular cartilage thickness ranges from 1500 to 3000 μm, and 78% of this is water. This amount of water is between 100 and 200 times the water required to effectively lubricate the joint. As the load increases in the joint, synovial fluid tends to be driven out of the gap between the surfaces. It is precisely under this condition that the interstitial fluid begins to move rapidly and to cause a replenishment of the required joint lubricant.

---

*References 1, 7, 22, 26, 29, 37, 40, 56, 59.

Interstitial fluid exudation and imbibition during joint motion were described by Mow and Lai.[40] The cartilage and an applied load were modeled as in Fig. 6-6. These authors predicted that, for normal cartilage matrix elastic moduli and permeability coefficients, fluid flow occurs in a manner that creates its own lubricant film. During joint articulation, the load transmission area on the joint surfaces moves to and fro. As new areas of the joint come into the contact zone, the interstitial fluid is expressed on and between the articulating surfaces to form the lubricant to support the required load. As the load moves off an area, the elastic solid matrix expands and imbibes the lubricant that was initially expressed (Fig. 6-7). This circulatory system is good for joint lubrication and also for cartilage nutrition. Joint motion is the pump required to provide a forced circulation of fluid through the avascular cartilage.[54,57] This circulatory-flow mechanism has been verified in an experiment using a microscopic flow visualization process at the articular surface.[39]

If animal joints are so well designed, why do they fail? Under certain loading conditions, such as jogging, automobile accidents (the dashboard knee syndrome), and falls, impact loads can cause microscopic damages to the various components of the tissue. (In addition, effects such as enzymatic degradation and infection can also damage cartilage.) There is a delicate balance of forces at the ultrastructural level between the constraining collagen network and the swelling proteoglycans.[36,43] A weakened collagen network would increase swelling and water content. If the collagen structure is disrupted by impact, the tissue would be expected to swell and increase its water content. Armstrong and Mow[2,3] have shown that the cartilage water content is a predominant factor governing the magnitude of both the solid matrix elastic modulus and the permeability coefficient. Increasing the water content by a few

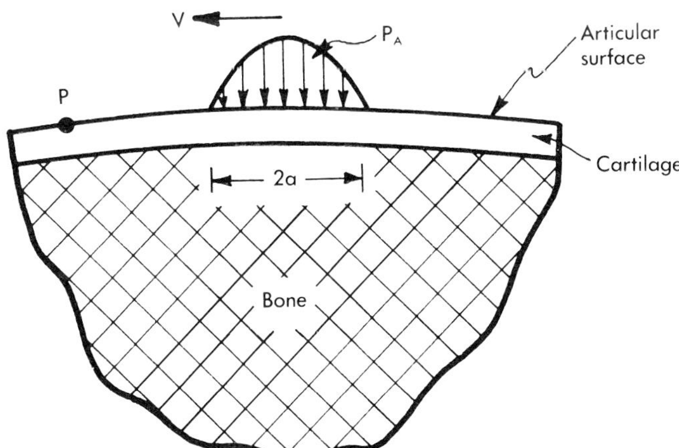

Fig. 6-6. System used to model compressive distributed load P_A moving across articular surface of joint with velocity V. Width of applied distributed load is 2a. Articular cartilage is modeled as layer of biphasic material attached to stiff underlying bone. Point P in Fig. 6-7 locates an observer on surface observing relative fluid motion as load passes over this point.

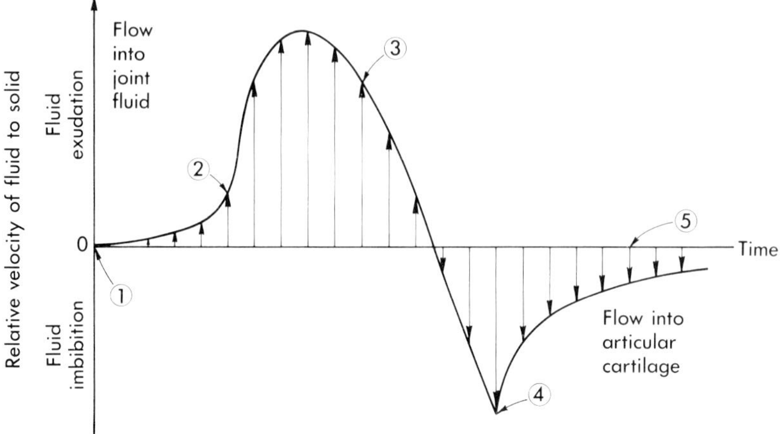

Fig. 6-7. Predicted fluid motion as distributed load P_A of Fig. 6-6 travels by the observer at point P on surface. Numbers correspond to following positions of moving load relative to observer at P: *1*, P_A is centered at distance of 2a in front of P; fluid exudation begins. *2*, The front edge of P_A is at P; fluid begins to exude in significant quantities. *3*, P_A is centered directly over P; fluid exudes underneath load and reaches maximum exudation as passed. *4*, The trailing edge of P_A is at P; elastic recovery of tissue occurs, and fluid is imbibed behind moving load. *5*, P_A is at a distance of 2a past P; the relative fluid motion begins to cease.

percentage points can drastically lower the elastic modulus of the solid matrix and increase the permeability coefficient. This simultaneous occurrence leads to a different flow pattern of the interstitial fluid in the tissue during joint articulation. Cartilage no longer has an effective means of pumping the interstitial fluid into the impending area of contact or of resorbing the fluid rapidly once it is lost from the tissue.[40] Thus the joint must rely on the other two probably less effective mechanisms of lubrication to function smoothly.

SUMMARY

In this chapter, the role of collagen, proteoglycan, and water in controlling the mechanical behavior of cartilage is examined. Normal cartilage properties ensure the interstitial fluid flow into the gap between the articulating surfaces during joint motion. Microdamage to the cartilage constituents will alter its properties through loss of proteoglycans and gain of water. Many unanswered questions remain. How is microdamage sustained? How do proteoglycans migrate through the tissue and eventually leach out? How do the cells perceive the changes, and how do they replenish the proteoglycans? Is there repair of the damaged collagen network? However, the most important question in sports medicine is how various traumas cause damage to articular cartilage. Little scientific information exists on this important aspect of sports medicine. Future researchers must find the answers to these and other questions.

ACKNOWLEDGMENT

The authors thank Ms. Rose Boshoff for her skillful editorial assistance in the preparation of this manuscript.

REFERENCES

1. Armstrong, C.G., and Mow, V.C.: Friction, lubrication and wear of synovial joints. In Owen, R., Goodfellow, J., and Bullough, P., editors: Scientific foundations of orthopaedics and traumatology, London, 1980, William Heinemann Medical Books, Ltd.
2. Armstrong, C.G., and Mow, V.C.: Biomechanics of normal and osteoarthritic articular cartilage. In Straub, L.R., and Wilson, Jr, P.D., editors: Clinical trends in orthopaedics, New York, 1982, Thieme-Stratton, Inc.
3. Armstrong, C.G., and Mow, V.C.: Variations in the intrinsic mechanical properties of human articular cartilage with age, degeneration, and water content, J. Bone Joint Surg. **64A**:88, 1982.
4. Askew, M.J., and Mow, V.C.: The biomechanical function of the collagen fibril ultrastructure of articular cartilage, J. Biomech. Eng. **100**:105, 1978.
5. Benninghoff, A.: Form und Bau der Gelenkknorpel in ihren Beziehungen zur Funktion 2. Der Aufbau des Gelenkknorpels in seinen Beziehungen zur Funktion, Z. Zellforsch. **2**:783, 1925.
6. Bodine, A.J., and others: The compression dependence of the shear modulus of articular cartilage, Trans. Orthop. Res. Soc. San Francisco **4**:142, 1979.
7. Charnley, J.: The lubrication of animal joints in relation to surgical reconstruction arthroplasty, Ann. Rheum. Dis. **19**:10, 1960.
8. Clarke, I.C.: Articular cartilage: a review and scanning electron microscope study. I. The interterritorial fibrillar architecture, J. Bone Joint Surg. **53B**:732, 1971.
9. Diamant, J., and others: Collagen: ultrastructure and its relation to mechanical properties as a function of aging, Proc. R. Soc. Lond. Biol. **180**:293, 1972.
10. Edwards, J.: Physical characteristics of articular cartilage, Proc. Inst. Mech. Eng. **181**:3, 1967.
11. Eyre, D.R.: Collagen: molecular diversity in the body's protein scaffold, Science **207**:1315, 1980.
12. Ferguson, A.B., and others: Relief of the patellofemoral contact stress by anterior displacement of the tibial tubercle, J. Bone Joint Surg. **61A**:159, 1979.
13. Ficat, R.P., and Hungerford, D.S.: Disorders of the patellofemoral joint, Baltimore, 1979, Williams & Wilkins Co.
14. Gardner, D.L., and MacGillivary, D.C.: Living articular cartilage is not smooth, Ann. Rheum. Dis. **30**:3, 1971.
15. Gardner, D.L., O'Connor, P., and Oates, K.: Surface structure of mammalian articular cartilage viewed at low temperature, Lancet **2**:538, 1979.
16. Ghadially, F.N.: Structure and function of articular cartilage, Clin. Rheum. Dis. **7**:3, 1981.
17. Grodzinsky, A.J., and others: The significance of electromechanical and osmotic forces in the non-equilibrium swelling behavior of articular cartilage in tension, J. Biomech. Eng. **103**:221, 1981.
18. Hayes, W.C., and Bodine, A.J.: Flow-independent viscoelastic properties of articular cartilage matrix, J. Biomech. **11**:407, 1978.
19. Hayes, W.C., and Snyder, B.: Towards a quantitative formulation of Wolff's law in trabecular bone, Proceedings of the American Society of Mechanical Engineers, symposium, New York, 1981, The Society.
20. Hirsch, C.: The pathogenesis of chondromalacia of the patella, Acta Chir. Scand. **90**(suppl. 83):1, 1944.
21. Hultkrantz, J.W.: Uber die Spaltrichtungen der Gelenkknorpel, Verh. Anat. Ges. **12**:248, 1898.
22. Jones, E.S.: Joint lubrication, Lancet **226**:1426, 1934.
23. Kempson, G.E., and others: The tensile properties of the cartilage of human femoral condyles related to the content of collagen and glycosaminoglycans, Biochim. Biophys. Acta, **297**:456, 1972.
24. Lane, J.M., and Weiss, C.: Review of articular cartilage collagen research, Arthritis Rheum. **18**:553, 1975.
25. Lemperg, R., and Larsson, S.E.: The glycosaminoglycans of bovine articular cartilage. I. Concentration and distribution in different layers in relation to age, Calcif. Tissue Res. **15**:237, 1974.
26. Linn, F.C.: Lubrication of animal joints, J. Bone Joint Surg. **49A**:1079, 1967.
27. Lipshitz, H., and Glimcher, M.J.: In vitro studies on wear in articular cartilage. II, Wear **52**:279, 1979.

28. Mak, A.F., and others: Assessment of proteoglycan-proteoglycan interactions from solution biorheological behavior, Trans. Orthop. Res. Soc. New Orleans 7:169, 1982.
29. Malcom, L.L.: An experimental investigation of the frictional and deformational responses of articular cartilage interfaces to static and dynamic loadings, Doctoral thesis, San Diego, 1976, University of California.
30. Mankin, J.H., Dorfman, H., and Lippiello, L.: Biochemical and metabolic abnormalities in articular cartilage from osteoarthritic human hips. II. Correlation of morphology with biochemical and metabolic data, J. Bone Joint Surg. 53A:523, 1971.
31. Maquet, P.G.J.: Biomechanics of the knee, Berlin, 1976, Springer-Verlag.
32. Maroudas, A.: Physicochemical properties of cartilage in the light of ion-exchange theory, Biophys. J. 8:575, 1968.
33. Maroudas, A.: Balance of swelling pressure and collagen tension in normal and degenerate cartilage, Nature 260:808, 1976.
34. Maroudas, A., Muir, H., and Wingham, J.: The correlation of fixed negative charge with glycosaminoglycan contents of human articular cartilage, Biochim. Biophys. Acta, 177:492, 1969.
35. Maroudas, A., and Thomas, H.: A simple physicochemical micromethod for determining fixed anionic groups in connective tissues, Biochim. Biophys. Acta 215:214, 1970.
36. Maroudas, A., and Venn, M.: Chemical composition and swelling of normal and osteoarthritic femoral head cartilage, Ann. Rheum. Dis. 36:399, 1977.
37. McCutchen, C.W.: The frictional properties of animal joints, Wear 5:1, 1962.
38. McDevitt, C.A., and Muir, H.: Biochemical changes in the cartilage of the knee in experimental and natural osteoarthrosis in the dog, J. Bone Joint Surg. 58B:94, 1976.
39. Mow, V.C., and Lai, W.M.: The optical sliding contact analytical rheometer (OSCAR) for flow visualization at the articular surface. In Wells, M.K., editor: Advances in bioengineering, New York, 1979, American Society of Mechanical Engineers.
40. Mow, V.C., and Lai, W.M.: Recent developments in synovial joint biomechanics, SIAM Rev. 22:275, 1980.
41. Mow, V.C., and Torzilli, P.A.: On the fundamental fluid transport mechanisms through articular cartilage, Ann. Rheum. Dis. 34(suppl. 2):82, 1975.
42. Mow, V.C., and others: Biphasic creep and stress relaxation of articular cartilage in compression: theory and experiments, J. Biomech. Eng. 102:73, 1980.
43. Mow, V.C., and others: Implications for collagen-proteoglycan interaction from cartilage stress relaxation behavior in isometric tension, Semin. Arthritis Rheum. 11(suppl. 1):41, 1981.
44. Mow, V.C., Lai, W.M., and Redler, I.: Some surface characteristics of articular cartilage. I. Scanning electron microscopy study and a theoretical model for the dynamic interaction of synovial fluid and articular cartilage, J. Biomech. 7:449, 1974.
45. Muir, H., Bullough, P., and Maroudas, A.: The distribution of collagen in human articular cartilage with some of its physiological implications, J. Bone Joint Surg. 52B:554, 1970.
45a. Muir, H.: Biochemistry. In Freeman, M.A.R., editor: Adult articular cartilage, Kent, England, 1979, Pitman Medical Publishing Co. Ltd.
46. Muir, I.H.M.: The chemistry of the ground substance of joint cartilage. In Sokoff, L., editor: The joints and synovial fluid, New York, 1980, Academic Press, Inc.
47. Powers, J.A.: Title IX knee. In Funk, F.J., editor: AAOS Symposium on the athlete's knee, St. Louis, 1980, The C.V. Mosby Co.
48. Radin, E.L., and others: Response of joints to impact loading. III. Relation between trabecular microfractures and cartilage degeneration, J. Biomech. 6:51, 1973.
49. Radin, E.L., and Paul, I.L.: Response of bone to impact loading. I. In vitro wear, Arthritis Rheum. 14:356, 1971.
50. Redler, I., and others: The ultrastructure and biomechanical significance of the tidemark of articular cartilage, Clin. Orthop. 112:357, 1975.
51. Roth, V., and Mow, V.C.: Finite element analysis of contact problems for indentation of articular cartilage. In Grood, E.S., and Smith, C.R., editors: Advances in bioengineering, New York, 1977, American Society of Mechanical Engineers.
52. Roth, V., and Mow, V.C.: The intrinsic tensile behavior of the matrix of bovine articular cartilage and its variation with age, J. Bone Joint Surg. 62A:1102, 1980.

53. Roth, V., Schoonbeck, J.M., and Mow, V.C.: Low frequency dynamic behavior of articular cartilage under torsional shear, Trans. Orthop. Res. Soc. New Orleans **7**:150, 1982.
54. Salter, R.B., and others: The biological effect of continuous passive motion on the healing of full-thickness defects in articular cartilage: an experimental investigation in rabbits, J. Bone Joint Surg. **62A**:1232, 1980.
55. Sokoloff, L.: Elasticity of articular cartilage: effects of ions and viscous solutions, Science **141**:1055, 1963.
56. Swann, D.A., and Radin, E.L.: The molecular basis of articular lubrication. I. Purification and properties of a lubricating fraction from bovine synovial fluid, J. Biol. Chem. **247**:8069, 1972.
57. Thompson, R.C., and Honner, R.: The nutritional pathways of articular cartilage, J. Bone Joint Surg. **53A**:742, 1971.
58. Viidik, A.: Interdependence between structure and function of collagenous tissues. In Viidik, A., and Vuust, J., editors: Biology of collagen, New York, 1980, Academic Press, Inc.
59. Walker, P.S., and others: Behavior of synovial fluid on surfaces of articular cartilage: A scanning electron microscope study, Ann. Rheum. Dis. **28**:1, 1969.
60. Weightman, B.: Tensile fatigue of human articular cartilage, J. Biomech. **9**:193, 1976.
61. Wirth, C.R., and others: Variation of tensile properties of human patellar cartilage with age and histological indices, Trans. Orthop. Res. Soc. Atlanta **5**:38, 1980.
62. Woo, S. L-Y., Akeson, W.H., and Jemmott, G.F.: Measurement of nonhomogeneous, directional mechanical properties of articular cartilage in tension, J. Biomech. **9**:785, 1976.

7. Biomechanics of impact-induced microdamage to articular cartilage: a possible genesis for chondromalacia patella

Cecil G. Armstrong
Van C. Mow
Carl R. Wirth

Chondromalacia of the patella is a nonspecific clinical term used to describe surface irregularities and softening of the articular cartilage of the patella. The clinical symptoms are palpable or audible patella crepitus, reactive synovitis, and pain.[1] However, surface irregularities and cartilage softening do not necessarily lead to clinically significant events. Owre[31] reported that 91.5% of patellas from patients over 20 years of age showed some alteration in the appearance of the cartilage surface. Scanning electron microscope studies of the cartilage ultrastructure have shown that even normal articular cartilage does not possess a smooth surface.[8,15] These normal irregularities may be important in the lubrication mechanisms found in diarthrodial joints.[3,27]

The surface region of articular cartilage is rich in collagen[16,35] and appears to serve as a biomechanical protective membrane against the loads of joint articulation. (For additional details see Chapter 6.) The surface region is protected by the magnificent lubrication mechanisms found in the diarthrodial joints.[3,46] If multiple lubricating factors were not found in the joint, that is, the lubricating glycoprotein fraction in synovial fluid[43] and the interstitial fluid of articular cartilage,[27] normal joint loads and motion would cause significant wear and rapid breakdown of the protective superficial tangential zones (STZ) on the opposing cartilaginous surfaces.[37]

This chapter describes how impact loading can damage the articular cartilage of the patella and possibly affect the biomechanical functional capacity of this tissue.

☐ Sponsored by General Motors Research Laboratories and the National Institute of Arthritis, Diabetes, and Digestive and Kidney Diseases grant no. AM19094.

70

This chapter will also detail the biomechanical causes for impact damage sustained at the STZ and at the tidemark of cartilage when the patellofemoral joint is subjected to an impact load.

BIOMECHANICS OF THE PATELLOFEMORAL JOINT

The patellofemoral joint is an essential component of the extensor mechanism of the human knee. The patella contributes to the extensor moment arm in all ranges of motion of the knee.[22] Thus it is essential that the articular cartilage surfaces of the patellofemoral joint function smoothly. High loads must be transmitted across this surface during knee flexion and extension.[10,17,18] Moreover, the loads experienced by the patella[24] are distributed over a relatively small surface area.[39] High stresses and strains are expected in the thin cartilage layers.[27] A knowledge of these stresses can immeasurably aid in the analysis of normal joint function, the patterns of patellar fracture, and the effects of malalignment on the bony structure.[13] Repeated loading of a joint with high stress concentrations,[30,31] malalignment of the joint,[13,24] trauma to the joint,[12,42,50] or even inherited qualities[38] may all contribute to the disruption of articular cartilage integrity. Mechanical fatigue failure of small specimens of articular cartilage has been demonstrated,[14,48] but more work needs to be done before the results of these small-specimen tests can be used to predict cartilage failure in the intact joint. Most of the factors just discussed probably contribute to the eventual degeneration of articular cartilage in the joint, and in particular to the degeneration of patellar cartilage.

INJURY TO THE PATELLOFEMORAL JOINT

Abnormal joint loadings during hyperflexions and the consequent abnormal internal stresses in the cartilage-bone structure can cause transverse and stellate fractures. Both defects could be initiated by great internal stresses in articular cartilage, and both are associated with a high incidence of subsequent cartilage degeneration.[9] Osteochondral fractures can occur following patellar subluxation. Patellar luxation is also common, and it usually occurs laterally. This lateral dislocation can shear off a portion of the odd or medial facet and may also cause a shear fracture of the lateral femoral condyle. Such injuries can be difficult to diagnosis, because only a small wafer of bone may be visible on radiography when cartilaginous shear injuries have occurred.[26]

Some investigators believe that such injuries can be biomechanically deleterious from two viewpoints: (1) the contact area at the joint surfaces is reduced, and during weight bearing the stresses at the joint surface are increased; (2) a protrusion at the joint surface could be produced that provides an abrasive region that may cause excessive cartilage wear. However, there are only two fundamental biomechanical mechanisms by which cartilage may be damaged during abnormal joint loading situations: (1) the tissue may be fractured by excessive tensile stress or strain or (2) the tissue may fail under the action of excessive shear stress. Under subtraumatic impact loading conditions (i.e., with no macroscopically observable bone fractures), the stresses and strains in the patellar cartilage can cause microdamage. Such microdamage can be quantified biomechanically and observed when dissected.

This chapter describes a series of detailed in vivo impact studies. These studies were aimed at investigating dashboard knee syndrome. However, these conclusions are equally valid for sports injuries sustained by athletes who experience blunt trauma to the patellofemoral joint.

Gross macroscopic studies on direct, nonpenetrating, blunt trauma to the knee have received a great deal of attention.[11,45] Most of these studies originate from the clinical condition of dashboard knee syndrome.[29,45] Blunt patellar injuries can also occur in athletes as a result of a fall, a collision with the boards during a hockey match, a bobsled crash, or other athletic event accidents. Most macroscopic studies have focused on the obvious gross anatomic fractures that cause the painful prepatellar and parapatellar syndromes accompanying these blunt impacts to the knee. These painful injuries may result in protracted discomfort, most do not cause permanent injury, but some do eventually lead to permanent change.

Therefore in what manner may impact loading cause a biomechanical injury of cartilage? How may these injuries be quantified by biomechanical methods, and what are the possible long-term consequences of these impact-induced injuries? This chapter is a report of a study performed on subtraumatic blunt impacts to the knee joints of pigs in vivo. Impact parameters were carefully adjusted to simulate a 15 to 20 mph collision. Detailed biomechanical tests and histologic-histochemical tests were performed to assess the microdamage caused by these subtraumatic impacts.

IMPACT OF THE PATELLOFEMORAL JOINT

A standardized, repeatable impacting device to be used with a single animal model had to be devised. To ensure that the stresses induced by impact were representative of natural events, the knee joints remained intact during the study. The use of rigid indenting devices[12,19,49] or small-cut specimens[36] may induce modes of failure that cannot be related to in vivo injury mechanisms. Thus a standardized experiment was developed to simulate blunt, subtraumatic impacts.

The knee of a domestic Yorkshire pig was the test model. The unimpacted contralateral knee of the animal served as control. The animal was anesthetized, and the femur was surgically exposed and transected perpendicular to the axis of the medullary canal. A stainless steel pin was implanted in the canal and held in place with polymethylmethacrylate (PMMA)[6] (Fig. 7-1). The femoral pin was fixed to the rigid base of a drop-tower impactor.* To provide the impact, a wire-guided mass of 6 kg was dropped from the height of 2 m. A load cell and accelerometer were mounted beneath a padded impacting surface made of materials similar to those used for padding dashboards of automobiles. The duration of the impact, the impact peak force, and the impactor position and deceleration were monitored on a high-speed tape recorder. With this system, titration of impact severity can be effectively controlled. The duration of impulse used ranged from 24 to 31 msec. Inertially com-

---

*From Biomedical Sciences Department of General Motors Research Laboratories.

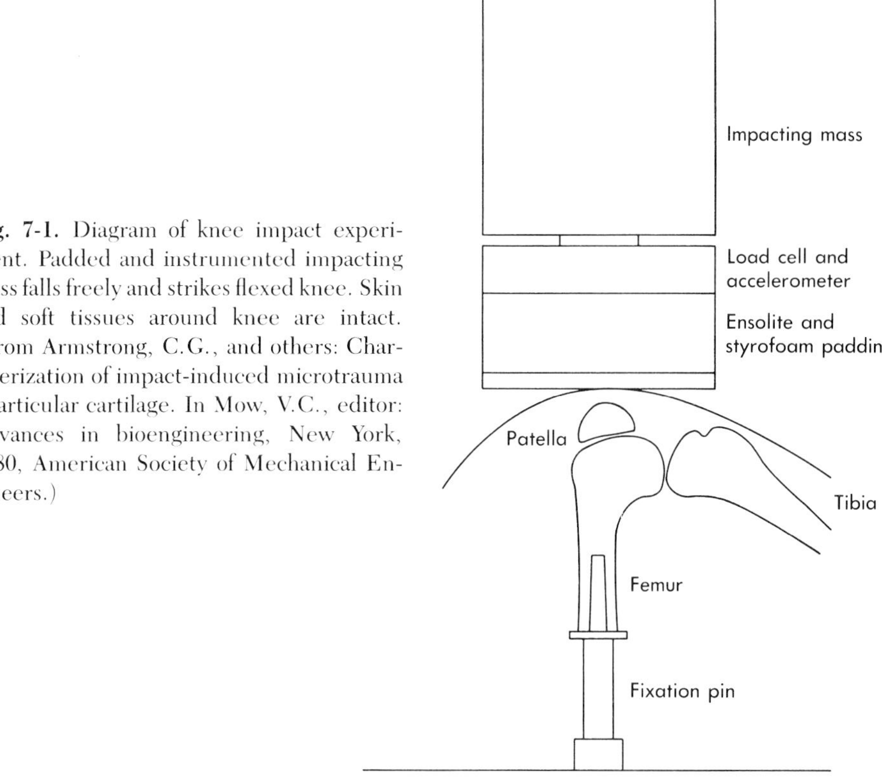

Fig. 7-1. Diagram of knee impact experiment. Padded and instrumented impacting mass falls freely and strikes flexed knee. Skin and soft tissues around knee are intact. (From Armstrong, C.G., and others: Characterization of impact-induced microtrauma to articular cartilage. In Mow, V.C., editor: Advances in bioengineering, New York, 1980, American Society of Mechanical Engineers.)

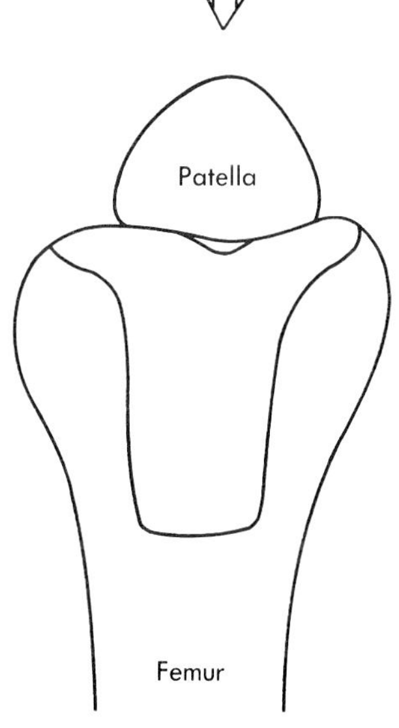

Fig. 7-2. Anterior *skyline* view of femur and patella positioned for impact loading.

pensated peak force ranged from 3.25 kN (715 lb) to 5.91 kN (1300 lb), and deceleration of the impacting mass ranged from 590 m/sec^2 to 830 m/sec^2.

The injuries produced during impact depend on the orientation of the joints in a line of action of the applied force. Viano and others[45] have shown that if the human knee is flexed to only 90 degrees, it is likely that the tibial tubercle will receive the impact, force the tibia posterior, and injure the posterior cruciate ligament. In this case the knees of the experimental pigs were flexed to 110 degrees. The impactor always struck at an angle normal to the long axis of the patella and drove the patella into the supporting femoral chondyles (Figs. 7-1 and 7-2).

BIOMECHANICAL PROPERTIES OF IMPACTED PATELLAR CARTILAGE

After impact the animals were immediatley sacrificed. This was done to avoid confusing effects of impact microdamage with biologic reactions subsequent to the impact. The knee joints were isolated, dissected free of soft tissues, macroscopically observed, and photographed. Articular cartilage was removed from the joint surfaces for mechanical testing. Tensile studies were pursued to assess tensile stiffness and strength of the collagen network. Confined compression creep studies were pursued to determine the permeability coefficient and equilibrium modulus of the proteoglycan-collagen solid matrix.[28] (Additional details of these biomechanical tests are found in Chapter 6.) The tensile stiffness and strength provide assessments of collagen network damage, while the permeability coefficient and equilibrium modulus provide indications of proteoglycan loss.[5,51]

Tensile test

Full-thickness rectangular strips of articular cartilage were removed from defined locations on both the control and impacted articular surfaces[6] (Fig. 7-3). The specimens were oriented so that the long axis lay parallel to the Hultkrantz split line patterns.[20,37] These strips were then microtomed into strips approximately 300 μm thick to permit assessment of the variation in tensile properties with the depth in the articular layer. From these rectangular slices, test specimens with a narrow gage section and enlarged ends were cut with a specially shaped dumbbell cutter. (See Fig. 6-4.) Both the extension and the lateral contraction of the specimen were measured during the testing procedure by a noncontacting electro-optical tracking device* that recorded the change in dimensions of a dark rectangular gage section painted on the central section of the specimen with nigrosin histologic stain. The tensile specimen was stretched in the Instron material testing machine at a constant rate until failure occurred. Tensile stiffness and strength were determined for the cartilage specimens obtained from the impacted and control knees. Statistical correlations were determined from 317 control specimens and 302 impacted specimens.

---

*Opton 511-B biaxial extensometer, United Technology Incorporated, Woodbridge, Conn.

Fig. 7-3. Diagram illustrating sites on control and impacted knees from which articular cartilage was harvested for testing. For tensile testing, full-thickness strips of cartilage were removed and cut into 300 μm thick slices.[37] Circular plugs of cartilage were full-thickness and were attached to subchondral bone. Specimens were tested in confined compression creep.[27] (From Armstrong, C.G., and others: Characterization of impact-induced microtrauma to articular cartilage. In Mow, C.V., editor: Advances in bioengineering, New York, 1980, American Society of Mechanical Engineers.)

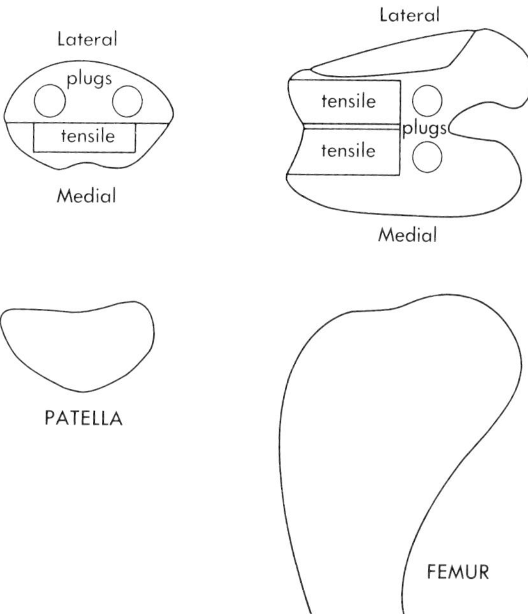

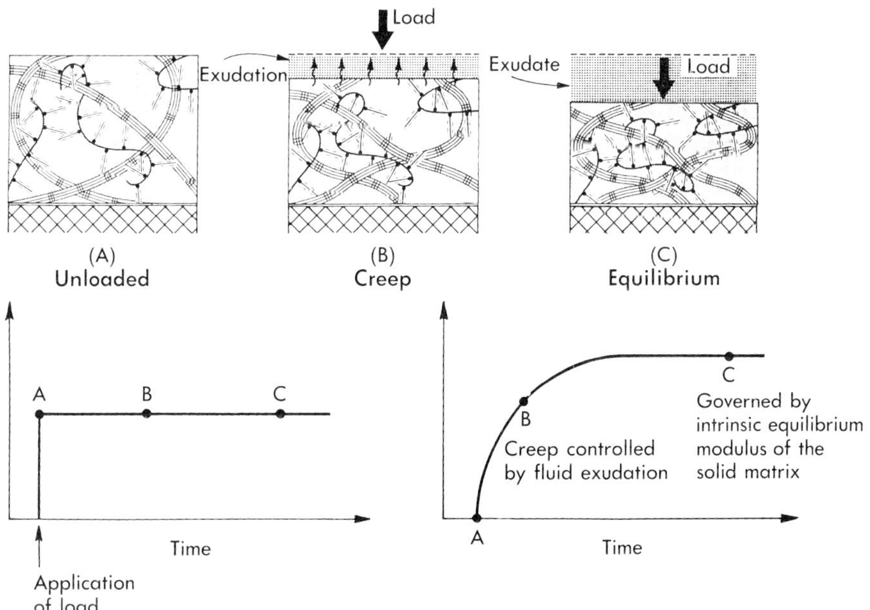

Fig. 7-4. Diagram of confined compression creep test. Compressive stress on cartilage surface causes fluid exudation and compaction of collagen-proteoglycan solid matrix. Rate of fluid exudation is controlled by matrix permeability, and modulus of solid matrix controls final equilibrium displacement.[28]

Compressive properties

To determine the compressive properties of articular cartilage, the confined compression creep test was used (Fig. 7-4). Cylindrical plugs of articular cartilage attached to a short length of subchondral bone were obtained from defined locations in both the impacted and control knees (Fig. 7-3). These plugs were mounted in rigid impermeable test chambers that prevented lateral expansion and lateral fluid flow from the specimen. The cartilage surface was loaded against a rigid porous filter. When the load was applied to the specimen, fluid could be squeezed out of the cartilage and the specimen would begin to creep or deform with time. (See Chapter 6 for additional details.)

Eventually, a compressive equilibrium was reached where no more fluid was exuded. This equilibrium deformation is controlled by the modulus of the solid organic matrix, while the creep of the material is controlled by the rate at which fluid is exuded, and thus by the permeability coefficient.[27] Armstrong and Mow[4,5,27] have shown that in human patellar cartilage these two material coefficients are primarily controlled by the tissue's water content and the proteoglycan concentration.

RESULTS
Gross anatomic effects

The in vivo impact experiments were performed on a total of 23 animals. In 3 animals, the impact caused fractures that extended to the joint space. These experiments have not been included in the results. In 4 other animals, fractures of the distal femur occurred near the tip of the implanted pin, but these fractures were remote from the knee joints. In several joints, the impacted cartilage appeared discolored. This seemed to be associated with separation of the articular cartilage from the subchondral bone at the cartilage-bone interface (Fig. 7-5). The separation was found immediately under the area of impact; it occurred in 7 of the 20 test knees and appeared to be a result of impaction. None of the contralateral control knees was observed to demonstrate this discoloration or separation. There was also an indication that the joints in which the separation occurred had experienced higher impact forces (Fig. 7-6).

The initial concerns were that the incidence of this injury might be related to the skeletal immaturity of the animals, but although the animals ranged in age from 14 to 24 weeks and in weight from 40 to 113 kg, the occurrence of cartilage-bone separation was not significantly associated with either age or weight.

Effects on tensile properties

The results show that a single impact will disrupt the mechanical properties of the cartilage surface layer. The tensile failure stress of the first cartilage slice incorporating the joint surface was statistically lower than the cartilage from the control joint (Table 7-1). This effect was especially pronounced in joints where cartilage-bone separation had occurred (Table 7-2). The tensile properties of the subsurface cartilage did not appear to be affected by the impact, and there were no significant differences

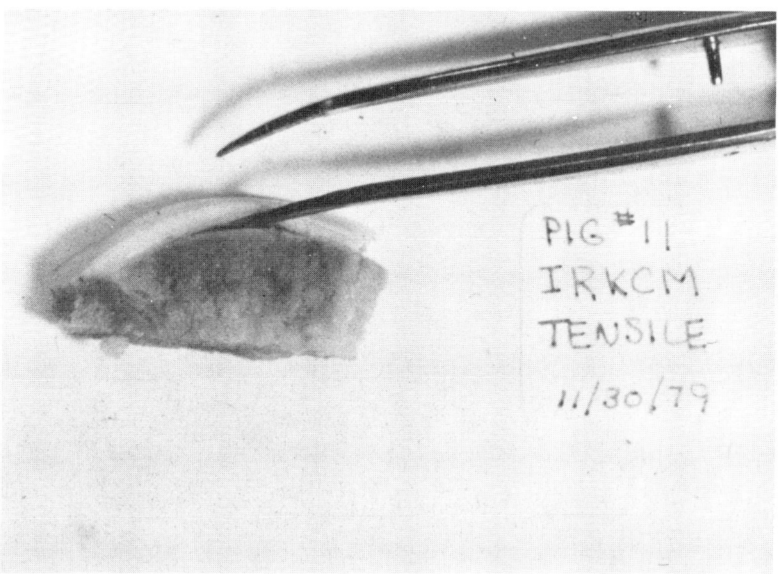

Fig. 7-5. Photograph of impacted pig patella sectioned along its long axis. Separation of articular cartilage from subchondral bone can be clearly seen. This was not a sectional artifact and was not noted in any control joints.[6]

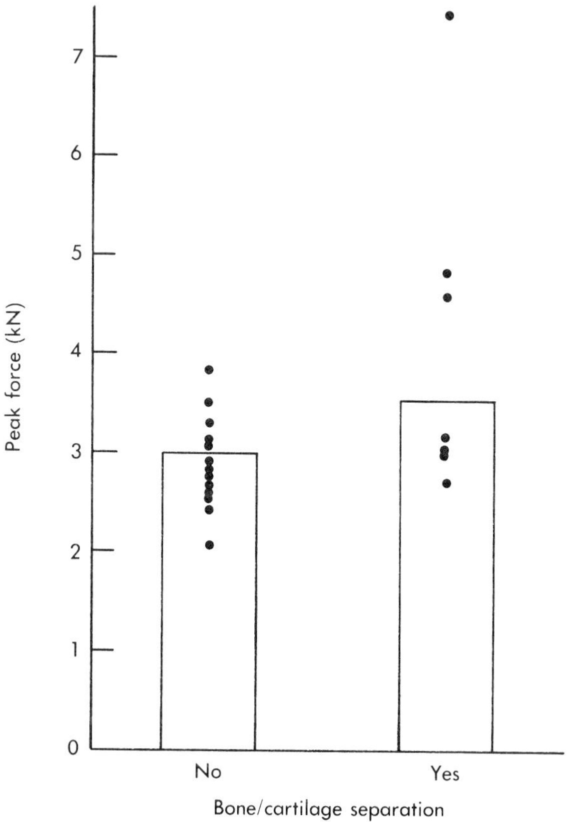

Fig. 7-6. Comparison of peak forces recorded in impact experiments that did not (*left*) and did (*right*) cause cartilage-bone separations. (In this plot, peak forces have not been corrected for inertia effects, which usually increased peak forces by approximately 20%.)

Table 7-1. Effect of single impact on ultimate tensile strength of articular cartilage specimens*

Variable	Control	Impact	Significance
Samples from slice 1			
Mean	10.5	9.3	$p < .02$
Variance	11.3	8.8	
N	77	77	
Samples from slice 2			
Mean	15.8	15.2	$p < .43$
Variance	17.9	23.2	
N	71	77	
Samples from slice 3			
Mean	16.9	17.1	$p < .76$
Variance	14.4	14.4	
N	66	68	

*Only the ultimate tensile strength of STZ slices was statistically significantly ($p < .02$) weakened by the blunt subtraumatic impact.

Table 7-2. Effect of single impact on the ultimate tensile strength of the STZ on joints suffering cartilage-bone separation*

Variable	Control	Impact	Significance
Samples from slice 1			
Mean	11.5	9.4	$p < .01$
Variance	7.9	7.9	
N	26	26	

*The differences between control and impacted articular cartilage are larger and more significant when cartilage-bone separation has occurred.

between cartilage from younger and older animals. This result is similar to the result on the variation of tensile properties of articular cartilage with age reported by Roth and Mow.[37] In these studies normal STZ tensile properties did not change with age. Thus subtraumatic impact of the patellofemoral joint appears to cause only STZ damage to the patellar cartilage-collagen ultrastructure. This result may be important in understanding further cartilage breakdown once the collagen network at the surface has been disrupted.[25]

Effects on compressive properties

The compressive properties, that is, equilibrium modulus and permeability, show no significant differences between the control and the impacted joints, (Table 7-3), but significant site-related differences were observed. This observation underlines the necessity for careful control of the sampling locations. The lack of difference

Table 7-3. Variation of equilibrium compression modulus and permeability coefficient between impacted and control specimens*

Variable	Control	Impact	Significance
Modulus (MPa)			
Mean	0.87	0.81	$p < .43$
Variance	0.19	0.17	
N	66	55	
Permeability ($\times 10^{-14}\,\mathrm{m^4/Ns}$)			
Mean	0.16	0.15	$p < .56$
Variance	0.01	0.01	
N	66	55	

*These biomechanical properties are controlled by the tissue proteoglycan content. No statistically significant variations were detected in specimens removed immediately after impact. This means that the proteoglycans have not had a chance to be lost from the tissue even though the superficial tangential zone has been disrupted by the impact.

between impacted and control cartilage compressive properties was initially surprising because it is well known that compressive properties do change with cartilage breakdown.[5,27]

DISCUSSION

During these knee impact experiments, the duration of the applied load is so short (30 msec) that there is no time for fluid to escape from the cartilage.[27] In this situation articular cartilage behaves like an incompressible elastic material. This behavior was modeled by Askew and Mow.[7] They showed that when the joint surfaces are forced rapidly together, the resulting radial expansion of cartilage can cause (1) substantial shear stresses at the tidemark where the cartilage becomes attached to the rigid subchondral bone and (2) large tensile strains at the cartilage surface immediately under the loaded area. Furthermore, the surface strains become increasingly large as the loading becomes more rapid.[2] However, if the load is maintained on the joint surface for any length of time, interstitial fluid flowing away from regions of high pressure will allow stress relaxation to occur and a more favorable contact geometry will be achieved. Thus it could be speculated that in impact or repetitive loading activities, such as falling or jogging, the range of mechanical damage to articular cartilage will be greatest if muscle action is not actively absorbing the shocks that result from these loading conditions. Radin and co-workers[32-34] have been major proponents of this concept of impact-induced articular cartilage degeneration. The studies in this chapter tend to confirm their observations, although the mechanisms of damage proposed are somewhat different.

Biomechanical mechanisms of impact-induced microdamage

Shear. High shear stress at the cartilage-bone junction appears to be a feasible mechanism for the separation of articular cartilage and subchondral bone seen in some of the impacted joints. Once this defect is introduced into the joint structure it will create local areas of stress concentration deep in the cartilage. These could be responsible for the eventual basal degeneration of the patella described by Goodfellow and others,[17] that is, a lesion that originates in the deep and middle zones of cartilage without first affecting the surface. The rupture of the cartilage-bone junction may also allow greater radial deformation of the cartilage layer and further increase the mechanical disruption of the collagen network.

Tension. The prediction of large tensile strains at the joint surface as a result of rapid loading of the joint agrees with the experimentally observed reduction in strength of the thin cartilage strips obtained from the joint surface. Large tensile strains will tend to break the relatively inextensible collagen fibrils.[37] In normal situations the stresses are probably much less important, since the interstitial fluid can support load without damage to the solid organic matrix. However, once a significant amount of surface damage has occurred, it is difficult for the interstitial fluid to support load, since it is easily exuded under compression, that is, the fluid escapes by the path of least resistance. Not only is this bad for load carriage, but it also defeats one of the three important lubricating mechanisms found in diarthrodial joints.[3] Thus damage to the collagen network at the articular surface can eventually impair the functional ability of the tissue.

Compression. The lack of any measurable effect on the confined compression properties as a result of impact loading was initially surprising. In this test no tensile strains are induced in the cartilage, and the collagen fibers are not called on to support the load. The resistance to compressive deformation is primarily controlled by the proteoglycan concentration in the tissue.[4] When testing is performed on specimens excised from joints immediately after a single impact, the collagen fibrous network may be disrupted. Since there has been little opportunity for any loss of proteoglycan from the tissue as a result of this disruption, no differences were observed.

Effect of rapid loading rates. The susceptibility of articular cartilage to impact loading has already been demonstrated in a number of studies. Radin and co-workers have conducted in vitro[33] and in vivo[34] studies of cartilage degeneration as a result of impact loading. Ficat[11] demonstrated cartilage fibrillation and degeneration as a result of a single impact by an hemispherical indenter on the joint surface. Repo and Finlay[36] conducted an extensive study of the effect of impact loading of small cylindrical specimens on chondrocyte viability and matrix disruption. In all of these studies rapid loading conditions during impact had the effect of reducing the compressive deformations of cartilage, since there was little or no time for appreciable fluid exudation to occur. However, impact loading does cause large tensile and shear strains in the cartilage, and such strains are potentially more damaging to the collagen fibrous ultrastructure at the surface and at the tidemark, respectively.

Effects of joint incongruity. Loading patterns in the patellofemoral joint have been studied by a number of researchers.[13,17,18,39] It is known that the patellar contact areas are relatively small. The effect of relative contact area size on loaded articular cartilage was also studied by Askew and Mow.[7] They found that the ratio of the radius of the loaded area on cartilage to the thickness of the articular cartilage, or the aspect ratio, plays a critical role on the deformation in articular cartilage. A decrease in the aspect ratio leads to an increase in the stresses, strains, and displacements in cartilage. Simon[40] has suggested that limb structures and synovial joint geometry are optimally designed to tolerate physiologic loading stresses. Although the impact study in this chapter did not address the points raised by Simon, it is suspected that increased joint incongruity, for example, during aging, will decrease the aspect ratio and therefore the ability of articular cartilage to sustain impact loading without damage.[7]

Long-term effects

The long-term effects of single-impact loading are potentially more serious. The weakened STZ of the cartilage may allow gradual proteoglycan loss and swelling of the matrix by increasing the water content, thus interfering with the natural load-bearing and lubrication processes.[3,27] However, studies to evaluate the long-term biologic effects need to be performed.

Lane and Bullough[23] have shown that the tidemark–calcified cartilage region is not biologically static, and chondral bone formation in the calcified zone continues throughout adult life. The rate of growth, however, declines over the years until, around 60 years of age, there is a sudden sharp increase in activity. This process results in an encroachment of the calcified zone into the noncalcified zone as shown by the increasing number of tidemarks in older specimens. The rate of encroachment of the calcified zone appears to be exceeded by the rate of enchondral bone formation resulting in a net thinning of the calcified zone that starts at 20 years of age. This thinning of the calcified zone could have significant detrimental effects on its ability to function as an interface between the two materials to withstand the large shear stresses generated by impact loading. It is known that the tensile strength of human articular cartilage decreases with age,[51] so we suspect that aging cartilage will have a decreased ability to survive the large tensile strains imposed by single-impact loads of the magnitudes used in our experiment. Therefore there could be speculation that the biomechanical consequences of impact-induced cartilage injury may be greater in older individuals. Again more investigations need to be done in this area.

Other biomechanical factors

There are many other factors that may contribute to chondrodegeneration. Direct blunt trauma to the articular surfaces is not the only pathway for joint degeneration following impact loading. The more common mechanism is through ligamentous injury. For example, the usual mechanism of dashboard knee injury occurs when an unrestrained occupant, who has his knees flexed at approximately 90 degrees, impacts the dashboard with the tibial tubercle. This causes the tibia to be driven back posteriorly and damages the posterior cruciate ligament.[45] A great deal of clinical[21,41] and experimental[25,47] evidence exists that abnormal joint laxity and the associated abnormal joint loadings and motions strongly predispose the joint to arthritic degeneration.[44]

SUMMARY

This study shows that single impact loads appear to cause disruption of the collagen network of the STZ in articular cartilage. This can be assessed by the tensile stiffness and strength tests performed on specimens excised from the surface layers. Immediately after injury there seems to be no significant change in the compressive properties of full-thickness articular cartilage specimens. Theoretic prediction of significant shear stresses at the cartilage-bone interface can explain the separation of articular cartilage from the subchondral cortical bone immediately under the impacted area. This separation is not visible on the surface of the articular cartilage except as a slight loss in the glistening white appearance of the apparently normal articular cartilage. These impact-induced microdamages could be the source of clinically significant cartilage degeneration problems found in chondromalacic patella.

ACKNOWLEDGMENTS

The authors wish to thank John Schoonbeck for his technical assistance during the course of our impact studies and Ms. Rose Boshoff for her skillful editorial assistance in the preparation of this manuscript. The authors also express their appreciation to Dr. D. C. Viano of the General Motors Research Laboratories for his support and encouragement, which made this study feasible.

REFERENCES

1. Aleman, O.: Chondromalacia posttraumatica patellae, Acta Chir. Scand. **63**:149, 1928.
2. Armstrong, C.G., Bahrani, A.S., and Gardner, D.L.: Changes in the deformational behavior of human hip cartilage with age, J. Biomech. Eng. **102**:214, 1980.
3. Armstrong, C.G., and Mow, V.C.: Friction, lubrication, and wear of synovial joints. In Owen, R., Goodfellow, J., and Bullough, P., editors: Scientific foundation of orthopaedics and traumatology, London, 1980, William Heinemann Medical Books, Ltd.
4. Armstrong, C.G., and Mow, V.C.: Biomechanics of normal and osteoarthrotic articular cartilage. In Wilson, Jr., P.D., and Straub, L.R., editors: Clinical trends in orthopaedics, New York, 1982, Thieme-Stratton, Inc.
5. Armstrong, C.G., and Mow, V.C.: Variations in the intrinsic mechanical properties of human articular cartilage with age, degeneration, and water content, J. Bone Joint Surg. **64A**:88, 1982
6. Armstrong, C.G., and others: Characterization of impact-induced microtrauma to articular cartilage. In Mow, V.C., editor: Advances in bioengineering, New York, 1980, American Society of Mechanical Engineers.
7. Askew, M.J., and Mow, V.C.: The biomechanical function of the collagen fibril ultrastructure of articular cartilage, J. Biomech. Eng. **100**:105, 1978.
8. Clarke, I.C.: Articular cartilage: a review and scanning electron microscope study. I. The interterritorial fibrillar architecture, J. Bone Joint Surg. **53B**:732, 1971.
9. Crawford, A.H.: Fractures about the knee in children, Orthop. Clin. North Am. **7**:639, 1976.
10. daSilva, O.L., and Bratt, J.F.: Stress trajectories in the patella, Acta Orthop. Scand. **41**:608, 1970.
11. Ficat, C.: Les contusions du cartilage articulaire etude experimentale, Rev. Chir. Orthop. **62**:493, 1976.
12. Ficat, P., Ficat, C., and Gedeon, P.: Arthrose post-traumatique et chondrose post-contusive: the relationship between cartilage contusion and chondrosis and between injury and arthrosis, Rev. Chir. Orthop. **64**:19, 1978.
13. Ficat, R.P., and Hungerford, D.S.: Disorders of the patellofemoral joint, Baltimore, 1977, Williams & Wilkins Co.

14. Freeman, M.A.R.: The fatigue of cartilage in the pathogenesis of osteoarthritis, Acta Orthop. Scand. **46**:323, 1975.
15. Gardner, D.L., and MacGillivary, D.C.: Living articular cartilage is not smooth, Ann. Rheum. Dis. **30**:3, 1971.
16. Ghadially, F.N.: Structure and function of articular cartilage, Clin. Rheum. Dis. **7**:3, 1981.
17. Goodfellow, J., Hungerford, D.S., and Woods, C.: Patellofemoral joint mechanics and pathology. II. Chondromalacia patellae, J. Bone Joint Surg. **58B**:291, 1976.
18. Goodfellow, J., Hungerford, D.S., and Zindel, M.: Patellofemoral joint mechanics and pathology. I. Functional anatomy of the patellofemoral joint, J. Bone Joint Surg. **58B**:287, 1976.
19. Hirsch, C.: The pathogenesis of chondromalacia of the patella, Acta Chir. Scand. **90**(suppl. 83):1, 1944.
20. Hultkrantz, J.W.: Uber die Spaltrichtungen der Gelenkknorpel, Verh. Anat. Ges. **12**:248, 1898.
21. James, S.L.: Chondromalacia of the patella in the adolescent. In Kennedy, J.C., editor: The injured adolescent knee, Baltimore, 1979, Williams & Wilkins Co.
22. Kaufer, H.: Mechanical function of the patella, J. Bone Joint Surg. **53A**:1551, 1971.
23. Lane, L.B., and Bullough, P.G.: Age-related changes in the thickness of the calcified zone and the number of tidemarks in adult human articular cartilage, J. Bone Joint Surg. **62B**:372, 1980.
24. Maquet, P.G.J.: Biomechanics of the knee, Berlin, 1976, Springer-Verlag.
25. McDevitt, C.A., and Muir, H.: Biochemical changes in the cartilage of the knee in experimental and natural osteoarthrosis in the dog, J. Bone Joint Surg. **58B**:94, 1976.
26. Morscher, E.: Cartilage-bone lesions of the knee joint following injury, Reconstr. Surg. Traumatol. **12**:2, 1971.
27. Mow, V.C., and Lai, W.M.: Recent developments in synovial joint biomechanics, SIAM Rev. **22**:275, 1980.
28. Myers, E.R., and Mow, V.C.: Variation of the intrinsic biomechanical properties of articular cartilage with age, degeneration, and composition. In Seminar on resources for basic science educators, American Academy of Orthopaedic Surgeons, San Diego, 1981.
29. Nagel, D., Burton, D., and Manning, J.: The dashboard knee injury, Clin. Orthop. **126**:203, 1977.
30. Outerbridge, R.E.: The etiology of chondromalacia patella, J. Bone Joint Surg. **43B**:752, 1961.
31. Owre, A.: Chondromalacia patella, Acta Chir. Scand. **77**(suppl. 41):entire issue, 1936.
32. Radin, E.L.: Etiology of osteoarthrosis, Clin. Rheum. Dis. **2**:509, 1976.
33. Radin, E.L., and others: Effect of repetitive impulsive loading on the knee joints of rabbits, Clin. Orthop. **131**:288, 1978.
34. Radin, E.L., and Paul, I.L.: Response of joints to impact loading. I. In vitro wear, Arthritis Rheum. **14**:356, 1971.
35. Redler, I., and Mow, V.C.: Biomechanical theories of ultrastructural alterations of articular surfaces of femoral heads. In Harris, W.H., editor: The hip, St. Louis, 1974, The C.V. Mosby Co.
36. Repo, R.U., and Finlay, J.B.: Survival of articular cartilage after controlled impact, J. Bone Joint Surg. **59A**:1068, 1977.
37. Roth, V., and Mow, V.C.: The intrinsic tensile behavior of the matrix of bovine articular cartilage and its variation with age, J. Bone Joint Surg. **62A**:1102, 1981.
38. Rybacky, G.E.: Inheritable chondromalacia of the patella, J. Bone Joint Surg. **54A**:1685, 1968.
39. Seedholm, B.B., and others: Mechanical factors in patellofemoral osteoarthrosis, Ann. Rheum. Dis. **38**:307, 1979.
40. Simon, W.H.: Scale effects in joints. I. Articular cartilage thickness and compressive stress, Arthritis Rheum. **13**:244, 1970.
41. Smillie, I.S.: Injuries of the knee joint, New York, 1978, Churchill Livingstone, Inc.
42. States, J.D.: Traumatic arthritis: a medical and legal dilemma, proceedings of the Annual Conference of the American Association Auto Med, 1970.
43. Swann, D.A., and Radin, E.L.: The molecular basis of articular lubrication. I. Purification and properties of a lubricating fraction from bovine synovial fluid, J. Biol. Chem. **247**:8069, 1972.
44. Thompson, R.C., and Bassettt, C.A.L.: Histological observations on experimentally induced degeneration of articular cartilage, J. Bone Joint Surg. **52A**:435, 1970.
45. Viano, D.C., et al.: Bolster impacts to the knee and tibia of human cadavers and an anthropomorphic dummy, Proceedings of the twenty-second Stapp Car Crash Conference of the Society of Automotive Engineers, Warrendale, Pa., 1978.

46. Walker, P.S., et al.: Modes of aggregation of hyaluronic acid protein complex on the surface of articular cartilage, Ann. Rheum. Dis. **29**:591, 1970.
47. Warren, L.F., Marshall, J.L., and Girgis, F.: The prime static stabilizer of the knee, J. Bone Joint Surg. **57A**:411, 1975.
48. Weightman, B.: Tensile fatigue failure of human articular cartilage, J. Biomech. **9**:193, 1976.
49. Weightman, B.O., Freeman, M.A.R., and Swanson, S.A.V.: Fatigue of articular cartilage, Nature **24**:303, 1973.
50. Wiberg, G.: Roentgenographic and anatomic studies on the femoropatellar joint, Acta Orthop. Scand. **12**:319, 1941.
51. Wirth, C.R., and others: Variation of tensile properties of human patellar cartilage with age and histological indices, Trans. Orthop. Res. Soc. Atlanta, **5**:38, 1980.

8. The effects of indirect blunt trauma on adult articular cartilage

J. Michael Donohue
Roby C. Thompson, Jr.
Theodore R. Oegema, Jr.

HYPOTHESIS

The correlation of joint surface injury and subsequent osteoarthritic changes is a common clinical observation. In the study of human articular cartilage samples from osteoarthritic joints, cystic degeneration deep in the radial zone without detectable communication with the surface has been noted. This observation led to the hypothesis that with trauma initial damage might reside in the radial zone and chondrocytes trapped in the matrix adjacent to the zone of calcified cartilage might be damaged by loads normally dissipated by the articular cartilage matrix. Previous studies have suggested an injury threshold for articular cartilage, but it is not known if progression to osteoarthritic changes is an absolute sequela to an injury exceeding this threshold.[1,2,3]

THE EXPERIMENT

To test this hypothesis, an experimental model with a drop tower delivering a single impact to the patellofemoral joint was used. Six adult male dogs (23 to 26 kg) had both patellofemoral joints impacted with a force of 25 N on the right (70% fracture load) and 16 N on the left (45% fracture load). Two nonimpacted animals served as controls.

The experimental animals were sacrificed in groups of two at 2, 4, and 6 weeks after impaction. Samples from the impacted patellas and femurs were removed and processed for both light and electron microscopy. Light microscopy sections were stained with safranin O and fast green FCF, and electron microscopy samples were stained with ruthenium red, uranyl acetate, and lead citrate.

☐ Supported by National Institutes of Health grant no. AM25606 and a grant from the Minnesota Arthritis Foundation.

Table 8-1. Transmission electron microscopy measurements: No. of proteoglycans along five consecutive A complex–B_1 bands

Variables	Fields counted	Number
Normal group	56	8.34 ± 0.37
Experimental groups	85	5.03 ± 0.46
Two-tailed T test		$p < .001$

RESULTS

Patellas from right and left knee joints in all experimental animals produced similar findings. Cartilage over the contact areas were elevated and dull in appearance when compared to noncontact areas. These changes were not observed in the gross femoral specimens. Sagittal sections of patellas confirmed a marked increase in cartilage thickness in contact areas. In the zone of calcified cartilage, there were no differences between the control and the 2-week group. Examinations 4 and 6 weeks after injury revealed an increase of safranin O staining on the zone of calcified cartilage and cloning of cells above and below the tidemark. There was also increased vascular invasion of the zone. These changes were present in both patellar and femoral specimens. Electron micrographs of impacted specimens revealed similar changes at 2, 4, and 6 weeks. Chondrocytes were rounded with a loss of cytoplasmic processes and territorial matrices. There was a marked increase in the number of necrotic cells.

The matrix of impacted animals also revealed differences. Globular structures identified as proteoglycans by ruthenium red staining had a constant relationship with the collagen fiber A complex–B_1 bands in controls. This was quantified by counting the number of particles associated with five consecutive A complex–B_1 bands. A statistically significant decrease of 40% was noted in all experimental animals (Table 8-1) when compared to the control group. In addition, collagen fibers in the radial zone of animals 4 and 6 weeks after impact were often increased in width, ranging from 1600 to 2300 Å. This response of articular cartilage to trauma appears to involve a loss of the normal relationship between collagen and proteoglycans with subsequent cell activation in the zone of calcified cartilage. In addition to confirming that alterations may occur in the hyaline cartilage matrix without joint surface disruption, this chapter provides evidence that a subfracture load delivered across the canine patellofemoral articulation can produce changes that may proceed to joint deterioration.

REFERENCES

1. Dekel, S., and Weissman, S.L.: Joint changes after overuse and peak overloading of rabbit knees in viva, Acta Orthop. Scand. **49:**519, 1978.
2. Repo, R.V., and Finlay, J.B.: Survival of articular cartilage after controlled impact, J. Bone Joint Surg. **59A:**1068, 1977.
3. Thompson, R.C.: An experimental study of surface injury to articular cartilage and enzyme responses within the joint, Clin. Orthop. **107:**239, 1975.

9. A summary of knee stability measurements

Keith L. Markolf

IN VITRO STUDIES
The meniscectomized knee

The primary function of the menisci is load bearing. By broadening the contact area between the tibia and femur, pressure on the cartilage is decreased as joint load is applied. Removal of the menisci in the intact knee has no significant effect on anterior-posterior or torsional laxity of either unloaded or loaded specimens. However, bilateral meniscectomy will increase varus-valgus laxity of the unloaded knee an average of 3 to 4 degrees at full extension and 20 degrees of flexion. These increases are best explained by a medial-lateral shift of the tibia with respect to the femur as varus-valgus force is applied to the ankle. As the buttressing effect of the menisci is lost, the pivot points for condyle lift-off move toward the edges of the tibial plateau and thus increase the tibial angulation for a unit moment applied to the joint.

Anterior cruciate ligament and medial collateral ligament deficiency in the knee

The anterior cruciate ligament provides the primary restraint to anterior translation of the tibia on the femur. Section of the anterior cruciate ligament in an intact, unloaded knee increases anterior-posterior laxity both at full extension and at 20 degrees of flexion (Fig. 9-1). This laxity increase is diminished when the tibia is internally rotated. Subsequent section of the medial collateral ligament in an unloaded knee with anterior cruciate ligament deficiency produces an additional anterior-posterior laxity increase, which is greatest for external rotation of the tibia. These additional laxity increases occur at large anterior tibial displacements where the medial collateral ligament acts as a secondary stabilizer. With 925 N of joint load applied to the knee, the absolute values of the measured laxities are reduced, but the patterns of change are similar (Fig. 9-2). Joint load acts to diminish the anterior-posterior laxity increase as a result of primary anterior cruciate ligament section in all foot rotation positions. In Fig. 9-2 the laxity increase caused by secondary section of the medial collateral ligament is eliminated at full extension by joint load.

In contrast, primary section of the medial collateral ligament produces no increase

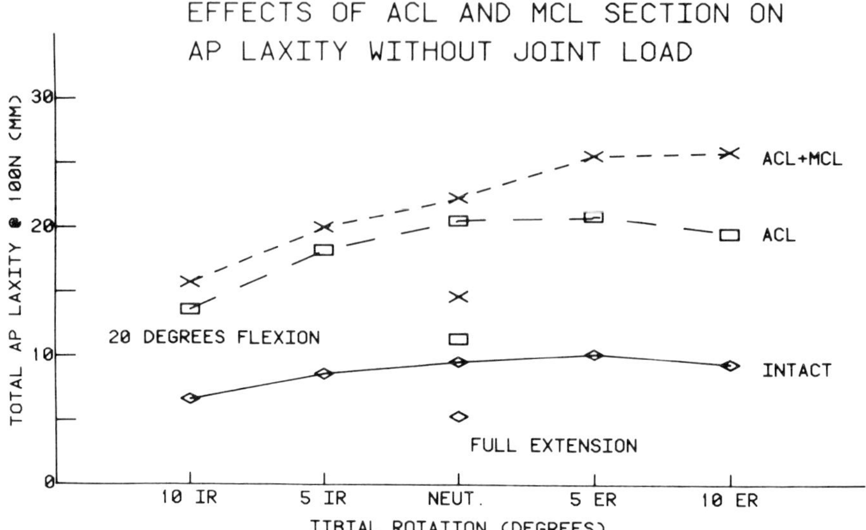

Fig. 9-1. Effects of serial anterior cruciate ligament–medial collateral ligament section on anterior-posterior laxity at various positions of tibial rotation without joint load. Symbols connected by solid or dashed lines represent laxity values at 20 degrees of flexion, and solitary symbols at neutral rotation represent values at full extension. Primary anterior cruciate ligament section increased laxity in all positions. Secondary medial collateral ligament section increased laxity, with greatest change occurring at 20 degrees of flexion and 10 degrees of external tibial rotation. Internal tibial rotation decreased laxity regardless of ligament status.

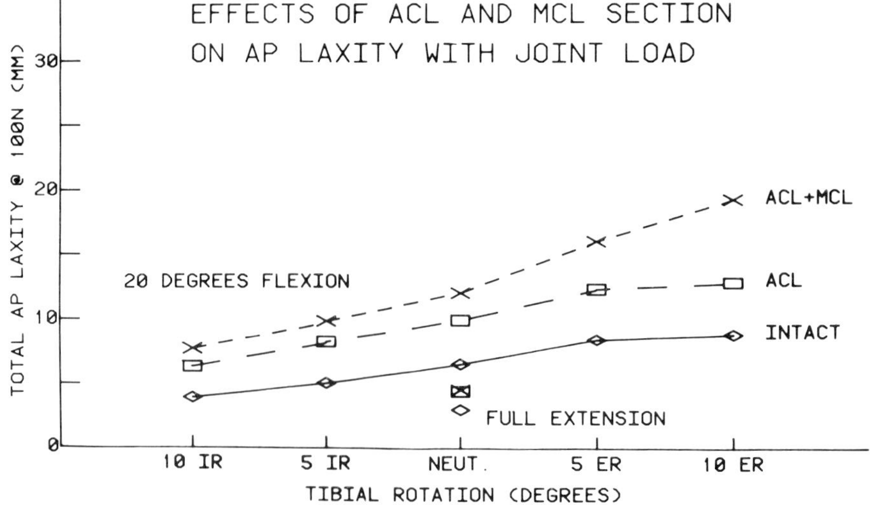

Fig. 9-2. Effects of serial anterior cruciate ligament–medial collateral ligament section on anterior-posterior laxity at various positions of tibial rotation under 925 N joint load. Primary anterior cruciate ligament section increased laxity significantly in all positions; however, these changes were smaller than those observed in unloaded conditions. Secondary medial collateral ligament section resulted in significant laxity increases at 20 degrees of flexion that were comparable to changes observed unloaded. At full extension, secondary medial collateral ligament section had no effect on laxity.

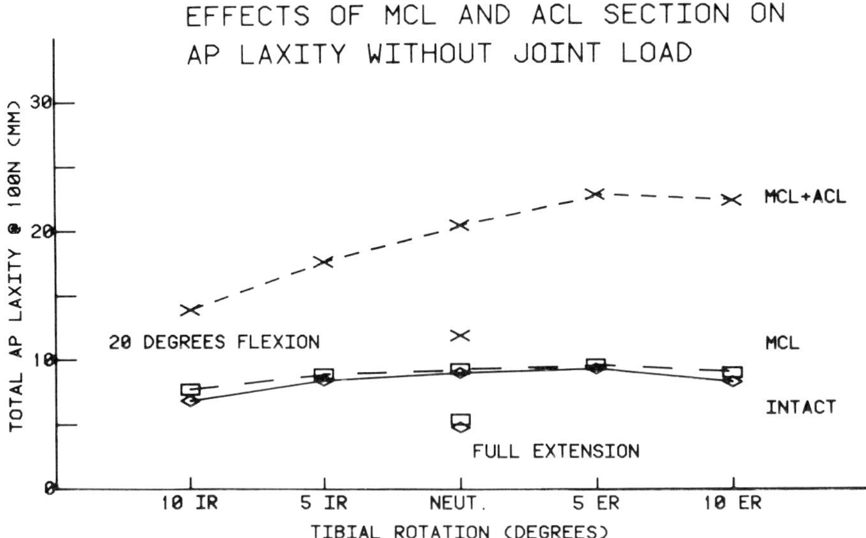

Fig. 9-3. Effects of serial medial collateral ligament–anterior cruciate ligament section on anterior-posterior laxity at various positions of tibial rotation without joint load. Primary medial collateral ligament section had little if any effect, whereas secondary anterior cruciate ligament section increased laxity significantly. Internal rotation of the tibia at 20 degrees of flexion decreased laxity regardless of ligament status, while external rotation of the tibia increased laxity in specimens with combined medial collateral ligament–anterior cruciate ligament deficit.

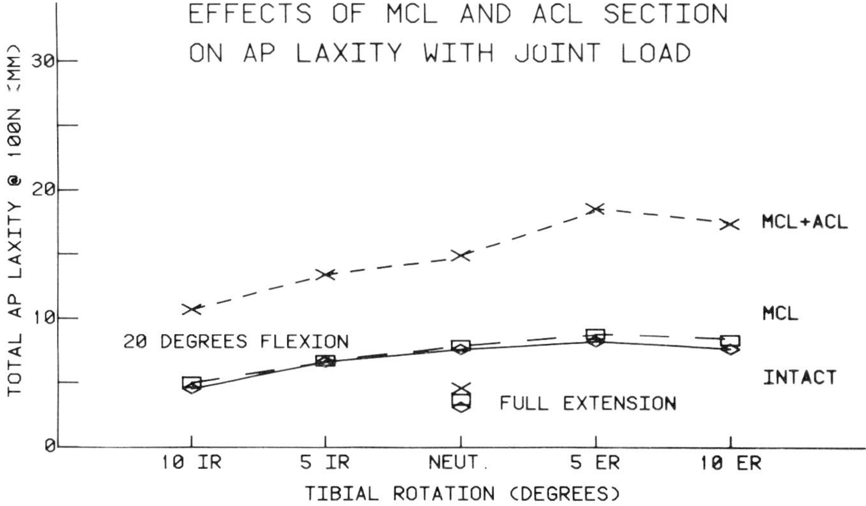

Fig. 9-4. Effects of serial medial collateral ligament–anterior cruciate ligament section on anterior-posterior laxity at various positions of tibial rotation under 925 N joint load. At 20 degrees of flexion laxity changes caused by ligament section followed a pattern similar to that seen without joint. Neither ligament section produced significant changes in laxity at full extension. Highly congruent surfaces, contact forces, and more complete compression of the menisci were probably responsible for ability of joint load to mask effects of ligament section at full extension.

in anterior-posterior laxity in either the unloaded or loaded states (Fig. 9-3 and 9-4). These figures also show that secondary section of the anterior cruciate ligament in a medial collateral ligament–deficient knee produces laxity increases comparable to primary anterior cruciate ligament section and that these laxity increases are greatest in external tibial rotation. In Fig. 9-4 joint load effectively eliminates the laxity increase at full extension from secondary anterior cruciate ligament section.

IN VIVO STUDIES

We used the UCLA instrumented clinical knee testing apparatus to measure anterior-posterior stiffness and laxity of patients who have had one or both menisci removed. Meniscectomized knees with an intact anterior cruciate ligament had anterior-posterior and varus-valgus laxities that were statistically indistinguishable from those of the contralateral uninjured limb. However, patients who had medial meniscectomies in combination with an absent anterior cruciate ligament had significantly increased laxity in their injured knees. This agrees with our observations of the effects of meniscectomy on anterior-posterior laxity in cadavers, but not for varus-valgus angulation of the tibia where laxity increases were observed in meniscectomized specimens. This discrepancy can perhaps be explained by passive muscle tension that tends to stabilize medial and lateral tibial translations of the tibia on the femur.

This test apparatus has also been used to measure anterior-posterior stability of 37 patients with documented absence of the anterior cruciate ligament. Fig. 9-5 illustrates that the injured-normal difference in anterior laxity is greater at 20 degrees of flexion than at 90 degrees of flexion and that this difference is best demonstrated with the tibia in slight external rotation. The problems with the 90-degree test are apparent in Fig. 9-6. The relative frequency distributions for the right versus left difference in a normal population and for the injured-normal difference in a population with anterior cruciate ligament deficiencies are shown. The high degree of overlap between these two distributions at 90 degrees makes this test inaccurate in detecting an absent anterior cruciate ligament. An estimate of the likelihood that a given patient has an absent anterior cruciate ligament can be obtained by comparing the relative heights of the distribution curves at a given laxity difference, that is, at any point on the x-axis the likelihood that a knee is injured is equal to the height of the injured curve divided by the sum of the heights of both curves. The likelihood curve in Fig. 9-6 approaches unity (100% certainty that the anterior cruciate ligament is absent) as the injured-normal laxity difference increases. Where the curves intersect the heights of the two curves are equal and the likelihood of injury is 50%.

Fig. 9-7 shows the injured and normal frequency distributions for the right-left differences in total laxity at 200 N of applied tibial force. These distributions show the best separation at 20 degrees of flexion. The steeper slope of the likelihood curve at 20 degrees indicates a better discrimination between injured and normal knees. Anterior stiffness difference also shows the best separation between injured and normal frequency distributions at 20 degrees of flexion (Fig. 9-8), with the likelihood curve also steepest in this position. It should be noted that the injured distribution

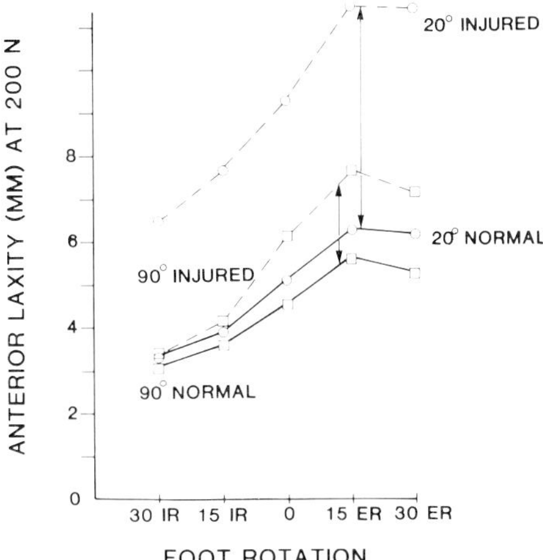

Fig. 9-5. Anterior laxity at 200 N as a function of foot rotation. Peak laxity for all knees tested occurred at approximately 15 degrees of external rotation of foot. Differences in laxity between injured and normal knees is greater at 20 degrees than at 90 degrees for all foot rotation positions.

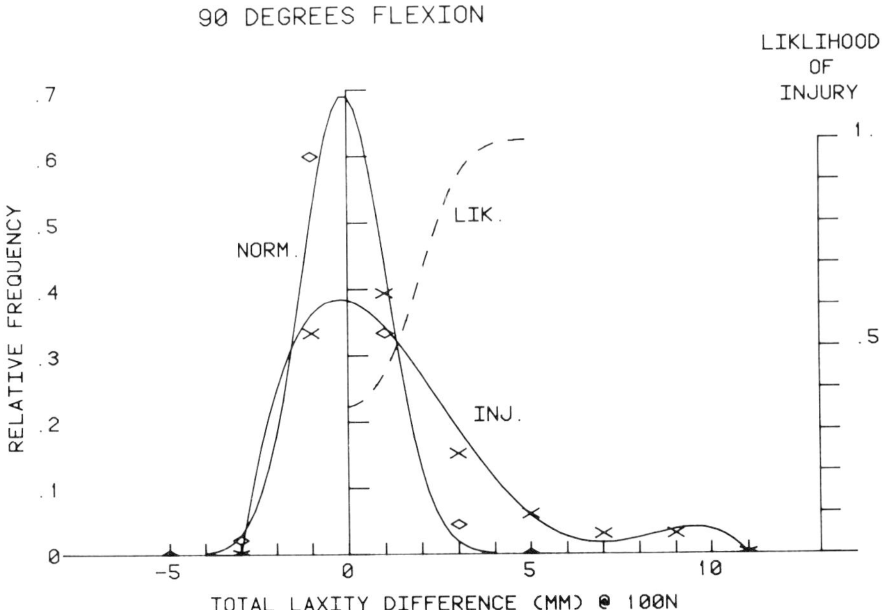

Fig. 9-6. Relative frequency distributions and likelihood of injury curve for total laxity difference at ± 100 N in 90 degrees of flexion position. Gaussian distribution curve (based on computed mean and standard deviation of normal uninjured knees) has been drawn, and comparison to actual frequency cell count *(diamond points)* reveals excellent theoretical agreement. Best fit polynomial regression curve has been drawn through frequency cell count points (✕) for injured knees. The likelihood of injury at specific laxity difference has been computed from relative heights of two distribution curves. At points where curves intersect (approximately 1.5 mm), heights are equal and likelihood of injury is 50% (as read from scale to right).

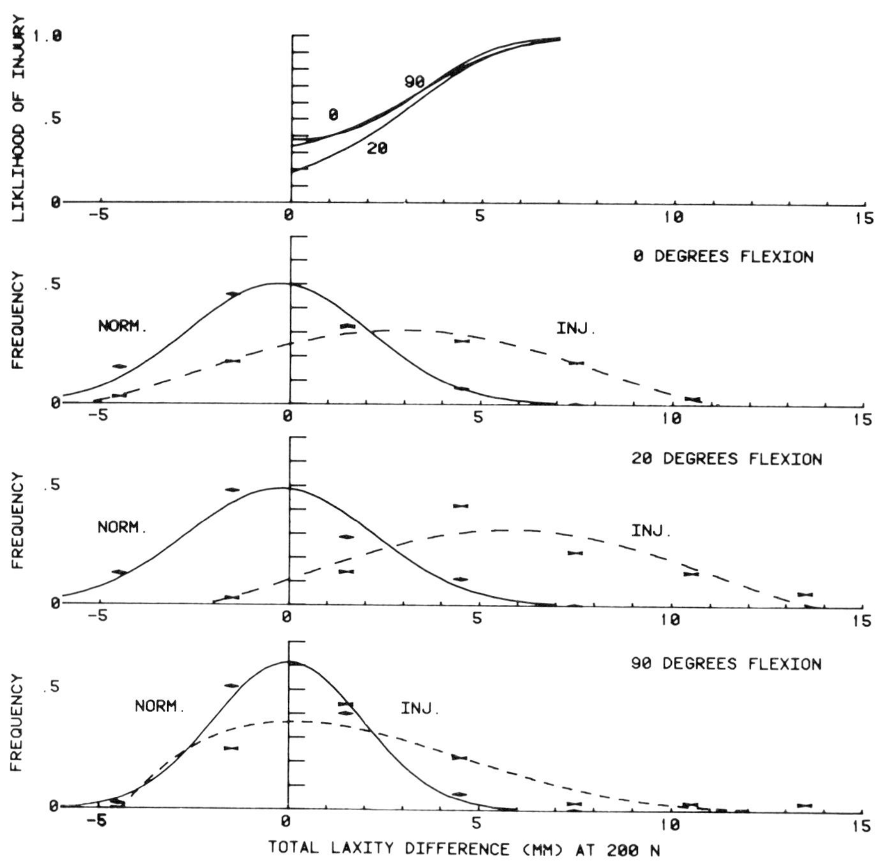

Fig. 9-7. Effects of knee flexion angle on injured and normal frequency distributions for total laxity difference at 200 N. Best separation between injured and normal populations is observed at 20 degrees, where a considerable portion of injured knee distribution lies outside normal band of right-left scatter.

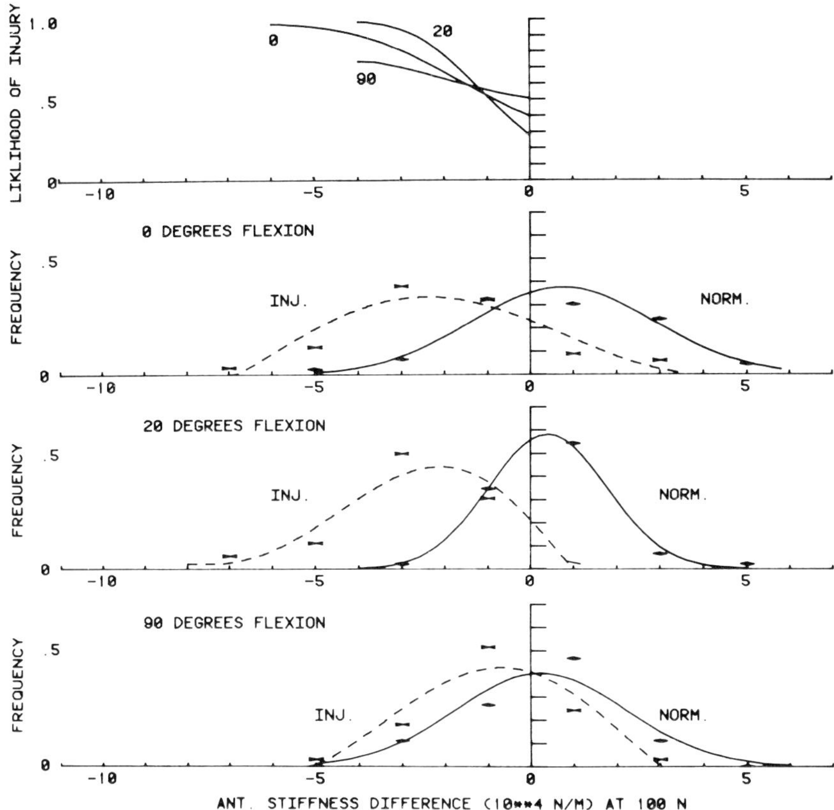

Fig. 9-8. Effects of knee flexion angle on injured and normal frequency distributions of anterior stiffness difference at 100 N. Excellent separation of two distributions is revealed at 20 degrees of flexion. Note likelihood of injury curve for 20 degrees is steepest, indicating higher degree of discrimination for measured changes in anterior stiffness difference.

falls to the left of the normal distribution, and reflects that a knee with anterior cruciate ligament deficiency is less stiff than a normal knee.

SUMMARY

1. Meniscectomy has relatively minor effects on the measured stability of the intact knee.
2. A knee with anterior cruciate ligament deficiency demonstrates decreased anterior stiffness and increased anterior laxity, which are best measured at 20 degrees of flexion.
3. The anterior drawer test at 90 degrees of flexion is not accurate for determining an absent anterior cruciate ligament.
4. Sacrifice of the medial collateral ligament in a knee with anterior cruciate ligament deficiency produces a further increase in anterior laxity, which is greatest in external tibial rotation.

10. The blood supply of the meniscus and its role in healing and repair

Steven Paul Arnoczky

The function, injury, and repair of the menisci have long been topics of interest and discussion among orthopaedic surgeons. Once described as the functionless remains of leg muscle,[21] the menisci are now realized to be integral components in the complex biomechanics of the knee.[8,11,14,16-19,22] This has stimulated many surgeons to consider primary repair of certain meniscal lesions over traditional meniscectomy.[7,10,12,23]

While Annandale[1] was credited with the first surgical repair of a torn meniscus in 1883, it was not until 1936 when King[15] published his classic experiment in dogs that the biologic limitations of meniscal healing were set forth. King stated that for meniscal lesions to heal they must communicate with the meniscal blood supply. Since the human meniscus has been considered an essentially avascular structure with a meager peripheral blood supply, relatively little has been written about its vascular anatomy[9] and the role of this vasculature in healing and repair.[5,6,13,15] This information predicates a rational approach to the surgical repair of meniscal lesions.

VASCULAR ANATOMY OF THE MENISCUS*

The vascular supply to the medial and lateral menisci of the human knee originates predominantly from the lateral and medial genicular arteries (both inferior and superior). Branches from these vessels give rise to a perimeniscal capillary plexus in the synovial and capsular tissues of the knee joint. The perimeniscal capillary plexus is an arborizing network of vessels that supply the peripheral border of the menisci throughout their attachment to the joint capsule (Fig. 10-1). These perimeniscal vessels are oriented in a predominantly circumferential pattern with radial branches directed toward the center of the joint (Fig. 10-2).

The middle genicular artery, along with a few terminal branches of the medial

---

*This information is based on a study[4] examining 20 cadaveric knees representing various ages from the sixth to the tenth decade of life. Twelve subjects were female and 8 were male; 14 were white and 6 were black.

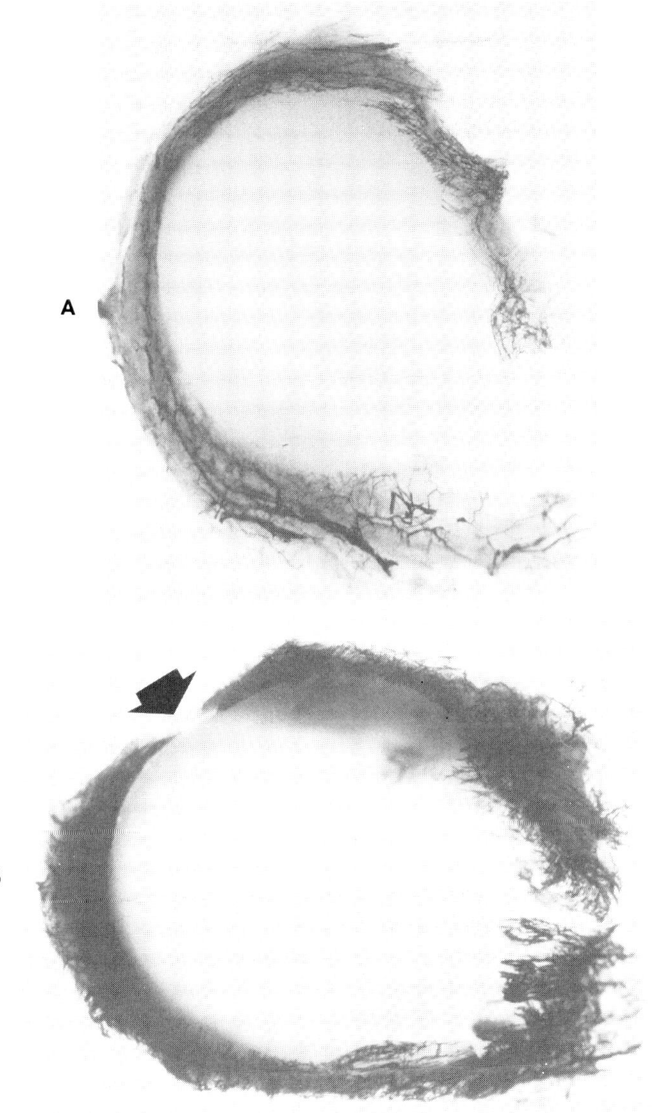

Fig. 10-1. Superior aspect of medial (**A**) and lateral (**B**) meniscus after vascular perfusion with India ink and tissue clearing using modified Spalteholz technique. Note vascularity at periphery of menisci and at anterior and posterior horn attachments. Absence of peripheral vasculature at posterolateral corner of lateral meniscus *(arrow)* represents area of passage of popliteal tendon. (From Arnoczky, S.P., and Warren, R.F.: Am. J. Sports Med. **10:**90, 1982.)

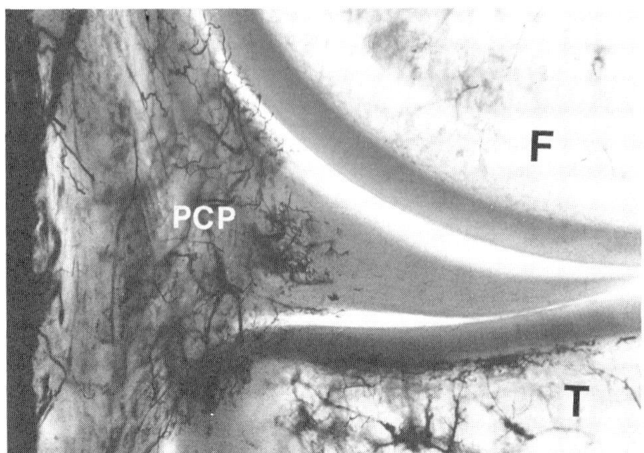

Fig. 10-2. Five-millimeter thick frontal section of medial compartment of knee (Spalteholz stain; × 3). Branching radial vessels from perimeniscal capillary plexus (PCP) can be seen penetrating peripheral border of medial meniscus. (From Arnoczky, S.P., and Warren, R.F.: Am. J. Sports Med. **10**:90, 1982.)

and lateral genicular arteries, also supplies vessels to the menisci through the vascular synovial covering of the anterior and posterior horn attachments. This synovial covering appears to be continuous in the vascular synovial sheath surrounding the cruciate ligaments[2] (Fig. 10-3).

Medial meniscus

The anterior horn attachment of the medial meniscus is covered with a layer of vascular synovial tissue. The vessels in this synovial covering supply branches to the ligamentous attachment of the anterior horn of the meniscus. These endoligamentous vessels penetrate the meniscal stroma of the anterior horn for a short distance (2 to 3 mm) and terminate in small capillary loops (Fig. 10-4). The vascular synovial covering of the anterior meniscal attachment extends over the femoral surface of the anterior horn of the meniscus for a short distance, but quickly recedes to the peripheral margin.

The body of the medial meniscus receives vessels from its peripheral attachment to the capsular and synovial tissues of the joint. Vessels from the perimeniscal capillary plexus course through this peripheral attachment and give off smaller radial branches that penetrate the meniscal stroma for a short distance and terminate in small capillary loops (Fig. 10-5). The degree of vascular penetration into the periphery of the medial meniscus varies between and within individual specimens and ranges from 10% to 30% of the meniscal width. No correlation could be established for this variation with regard to age, sex, race, or anatomic location.

A small reflection of vascular synovial tissue is present throughout the peripheral border of the medial meniscus on both its femoral and tibial surfaces. This *synovial fringe* extends a short distance (1 to 3 mm) over the articular surfaces of the meniscus

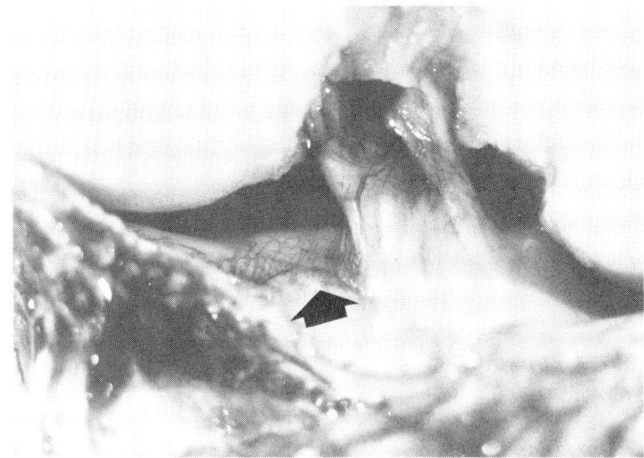

Fig. 10-3. Anterior view of India ink–perfused knee showing vascular covering of anterior cruciate ligament and anterior horn attachment of lateral meniscus (*arrow*). (From Arnoczky, S.P., and Warren, R.F.: Am. J. Sports Med. **10:**90, 1982.)

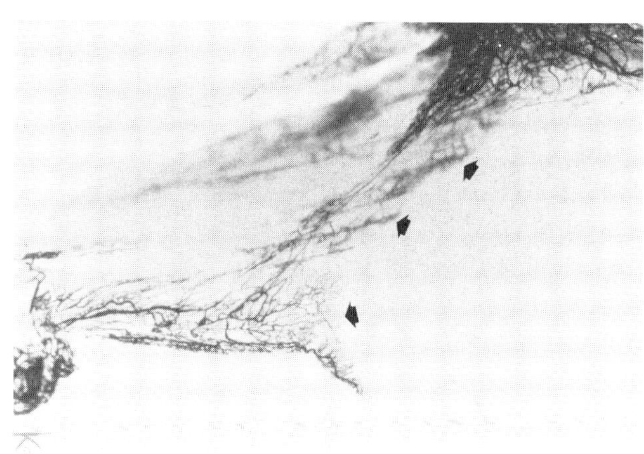

Fig. 10-4. Anterior horn attachment of medial meniscus (Spalteholz stain; × 5) demonstrating capillary vessels that penetrate anterior horn of medial meniscus (*arrows*). (From Arnoczky, S.P., and Warren, R.F.: Am. J. Sports Med. **10:**90, 1982.)

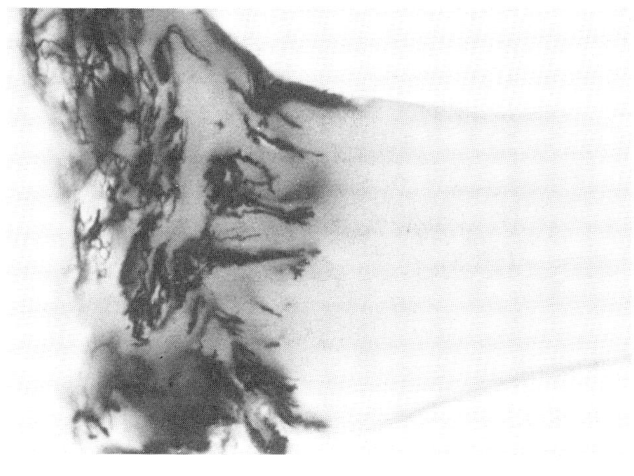

Fig. 10-5. Three-millimeter thick transverse section of medial meniscus (Spalteholz stain; × 8) demonstrating terminally looped capillary vessels and their penetration into peripheral border of meniscus. (From Arnoczky, S.P., and Warren, R.F.: Am. J. Sports Med. **10:**90, 1982.)

and contains small, terminally looped vessels (Fig. 10-6). Although this vascular synovial tissue intimately adheres to the articular surfaces of the menisci, histologic and cleared-tissue injection specimens reveal that it does not contribute vessels into the meniscal tissues. In some specimens the synovial fringe recedes markedly in the area of the medial collateral ligament and posterior medial aspect of the meniscus. On the femoral surface of the medial meniscus, this synovial fringe appears to be continuous with the synovial covering of the anterior horn and anterior horn attachment (Fig. 10-7).

The posterior horn attachment of the medial meniscus is also covered with a smooth layer of synovial tissue. As with the anterior horn, these synovial vessels penetrate the posterior attachment and result in endoligamentous vessels that enter the posterior horn of the meniscus for a short distance and end in capillary loops.

Lateral meniscus

The microvascular anatomy of the lateral meniscus is similar to that observed in the medial meniscus. Both anterior and posterior horn attachments are covered with a layer of vascular synovial tissue that appears to be continuous with the vascular synovial sheath that surrounds the cruciate ligaments.[2] Vessels in these horn attachments penetrate the meniscal tissue for a short distance and end in terminal capillary loops (Fig. 10-8).

The body of the lateral meniscus is supplied by circumferential and radial branches of the lateral inferior genicular artery that courses adjacent to the peripheral border of the lateral meniscus and deep to the lateral collateral ligament (Fig. 10-9). (The lateral inferior genicular artery at this location is a fairly large caliber vessel, and, because of its proximity to the peripheral border of the lateral meniscus, extreme care should be taken when performing a total lateral meniscectomy.) As in the medial meniscus, these radial vessels penetrate the peripheral meniscal stroma for a short distance and end in terminal capillary loops. The degree of vascular penetration in the lateral meniscus ranges from 10% to 25% of the meniscal width. This peripheral vascular supply is altered at the posterolateral aspect of the lateral meniscus. In this area the popliteal tendon lies adjacent to the peripheral border of the meniscus and in between the meniscus and the lateral capsular tissues. This posterolateral corner of the lateral meniscus is supplied by a ventral pedicle of synovial tissue that provides small vascular branches to the lateral wall of the meniscus (Fig. 10-10). Circumferential vessels from the capsular tissues anterior and posterior to this segment also extend along the lateral wall of the meniscus in a horizontal fashion, but do not appear to penetrate the meniscal stroma. In all lateral menisci examined there exists an avascular area on the peripheral wall of the meniscus immediately adjacent to the popliteal tendon (Fig. 10-11). It has been suggested that this avascular area is a result of intermittent reciprocal pressures between the tendon and the meniscus.[9]

A synovial fringe is also present on the femoral and tibial surfaces of the lateral meniscus. This fringe extends a short distance over the articular surfaces of the meniscus and appears to be continuous with the vascular synovial covering of the

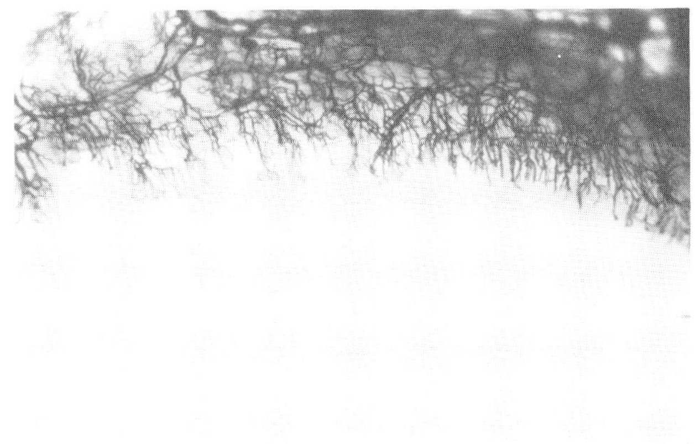

Fig. 10-6. Superior aspect of medial meniscus (Spalteholz stain; × 5) demonstrating terminally looped capillary vessels in synovial fringe as they extend out from peripheral border of meniscus. (From Arnoczky, S.P., and Warren, R.F.: Am. J. Sports Med. **10:**90, 1982.)

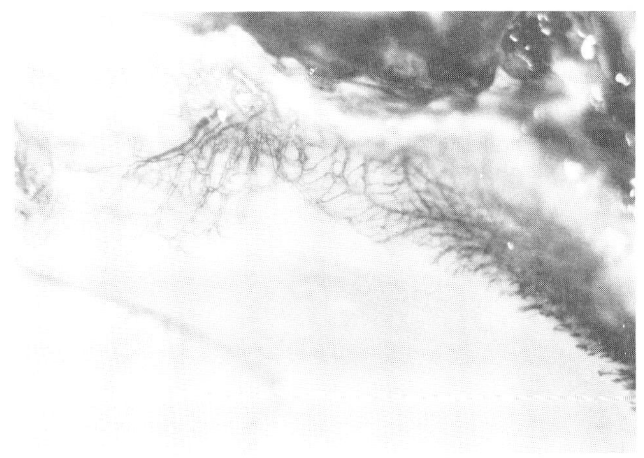

Fig. 10-7. Anterior horn of India ink–perfused medial meniscus showing extension of vascular synovial fringe into synovial covering of anterior horn attachment. (From Arnoczky, S.P., and Warren, R.F.: Am. J. Sports Med. **10:**90, 1982.)

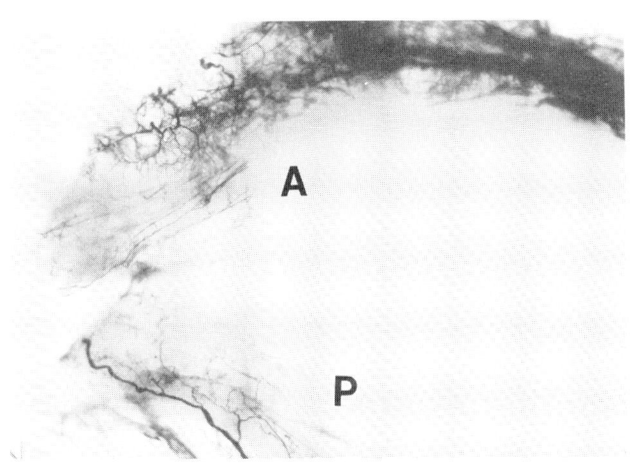

Fig. 10-8. Anterior (A) and posterior (P) horn attachments of lateral meniscus (Spalteholz stain; × 2) showing vascularity of attachments and penetration into horns of meniscus. (From Arnoczky, S.P., and Warren, R.F.: Am. J. Sports Med. **10:**90, 1982.)

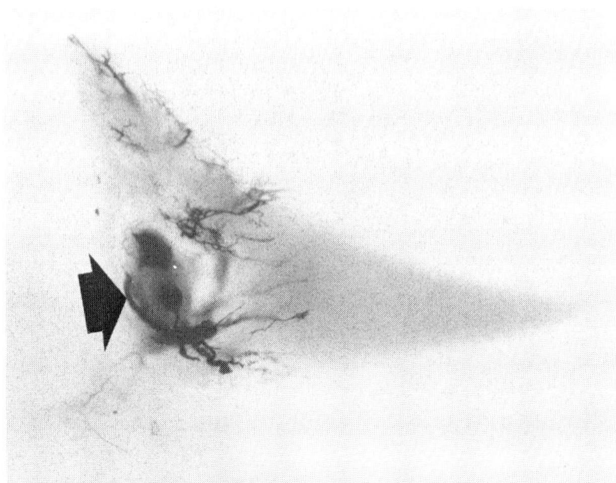

Fig. 10-9. Tranverse section of lateral meniscus just anterior to level of politeal tendon (Spalteholz stain; × 2) showing locatoin of lateral inferior genicular artery *(arrow)* adjacent to peripheral border of lateral meniscus. Note penetration of small capillary vessels into meniscus. (From Arnoczky, S.P., and Warren, R.F.: Am. J. Sports Med. **10**:90, 1982.)

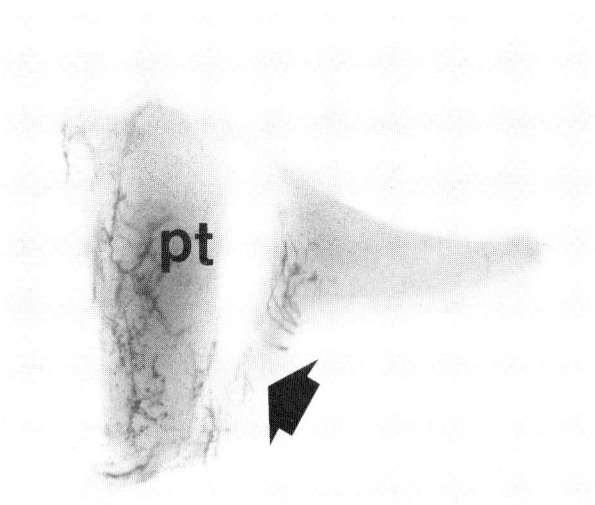

Fig. 10-10. Transverse secton of lateral meniscus adjacent to popliteal tendon *(PT)* (Spalteholz stain; × 2) showing ventral capsular attachment in this area and vascular pedicle *(arrow)* that supplies surface vessels to periphery of meniscus in this area. (From Arnoczky, S.P., and Warren, R.F.: Am. J. Sports Med. **10**:90, 1982.)

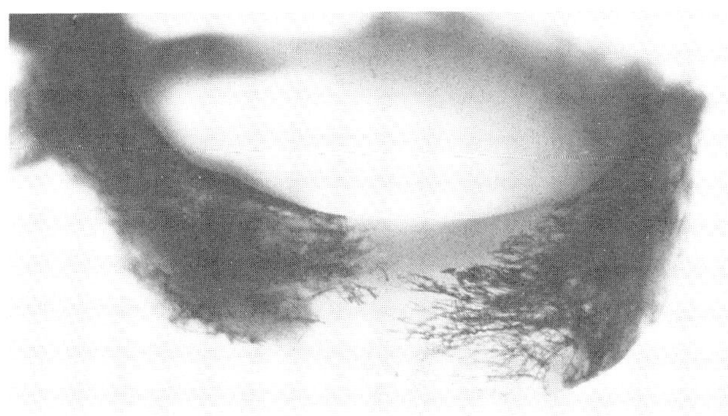

Fig. 10-11. Peripheral surface of lateral meniscus immediately adjacent to popliteal tendon (Spalteholz stain; × 2). Note avascular area on peripheral surface of meniscus where tendon passes across meniscus. (From Arnoczky, S.P., and Warren, R.F.: Am. J. Sports Med. **10**:90, 1982.)

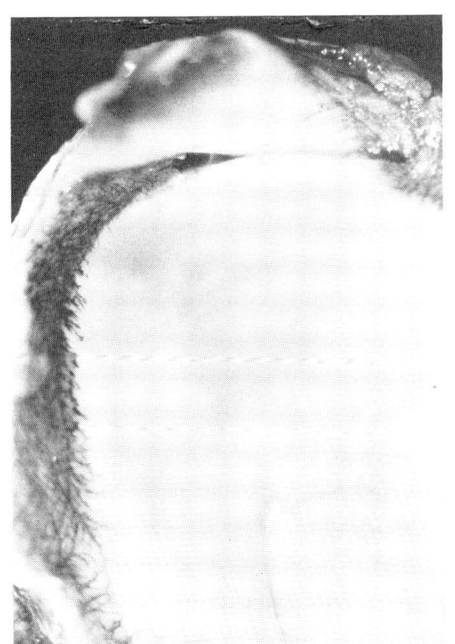

Fig. 10-12. Photograph of India ink-injected specimen showing absence of synovial fringe in area of popliteal tendon. (From Arnoczky, S.P., and Warren, R.F.: Am. J. Sports Med. **10**:90, 1982.)

anterior and posterior horn attachments. As in the medial meniscus, this vascular fringe is intimately attached to the meniscal surface, but does not contribute vessels into the meniscal tissue. This synovial fringe is absent in the area of the popliteal tendon (Fig. 10-12). There is no apparent difference in the microvascular anatomy of the menisci with regard to age, sex, or race.

The importance of the peripheral meniscal vasculature in healing and repair in animals has been stressed by King[15] and others.[5,6,13] Several cases of naturally healed

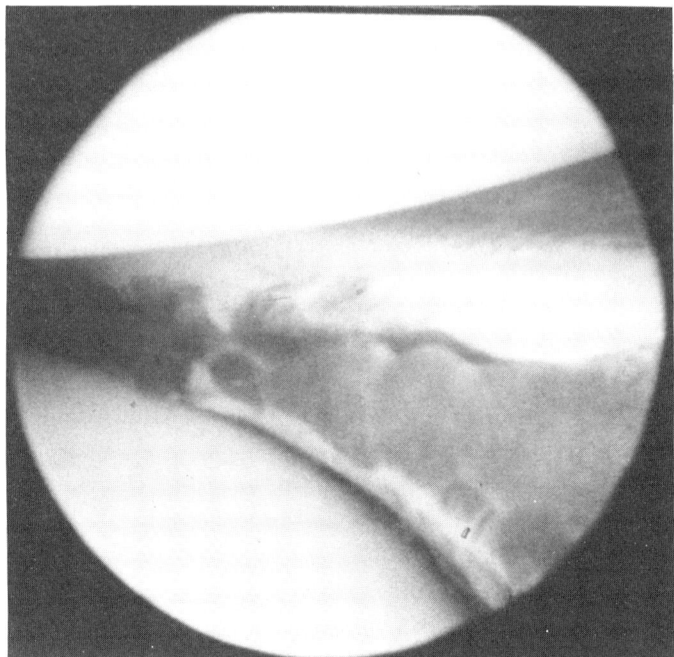

Fig. 10-13. Arthroscopic view of peripheral tear of human meniscus. Note granulation tissue present at margin of lesion and synovial fringe over femoral surface of meniscus. (Courtesy R. Jackson, Toronto.)

meniscal lesions that have communicated with the peripheral meniscal vasculature have also been reported in humans.[20,23] From this description it appears that lesions of the peripheral attachment of the menisci, and those involving the anterior or posterior horn attachments, have access to a vascular supply that may be adequate enough to support a healing response (Fig. 10-13). Lesions in the posterolateral aspect of the lateral meniscus where the blood supply is tenuous would be an exception. These observations have led to increasing efforts by orthopaedic surgeons to repair certain meniscal lesions.[7,10,12,23]

VASCULAR RESPONSE TO INJURY

Although the identification of a blood supply is essential in determining the ability of a meniscal lesion to heal, the role of this blood supply in the reparative response is equally important. A recent study examined the role of the peripheral vasculature in meniscal healing in dogs.[5] The dog was used as a model because its meniscal blood supply is similar to that in humans.[4,5]

In this study the medial meniscus was completely bisected by a radial incision (Fig. 10-14). Following transection, a small gap of 1 to 2 mm formed between the meniscal segments. By 2 weeks this gap was filled with an organized fibrin clot. Vessels from the perimeniscal capillary plexus proliferated through this fibrin *scaffold* accompanied by a proliferation of mesenchymal cells (Fig. 10-15).

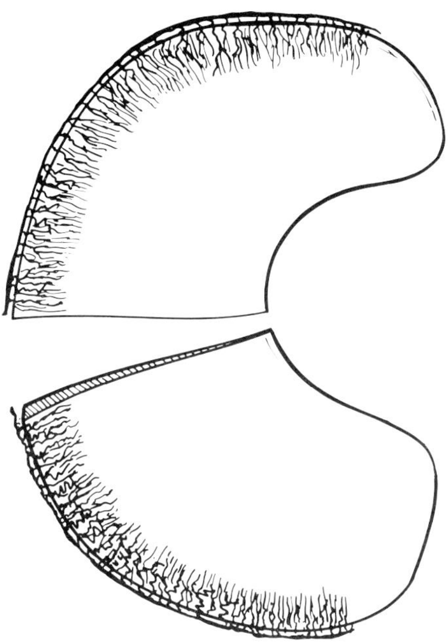

Fig. 10-14. Schematic drawing of medial meniscus illustrating location and extent of transverse incision. (From Arnoczky, S.P., and Warren, R.F.: Am. J. Sports Med. **11:**131, 1983.)

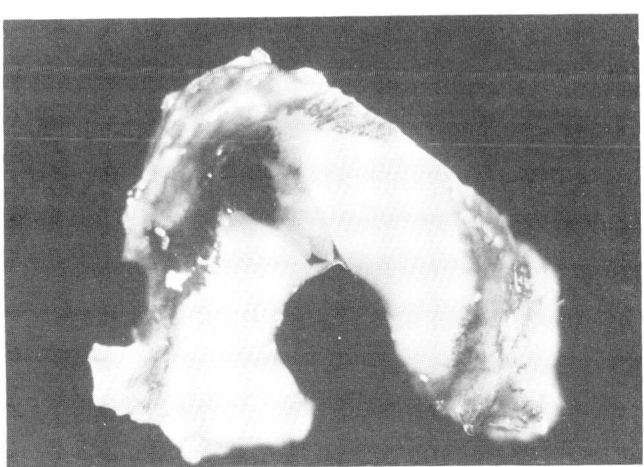

Fig. 10-15. India ink–perfused medial meniscus 2 weeks after complete transection. Note proliferation of vessels from perimensical capillary plexus into fibrous clot. (From Arnoczky, S.P., and Warren, R.F.: Am. J. Sports Med. **11:**131, 1983.)

This vascular and cellular proliferation continued through the fourth week, and by the sixth week the gap between the meniscal segments was completely filled with a fibrovascular scar. This scar tissue was cellular and appeared to be continuous with the normal adjacent fibrocartilage of the meniscus (Fig. 10-16). Also noted was the presence of a vascular synovial pannus over the area of the fibrovascular scar (Fig. 10-17), which appeared to be a proliferation of the synovial fringe immediately adjacent to the lesion. Vessels from this synovial proliferation extended over both the femoral and tibial articular surfaces of the lesion and penetrated the fibrovascular scar to anastomose with vessels from the perimeniscal capillary plexus (Fig. 10-18).

At 8 weeks the vascular response of both the synovial fringe and the perimeniscal capillary plexus had begun to subside. Histologic examination revealed a normal circumferential orientation of the collagen fibers in the scar tissue.

By 10 weeks the fibrovascular scar had remodeled to reflect the contours of the normal meniscus (Fig. 10-19). While the synovial fringe had receded to the peripheral border of the lesion, vessels in the fibrous tissue remained throughout most of the scar. Histologically the scar tissue was cellular and, with the exception of its collagen orientation, showed little resemblance to the adjacent fibrocartilage. Modulation of this scar tissue into normal-appearing fibrocartilage requires several months.

The ability of the peripheral vasculature to support a reparative response has provided the rationale for the repair of peripheral meniscal injuries, and several reports have demonstrated excellent results following primary repair of peripheral meniscal lesions.[7,10,12,23] Postoperative examination of these peripheral repairs reveals a process of repair similar to that just described (Fig. 10-20).

While meniscal repair to date has been limited to the peripheral vascular area of the meniscus, a significant number of meniscal lesions occur in the central, avascular portion of the meniscus. Experimental[5,15] and clinical observations have shown that these lesions are incapable of healing and thus provide the rationale for partial meniscectomy. Recent experimental evidence has demonstrated, however, that if longitudinal lesions in the avascular portion of the meniscus are connected to the peripheral vasculature by a *vascular access channel*, these lesions are capable of healing through a process of fibrovascular scar proliferation similar to that just described.[5] In this technique, a full-thickness vascular access channel was made at the midportion of longitudinal lesions in the avascular portion of the medial meniscus of dogs connecting the lesions to the vasculature of the perimeniscal capillary plexus (Fig. 10-21).

In this study it was observed that 2 weeks after creation of a vascular access channel a fibrin clot was present throughout the vascular access channel and most of the longitudinal lesion. Also, vessels from the perimeniscal capillary plexus had begun to proliferate into the clot, and the synovial fringe could be seen extending over the vascular access channel.

This vascular response continued, and by 4 weeks fibrovascular scar tissue could be seen proliferating in the longitudinal lesion (Fig. 10-22). The vascular pannus from the synovial fringe did not extend over the longitudinal aspect of the lesion and was limited to the area over the vascular access channel.

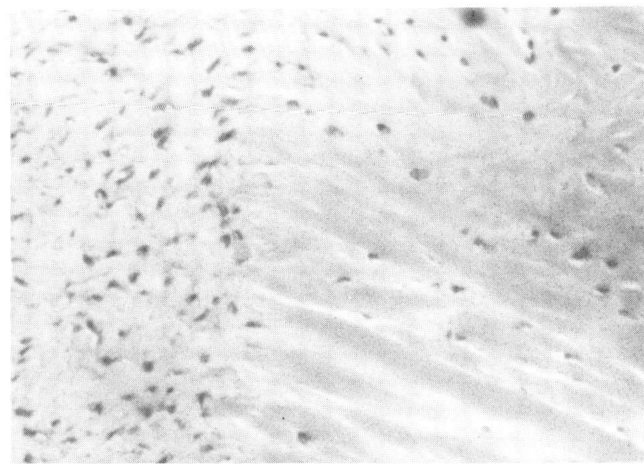

Fig. 10-16. Photomicrograph of healing meniscus at junction of fibrovascular scar and normal adjacent meniscal tissue. (Hematoxylin-eosin-stain; × 100.) (From Arnoczky, S.P., and Warren, R.F.: Am. J. Sports Med. **11**:131, 1983.)

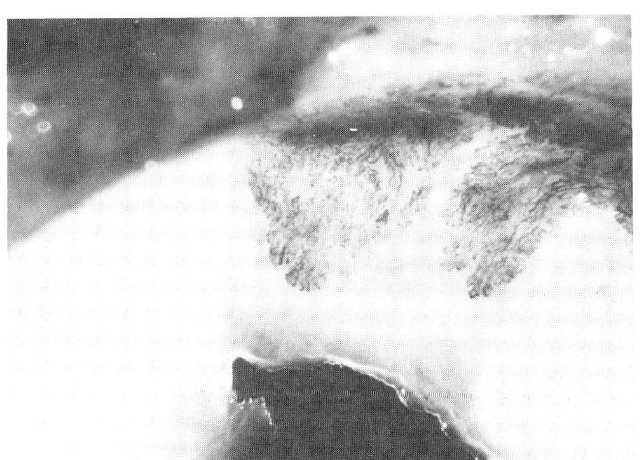

Fig. 10-17. India ink–perfused specimen showing fibrovascular scar 6 weeks after complete transection of medial meniscus. Notice proliferation of vascular synovial tissue over fibrovascular scar. (From Arnoczky, S.P., and Warren, R.F.: Am. J. Sports Med. **11**: 131, 1983.)

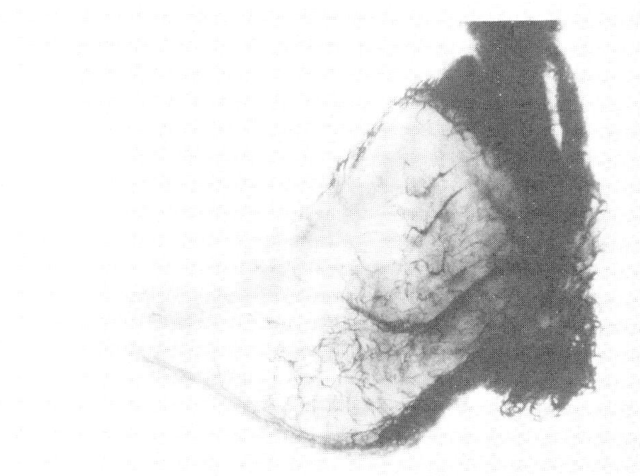

Fig. 10-18. Two-millimeter thick transverse section through fibrovascular scar seen in Fig. 10-17 (Spalteholz stain; × 8). Note proliferation of vessels of synovial fringe and their anastomosis with proliferating vessels of perimeniscal capillary plexus. (From Arnoczky, S.P., and Warren, R.F.: Am. J. Sports Med. **11**:131, 1983.)

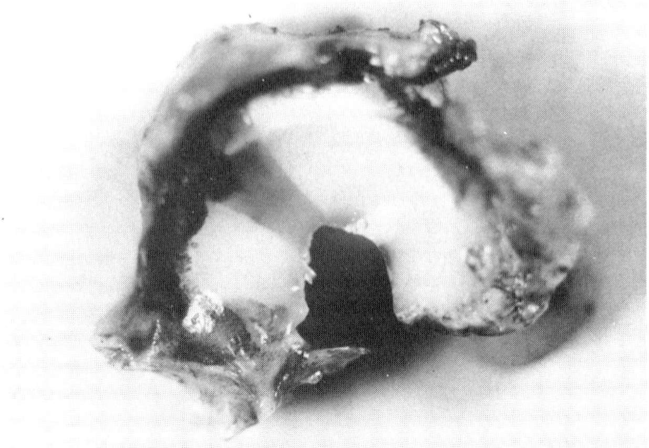

Fig. 10-19. India ink–perfused medial meniscus 10 weeks after complete transection. Fibrovascular scar has completely filled lesion and remodeled to normal contours of meniscus. Note that response of synovial fringe has subsided, but injected vessels from perimeniscal capillary plexus are still visible in fibrovascular scar. (From Arnoczky, S.P., and Warren, R.F.: Am. J. Sports Med. **11:**131, 1983.)

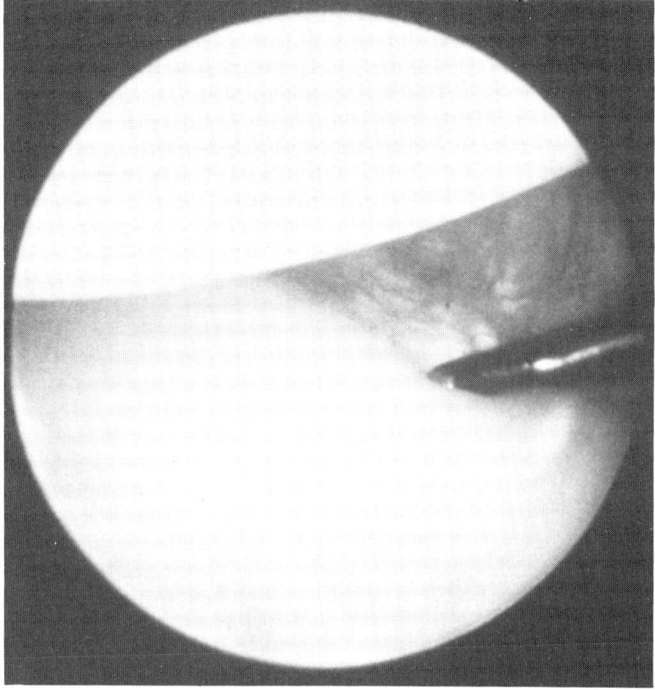

Fig. 10-20. Arthroscopic view of human meniscus 18 months after repair of peripheral lesion. Note synovial pannus present in area of repair (probe). (Courtesy K. DeHaven, Rochester, N.Y.)

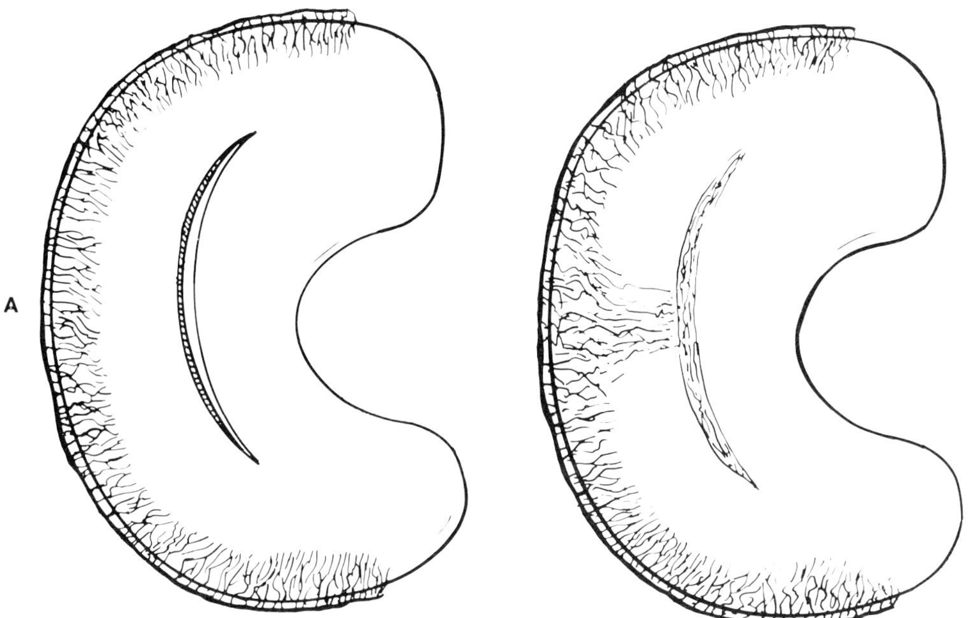

Fig. 10-21. Schematic drawing of medial meniscus illustrating **A,** location and extent of longitudinal lesion, and **B,** location of full-thickness vascular access channel and vascular responses associated with it. (From Arnoczky, S.P., and Warren, R.F.: Am. J. Sports Med. **11:**131, 1983.)

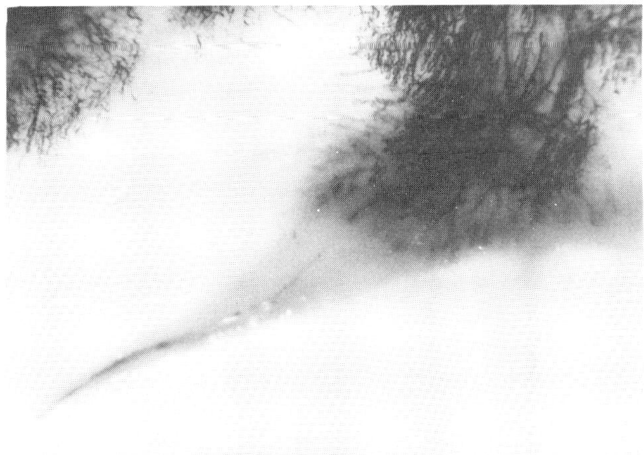

Fig. 10-22. India ink–perfused medial meniscus 4 weeks after longitudinal incision and creation of vascular access channel. Vessels can be seen progressing in fibrin clot in anterior limb of longitudinal lesion. (From Arnoczky, S.P., and Warren, R.F.: Am. J. Sports Med. **11:**131, 1983.)

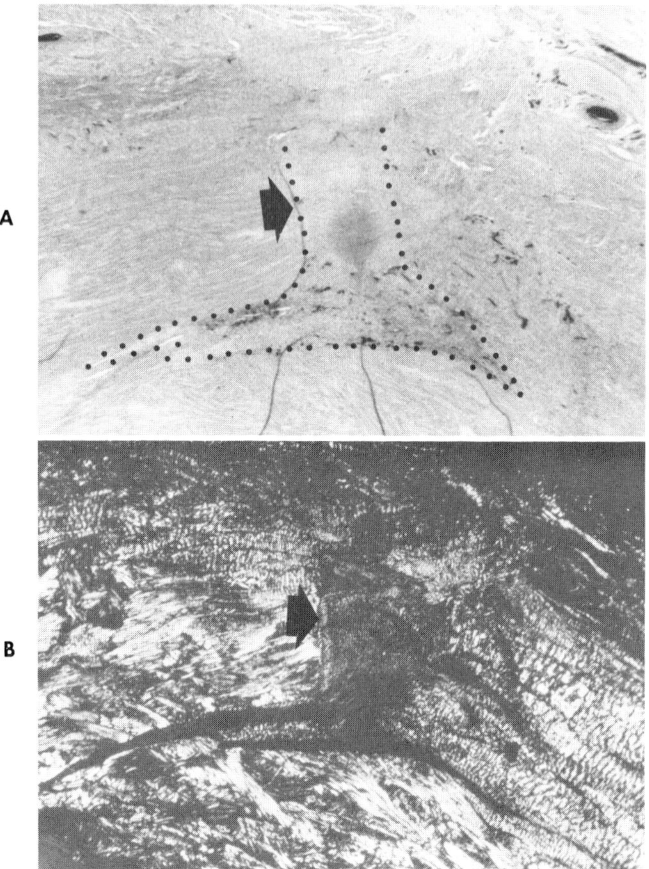

Fig. 10-23. A, Photomicrograph of horizontal section of medial meniscus 10 weeks after creation of longitudinal lesion and vascular access channel *(arrow)*. Note entire longitudinal lesion is filled with fibrovascular scar tissue. (Vessels are black because of India ink perfusion) **B,** Polarized-light photomicrograph of same section illustrating extent of lesion and location of vascular access channel *(arrow)*. (Hematoxylin-eosin stain; × 40.) (From Arnoczky, S.P., and Warren, R.F.: Am. J. Sports Med. **11:**131, 1983.)

The proliferation of the fibrovascular scar in the longitudinal lesion continued through the eighth postoperative week, and by 10 weeks the entire longitudinal lesion was filled with fibrovascular scar tissue (Fig. 10-23 and 10-24). Although this tissue appeared continuous with the adjacent meniscal fibrocartilage, examination under polarized light microscopy revealed no orientation of the collagen fibers in the scar.

This technique has been limited to investigation in animal models. However, as experience with meniscal repair increases such modifications may optimize the potential for meniscal healing and increase the scope of meniscal repair.

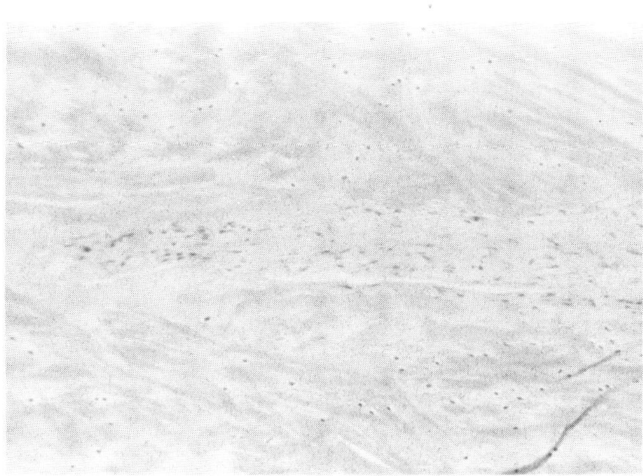

Fig. 10-24. Photomicrograph of anterior limit of longitudinal incision 10 weeks after creation of vascular access channel. Note lesion is completely healed by fibrous tissue. (Hematoxylin-eosin stain; × 100.) (From Arnoczky, S.P., and Warren, R.F.: Am. J. Sports Med. 11:131, 1983.)

SUMMARY

The menisci are supplied by branches of the lateral, medial, and middle genicular arteries. A perimeniscal capillary plexus originating in the capsular and synovial tissues of the joint supplies the peripheral 10% to 25% of the menisci. A peripheral vascular synovial fringe extends a short distance over both the femoral and tibial surfaces of the menisci, but does not contribute any vessels to the meniscal stroma. The posterolateral aspect of the lateral meniscus adjacent to the popliteal tendon is devoid of penetrating vessels and a synovial fringe. The anterior and posterior horn attachments of the menisci are covered with vascular synovial tissue and appear to have a good blood supply.

The peripheral vasculature of the meniscus appears to be sufficient to support a reparative response. This response is in the form of a fibrovascular scar that originates in the vasculature of the perimeniscal capillary plexus and the synovial fringe. These peripheral soft tissues provide a vascular response similar to that observed in the synovial covering of the cruciate ligaments.[3] Experimental evidence suggests that lesions in the avascular portion of the meniscus can heal through a similar process by the creation of a vascular access channel that joins the avascular lesion to the peripheral blood supply.

REFERENCES

1. Annandale, T.: An operation for displaced semilunar cartilage, Br. Med. J. **1:**779, 1885.
2. Arnoczky, S.P.: The anatomy of the anterior cruciate ligament, Clin Orthop. **172:**19, 1983.
3. Arnoczky, S.P., Rubin, R.M., and Marshall, J.L.: The microvasculature of the cruciate ligaments and its response to injury, J. Bone Joint Surg. **61A:**1221, 1979.

4. Arnoczky, S.P., and Warren, R.F.: Microvasculature of the human meniscus, Am. J. Sports Med. **10**:90, 1982.

5. Arnoczky, S.P., and Warren, R.F.: The microvasculature of the meniscus and its response to injury: an experimental study in the dog, Am. J. Sports Med. **11**:131, 1983.

6. Cabaud, H.E., Rodkey, W.G., and Fitzwater, J.E.: Medial meniscus repairs: an experimental and morphological study, Am. J. Sports Med. **9**:129, 1981.

7. Cassidy, R.E., and Shaffer, A.J.: Repair of peripheral meniscal tears: a preliminary report, Am. J. Sports Med. **9**:209, 1981.

8. Cox, J.S., and others: The degenerative effects of partial and total resection of the medial meniscus in dog's knees, Clin. Orthop. **109**:178, 1975.

9. Davies, D.V., and Edwards, D.A.W.: The blood supply of the synovial membrane and intra-articular structures, Ann. R. Coll. Surg. Engl. **2**:142, 1948.

10. DeHaven, K.E.: Peripheral meniscal repair: an alternative to meniscectomy, Trans. Orthop. Res. Soc., Las Vegas, **5**:399, 1981.

11. Fairbanks, T.J.: Knee joint changes after meniscectomy, J. Bone Joint Surg. **30B**:664, 1948.

12. Hamberg, P., Gillquist, J., and Lysholm, J.: Suture of new and old peripheral meniscal tears, J. Bone Joint Surg. **65A**:193, 1983.

13. Heatley, F.W.: The meniscus: can it be repaired? An experimental investigation in rabbits, J. Bone Joint Surg. **62B**:397, 1980.

14. King, D.: The function of semilunar cartilages, J. Bone Joint Surg. **18**:1069, 1936.

15. King, D.: The healing of semilunar cartilages, J. Bone Joint Surg. **18**:333, 1936.

16. Krause, W.R., and others: Mechanical changes in the knee after meniscectomy, J. Bone Joint Surg. **58A**:599, 1976.

17. Levy, I.M., Torzilli, P.A., and Warren, R.F.: The effect of medial meniscectomy on anteroposterior motion of the knee, J. Bone Joint Surg. **64A**:883, 1982.

18. Seedhom, B.B.: Loadbearing function of the meniscus, Physiotherapy **62**:223, 1976.

19. Seedhom, B.B., Dowson, D., and Wright, V.: Functions of the menisci: a preliminary study, J. Bone Joint Surg. **56B**:381, 1974.

20. Smillie, I.S.: Injuries of the knee joint, Edinburgh, 1946, E.S. Livingstone.

21. Sutton, J.B.: Ligaments: their nature and morphology, London, 1897, H.K. Lewis & Co., Ltd.

22. Tapper, E.M., and Hoover, N.W.: Late results after meniscectomy, J. Bone Joint Surg. **51A**:517, 1969.

23. Wirth, C.R.: Meniscus repair, Clin. Orthop. **157**:153, 1981.

11. Ligament biology and biomechanics

Wayne H. Akeson
Cyril B. Frank
David Amiel
Savio L.-Y. Woo

This chapter summarizes present knowledge of ligament biology and biomechanics. It updates material reviewed elsewhere[7] on the effects of stress enhancement and stress deprivation on connective tissue and details present knowledge of ligament healing. The scientific basis for clinical practice in this field is weak and requires reinforcement with well-controlled basic and clinical studies.

MORPHOLOGY
Definition

Ligaments are short bands of tough, flexible fibrous tissue that bind the bones of the body together and support the organs in place.[48] Ligaments are relatively unyielding with regard to the joints and are only pliant enough to allow restricted ranges of movement. Ligaments supply static support and guidance and supplement both bony geometry and the dynamic effects of muscle and tendon.[74,81]

Embryology

Derived mainly from portions of differentiating interzonal mesenchyme,[110] ligaments commonly contribute to cuffs of dense tissue known as the *fibrous capsular* components of the synovial joints. A fibrous capsule is a membrane that unites two bones and is distinct from tendon aponeuroses.[51] Although sometimes the structure remains almost indistinguishable, it is common for functionally distinct specialized thickening of capsules to form. As joint development proceeds (apparently dependent on the beginning of intrauterine movements[110]), strengthened parallel arrangements of fibers orient to resist tension in particular directions and usually become more distinct and allow specific anatomic subclassification. These, along with both extra-

☐ Supported by the Alberta Heritage Foundation for Medical Research, National Institutes of Health grant no. AM14918 and grant no. AM00304 (Research Career Development Award), the Veterans Administration Medical Research Service, and the Bone and Joint Disease Foundation.

capsular *accessory* and intraarticular homologues (intraarticular ligaments may form from condensations of synovial interzonal mesenchyme[110]), are named according to position (e.g., collateral) or attachments (e.g., coracoclavicular).

Appearance

On gross examination, ligaments belong to a family of dense regular connective tissues (including tendons, fascia, and aponeuroses) with closely packed parallel collagenous bundles having a shining white appearance.[20] Under microscopic examination, these tissues contain a meshwork of interlacing fibers, flattened cells, and ground substance (including water). Polarized light and specialized stains are used to differentiate and isolate the fibrous elements (collagen, elastin and reticulin) and similarly distinguish ground substance and fibroblasts in the interfibrillar spaces (Fig. 11-1).

Ultrastructural methods are used to define detailed hierarchies of arrangement down to microfibril size in tendons[15] with presumably similar arrangements in ligaments. Fasciae and aponeuroses are arranged regularly in multiple sheets or la-

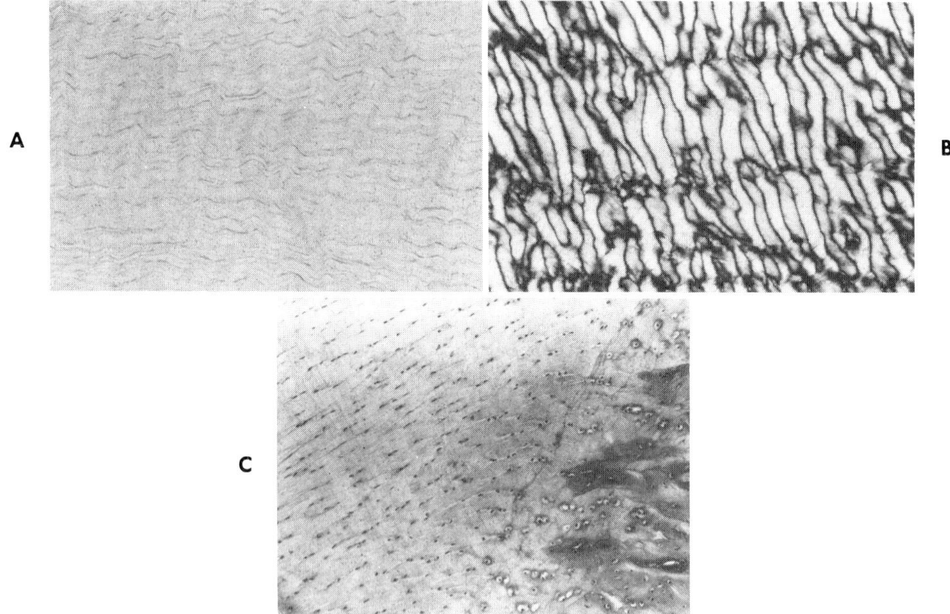

Fig. 11-1. **A,** Normal medial collateral ligament. Note longitudinal orientation of matrix seen under low power magnification. (Hematoxylin-eosin stain; × 100.) **B,** Polarizing light of low power section of normal medial collateral ligament demonstrates undulating pattern of matrix (crimp). (× 100.) **C,** Insertion of normal anterior cruciate ligament demonstrates progression from normal ligament *(left)* through fibrocartilage and mineralized fibrocartilage to bone *(right)*. Note line separating fibrocartilage and mineralized fibrocartilage passing obliquely through this specimen.

mellae, which may or may not have similar orientation. Tendons and ligaments, however, are regularly arranged with bundles of fibers oriented in the direction of *functional need*.

Insertions

The insertions of ligaments and tendons progress from fibril through fibrocartilage (usually less than 0.6 mm) to mineralized fibrocartilage (less than 0.4 mm) and finally to bone[32,64] (Fig. 11-1, *C*). Zones of fibrocartilage and calcified fibrocartilage are separated by a narrow line of unknown significance, which stains blue in hematoxylin and eosin. Transmission electron microscopy shows two types of insertion of collagen fibers into bone with the more common crossing the mineralization front previously described, and the second, less common, inserting directly into bone in relation to the periosteum.[32,64,73] Combinations of these insertion patterns serve to dissipate force and minimize insertional failures. Stress is important in maintaining the functional integrity of the insertion sites.[76,99]

Blood supply

Ligaments normally receive blood vessels from periarticular arterial plexuses, from which numerous offsets also supply synovium and loose areolar tissue in the region. Intraligamentous vessels are relatively sparse, which implies that at least some degree of diffusion is necessary for midsubstance cellular nutrition. Insertion sites are nearly avascular in a number of ligaments, and tenuous vascular connections are easily damaged.[81] Lymphatics form a plexus in the subintima of the synovium and drain along blood vessels to regional lymph nodes.[110] The details of blood supply to each joint are, however, both complex and variable and must be studied individually, for example, the knee joint.[13,93]

The importance of blood supply to the anterior cruciate ligament is currently being debated. Evidence has been presented that points to synovial fluid as a principal source of nutrients of this ligament.[112]

Nerve supply

The nerve supplies of the ligaments come from the nerves to the muscles acting on that joint. Reflex arcs to antagonistic muscle groups prevent overstretching of capsules and harmful or abnormal posturing.[110] There are numerous free nerve endings in the ligaments with both nonmyelinated and finely myelinated fibers believed to moderate pain sensation.[46] Combinations of nonencapsulated and specialized encapsulated endings mediate position sense. Intraligamentous pacinian corpuscles, Ruffini endings, and Golgi end organs collectively assist in mediation of proprioception, including speed and direction of joint movement.[18]

BIOMECHANICS

Ligaments demonstrate complex rheologic behavior similar to that previously described for other soft tissues.[41,42] Different components of the tissue take up loads at different stress levels and contribute to a nonlinear mechanical behavior. Ligaments are anisotropic, being oriented primarily for the resistance of tensile stress. They are also similar to other soft tissues, since they possess time- and history-dependent viscoelastic properties.

The fibrillar components of ligaments (predominantly collagen) are arranged in an undulating path or *crimp* between origin and insertion in their physiologic relaxed state. During movements in which tensile stretch is applied, progressive straightening and stretching of an increasing number of fibers occurs (recruitment) and contributes to a nonlinear stress-strain relationship that can be illustrated by a simplified mechanical model[40] (Fig. 11-2).

The stress-strain relationship of ligaments is initially concave upward, demonstrating increasing slope with increasing strain, but this slope becomes near linear in the prefailure phase of tensile loading.

When compared with relatively loose and disorganized fiber arrangements such as skin, recruitment in ligament structures (indicated by increasing stress and stiffness) takes place much sooner, that is, at much smaller strain levels (Fig. 11-3). The densely packed and nearly parallel pattern of fibers in ligaments is well suited to the functional roles that ligaments play, offering early and increasing resistance to tensile loading in relatively narrow ranges of joint displacement.

Ligaments, however, are more than just an aggregation of collagen fibers of different length. A complex interaction of collagen with surrounding proteins and ground substance results in a mechanical behavior that is considerably different from that of isolated fibrillar material. Ligaments are viscoelastic and possess both time- and history-dependent properties. For example, their loading and unloading curves do not follow the same path, describing instead a *hysteresis loop* with a net loss of energy (caused by internal friction) during each cycle (Fig. 11-4). This behavior has

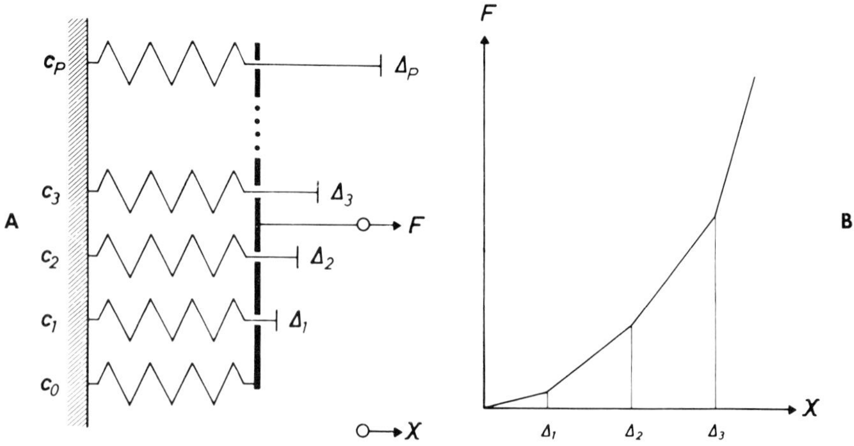

Fig. 11-2. A, and **B,** Model of nonlinear elasticity demonstrates different components coming into action at different stages of deformation, resulting in nonlinear load deformation curve. (From Frisen, M., and others: J. Biomech. 2:13, 1969.)

been likened to that of nylon hose[26]: an organized material that behaves with a similar nonlinear elastic stretch and recovery (Fig. 11-5).

Significant viscoelastic properties of ligaments include creep (increasing deformation with time under constant load) (Fig. 11-6) and stress relaxation (decreasing stress with time under constant deformation) (Fig. 11-7). Through a combination of these nonlinear viscoelastic properties, the originally described stress-strain relationship for the medial collateral ligament at various strain rates has been predicted mathematically and shown to conform to experimental data[118] (Fig. 11-8).

Viscoelastic properties not only influence the case of single-cycle loading and unloading, but more complex loading states as well, both in vitro and in vivo. Cyclic

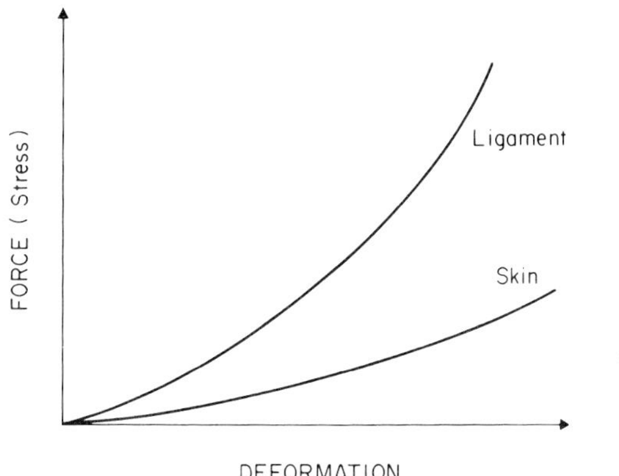

Fig. 11-3. Schematic representation of force-displacement relationship of ligament (highly organized fibrillar material) and skin (loose meshwork). Ligament fibers take up loads at much earlier stages of deformation than more randomly organized structures exemplified by skin.

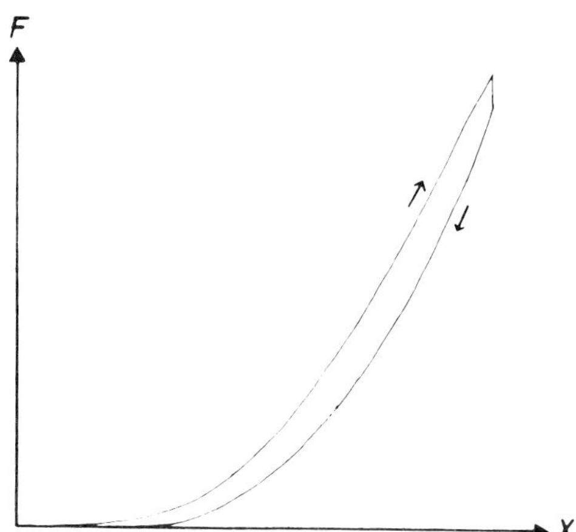

Fig. 11-4. Schematic load deformation diagram for cycle of loading and unloading of ligament, showing hysteresis loop typical of viscoelastic material. (From Viidik, A.: J. Biomech. 1:3, 1968.)

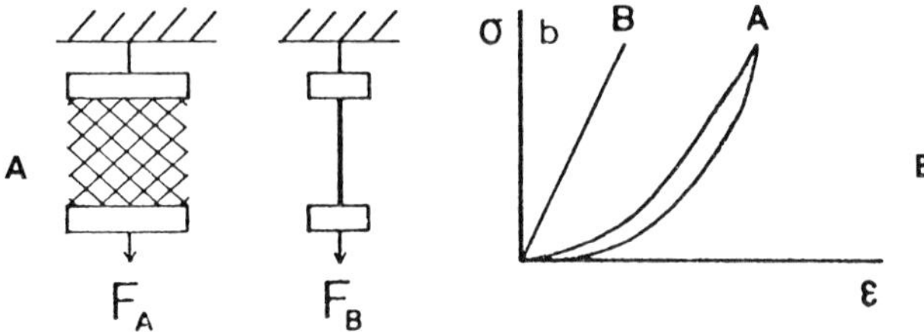

Fig. 11-5. Schematic representation of nylon hose model demonstrating nonlinear hysteresis behavior (**A**) as opposed to linear stress-strain behavior of uniform material (**B**).

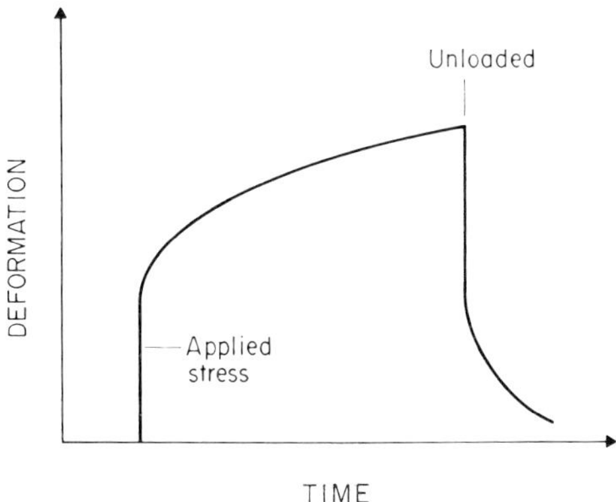

Fig. 11-6. Schematic representation of creep behavior (increasing deformation with time under constant load) of viscoelastic material.

loading, such as during walking or exercise, has been shown to cause several important, but notably transient property changes in ligament complexes. Transient *softening* of ligament substance occurs as cycling proceeds, with slight decreases in peak loads being noted while the applied strains and strain rates are constant[114] (Fig. 11-9). Similarly, deformation increases slightly during early cycles to a constant load showing creep effects on the ligament (Fig. 11-10).

These changes have been noted clinically with temporary *softening* and increases of test excursion in exercised joints. There is also a return to normal stiffness and apparent length after a short recovery period. The ultimate strength of bone-ligament-bone complexes may also be decreased during such repeated cycling and may thus relatively predispose such joints to failure during ongoing exercise.[111]

A similarly interesting phenomenon is the temperature sensitivity of ligament tissue. It has been shown that peak stresses are influenced by ambient temperature, which is a finding of considerable significance with respect to in vitro testing and of some clinical importance[63] (Fig. 11-11).

Although peripheral joints are probably maintained near the core temperature

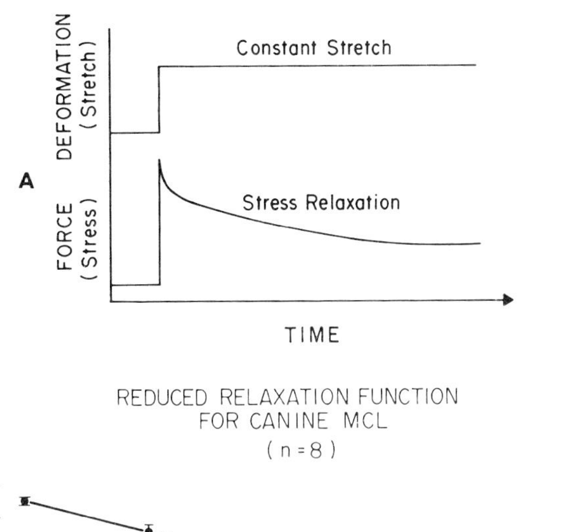

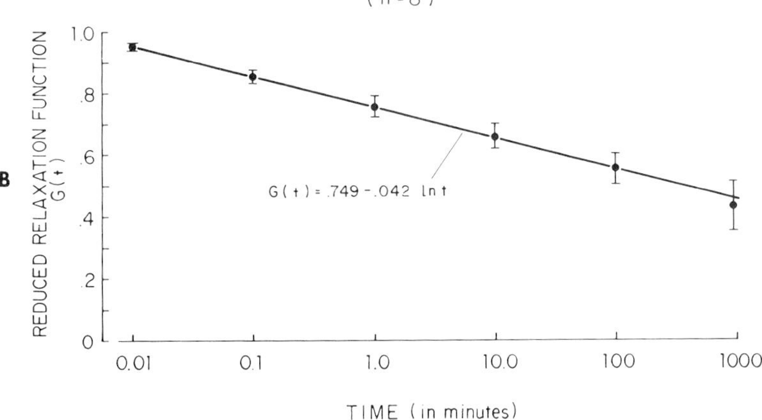

Fig. 11-7. A, and **B,** Stress relaxation (decreasing stress with time under constant deformation) in schematic form with typical stress relaxation curve for medial collateral ligament. (From Woo, S. L.-Y., and others: J. Biomech. Eng. **103**:293, 1981.)

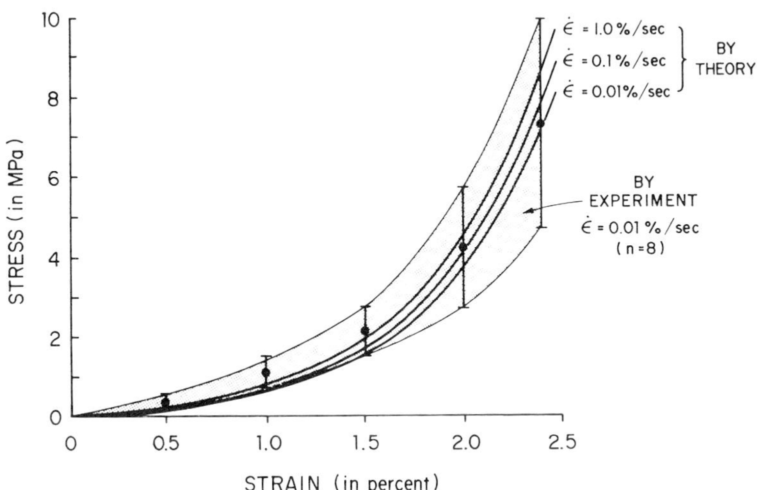

Fig. 11-8. The stress-strain curves of medial collateral ligament at various strain rates are calculated by quasi-linear viscoelastic theory and found to be in range of stress-strain curves obtained by experiment. (From Woo, S. L.-Y., and others: J. Biomech. Eng. **103**:293, 1981.)

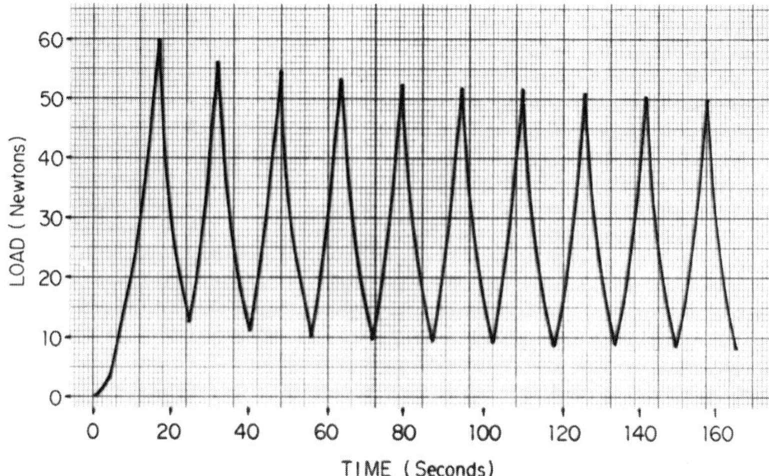

Fig. 11-9. Cyclic loading of medial collateral ligament with strains between 1.6% and 2.4% and strain rate of 0.1%/sec. Note decreasing peak loads as cyclic softening occurs. (From Woo, S. L.-Y.: Biorheology **19**:385, 1982.)

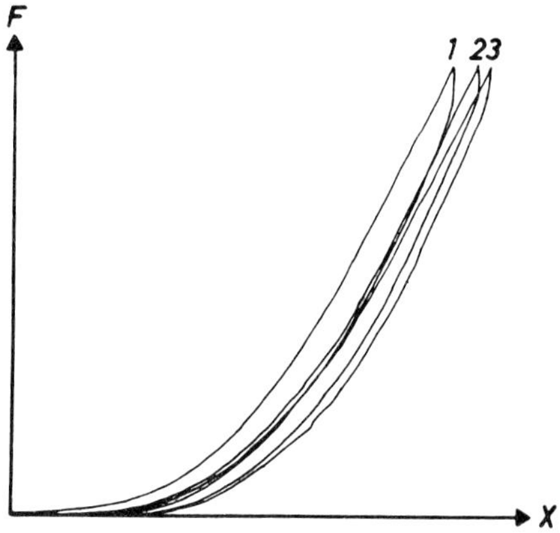

Fig. 11-10. Schematic load deformation diagrams of three successive cycles of loading and unloading of same specimen showing viscoelastic creep effect of ligament. (From Viidik, A.: J. Biomech. **1**:3, 1968.)

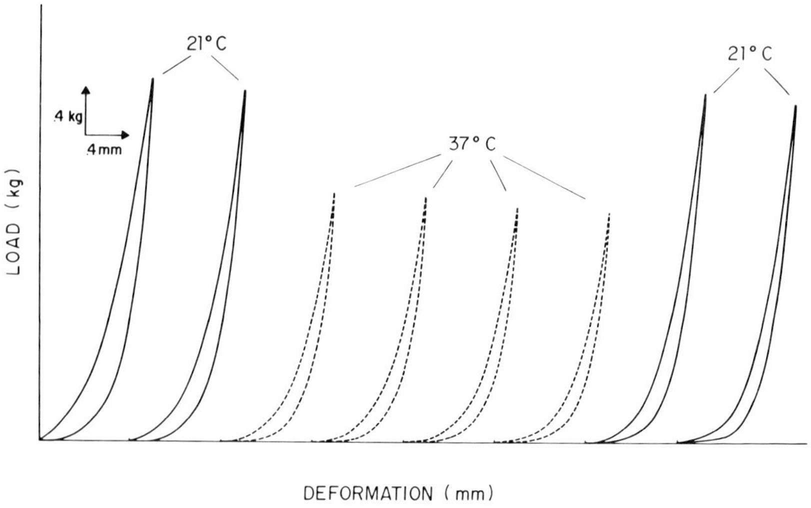

Fig. 11-11. Loading of single bone-ligament-bone preparation under different temperature conditions (allowing recovery time between each test) demonstrates decreased peak stress at 37° C as compared with 21° C.

of 37° C under normal circumstances, many alterations in their temperature can occur. Superficial wrapping, heat, or ice, for example, may significantly alter the joint temperature and the mechanical characteristics of the ligaments. Similarly, in any number of pathologic conditions such as trauma, infection, or inflammation, joint temperatures can be considerably altered[54] and perhaps secondarily affect joint ligament biomechanics.

Of major clinical interest are the failure properties of ligament tissue. When elongation limits are exceeded a characteristic failure pattern occurs. The typical force elongation to failure diagram for ligaments can be arbitrarily divided into four major parts[40,73]: (1) toe region (crimp straightening), (2) linear midportion (fiber resistance), (3) early failure region (microscopic disruption), and (4) complete failure region (macroscopic disruption). This possibility of microscopic failure or partial injury poses difficult clinical problems of diagnosis and treatment.[60]

A considerable amount of work has been done on the definition of the biomechanical limits of various ligaments, particularly those in and around the knee. The strain rate (the speed at which deformation occurs) has been implicated as a determinant of the failure pattern in certain ligamentous injuries.[33]

Experimentally, however, when medial collateral ligament substance was subjected to tensile tests through several decades of strain rates, it was noted that only slight variations in the stress-strain characteristics occurred[114] (Fig. 11-12). With increasing rates there are slight increases in stiffness and peak failure loads of the ligament substance. This is probably an adaptive feature in resisting sudden or abnormal movements.

Peri-insertional bone, however, demonstrates considerable viscoelastic stiffening with increasing loading rates and becomes extremely strong under fast loading conditions. Ligaments therefore are often the *weak link* of the bone ligament-bone complex under rapid loading conditions and become the most predictable site of failure (Fig. 11-13).

A spectrum of bone-ligament-bone failure modes from rapid conditions (with predominant ligament tearing and combined failures) to the alternative slower loading conditions (predisposed to a higher percentage of bony avulsion failures) has been produced experimentally.[33,60] Although a similar spectrum may be operative clinically, the loading rates involved are difficult to define, and the analysis of failure modes is therefore less clear-cut. As a further complication, recent work has indicated that strain distribution may not be symmetrical throughout the ligament.[119] Large and nonuniform deformations appear to occur near insertional areas and may therefore predispose them to an increased frequency of failure under proper conditions. This asymmetry has also been important for the explanation of experimental variability in reported strain analyses of prefailure test specimens.

Finally it should be emphasized that many of the mechanical properties of ligaments previously mentioned probably depend on a number of variables including sex,[99] body weight (Fig. 11-14), age*, and local conditions including drug adminis-

---

*References 8, 21, 33, 98, 104, 108.

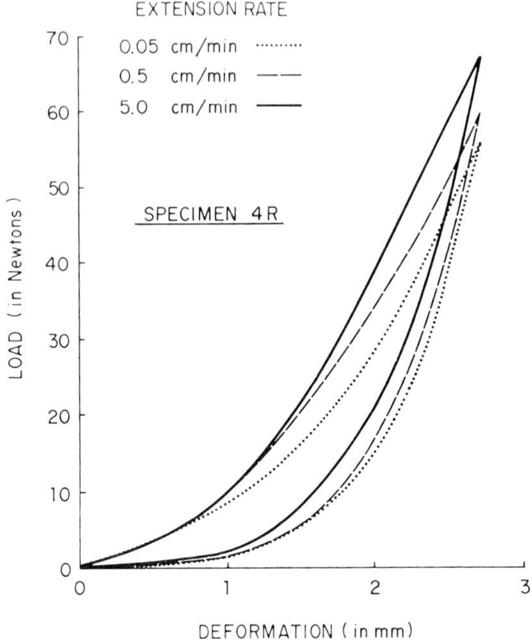

Fig. 11-12. Hysteresis loop of canine medial collateral ligament subjected to tensile tests through three decades of stretch rates, demonstrating minimal strain rate sensitivity of ligament substance. (From Woo, S. L.-Y., and others: J. Biomech. Eng. **103**:293, 1981.)

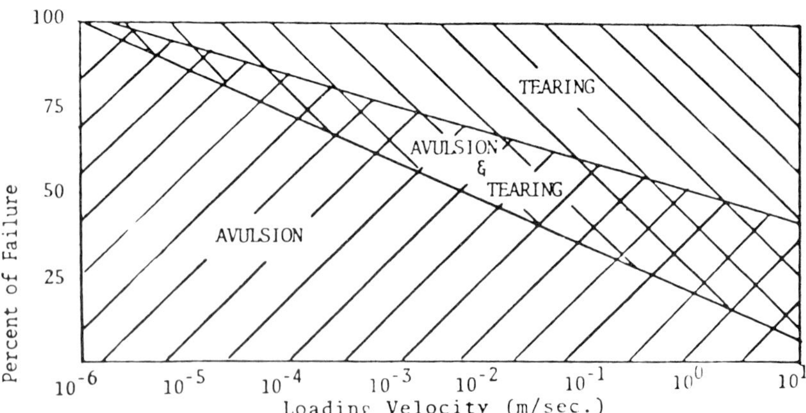

Fig. 11-13. Experimental results of probability of failure mode of bone-ligament-bone complex according to loading velocity. (From Crowninshield, R.D., and Pope, M.P.: J. Trauma **16**:99, 1976.)

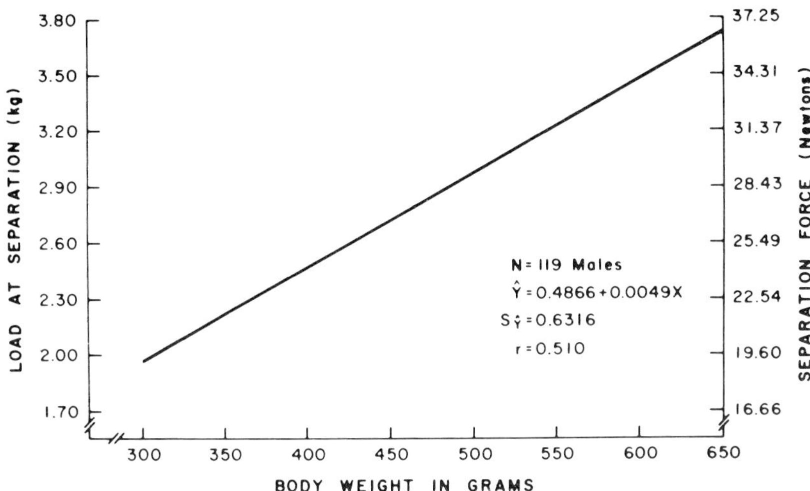

Fig. 11-14. Importance of body weight in determining separation force of bone-ligament-bone preparations. (From Tipton, C.M., and others: Med. Sci. Sports Exerc. 7[3]:165, 1975.)

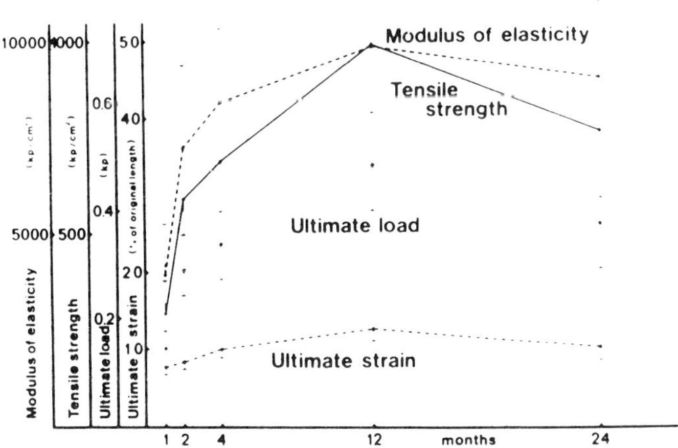

Fig. 11-15. Age dependence of mechanical parameters of rat tail tendons showing peak values near maturity. (From Vogel, H.G.: Connect. Tissue Res. 6:161, 1978.)

tration.[75] Peak properties of stiffness and ultimate failure strength of the dense connective tissues occur when maturity of the individual[109] is attained (Fig. 11-15). Strength and other ligament properties are, however, almost equal bilaterally in the same individual. This is a significant convenience in clinical comparative testing and design of animal experiments.[73,97,101]

BIOCHEMISTRY

Ligaments consist of functional complexes of interdependent aggregations of collagen, elastin, glycoproteins, protein polysaccharides, glycolipids, water, and cells. Ligaments share these constituent characteristics with other fibrous connective tissues. The nature of the constituents is complex, and our understanding of their chemistry and interaction continues to evolve. For practical purposes the physical behavior of ligaments can be predicted on the basis of content and organization of collagen and ground substance (water and proteoglycans), since other components are present in relatively minute quantities. Detailed reviews of collagen chemistry[45,53,72,87,105], proteoglycan chemistry[47,55,70,89], and their interaction[14,19,27,29,35] are available for more complete discussions of structure and function. A detailed discussion would be too lengthy, but an overview of the major constituents will provide useful background for understanding subsequent discussions of stress effects and ligament healing.

Collagen

Roughly 70% to 80% of normal ligament is composed of collagen by dry weight. The collagen is mainly Type I (also found in tendon, skin, and bone) and is the principal tensile resistant substance present. Type I collagen has an amino acid profile[85] and can be cleaved into characteristic, recognizable peptide units by various agents.[22] Hydroxyproline, an imino acid, has been useful as an index of collagen content as a result of the relatively consistent proportion in the molecule.[50,94] The collagen in ligament is thought to remain relatively inert metabolically with a half-life of 300 to 500 days[71] (a turnover rate even slower than that of bone collagen). Certain components of the collagen molecule, however, may turn over faster than others[49] and may therefore be of greater functional importance in adaptations to environmental, traumatic, or pathologic processes.

The collagen of ligaments obtains its structural stability from its unique molecular coil configuration and the quarter staggered packing of tropocollagen units.[84] It also has the ability to form covalent intramolecular and intermolecular cross-links.* The functional importance of glycosylation of hydroxylysine residues is uncertain, but various effects have been postulated, including aiding in stability, regulation of synthesis, control of fiber diameter, and effects on collagen-proteoglycan interaction.

However, since the cross-links are key to tensile strength characteristics and resistance to chemical or enzymatic breakdown, they deserve greater emphasis. Absence of these cross-links causes the collagen fibers to be extremely weak and

---

*References 16, 17, 44, 67, 82, 95, 105.

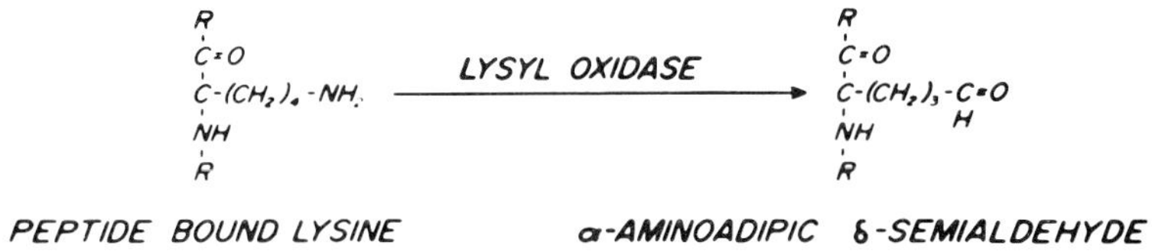

Fig. 11-16. Oxidative deamination of peptide-bound lysine by enzyme lysyl oxidase generates aldehydes associated with collagen molecule.

friable. Chemical studies of purified collagens showed the presence of aldehyde groups in these polypeptides. These aldehydes are derived from an enzymatic modification of the amino acids lysine and hydroxylysine. An enzyme, lysyloxidase, has been isolated from connective tissues, which is known to convert specific lysine and hydroxylysine residues in collagen and elastin into peptide-bound aldehydes. The reaction involves an oxidative deamination of the ϵ amino carbon yielding the corresponding δ-semialdehyde (Fig. 11-16).

The aldehydes found on collagen are the precursors of both the intramolecular and intermolecular cross-links in collagen. Intramolecular cross-links of the aldol type seem to be restricted to the N-terminal region of the collagen molecules in which they occur. In collagen from ligament there is a good correlation between the amount of β components seen after denaturation and the concentration of α-β unsaturated aldol.

The reactions leading to the formation of the intramolecular (aldol) and intermolecular cross-links (Schiff base) are shown in Fig. 11-17 and 11-18. In addition to lysinonorleucine, a compound first identified in elastin, other important Schiff bases in ligaments are hydroxylysinonorleucine (HLNL), which results from the association of a lysine-derived aldehyde with hydroxylysine residue, and dihydroxylysinonorleucine (DHLNL), which originates from a hydroxylysine-derived aldehyde and an unmodified hydroxylysine residue (Fig. 11-19). Although these cross-links containing hydroxylysine are the most prevalent intermolecular cross-links in native insoluble collagen, other more complex combinations also exist, including hydroxymerodesmosine (HMD) and histidinohydroxymerodesmosine (HHMD) (Fig. 11-20). These hydroxylysine-derived cross-links have resonating forms with the initial imminium forming on enamine, which can tautomerize to the more stable ketoimine (Fig. 11-21).

A significant difference is that tendons ahave been shown to contain relatively large amounts of the intermolecular cross-links of HLNL and HHMD, while ligaments contain mainly DHLNL and lesser amounts of both HLNL and HHMD.[11] The significance of these differences is not known.

Ground substance

On a dry weight basis, the ground substance constituents of ligaments comprise less than 1% of the total tissue. Water, however, comprises 60% to 80% of the total wet weight, and a significant part of that water is associated with the ground substance. The water and proteoglycan probably provide lubrication and spacing that

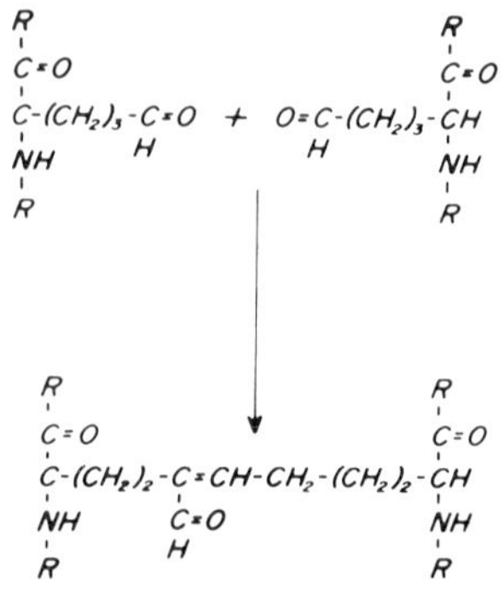

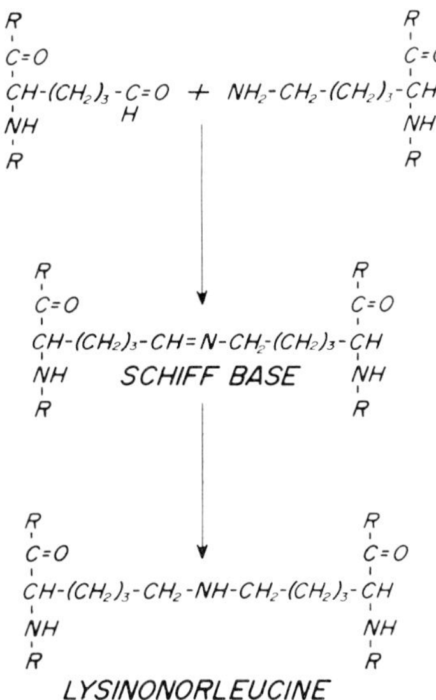

Fig. 11-17. Aldol condensation reaction involving lysine-derived aldehydes located near N terminal of molecule. This aldol condensation is responsible for formation of intramolecular cross-link.

Fig. 11-18. Schiff base reaction occurring between lysine-derived aldehyde and unmodified amino group, responsible for intermolecular cross-link formation involving either lysine or hydroxylysine.

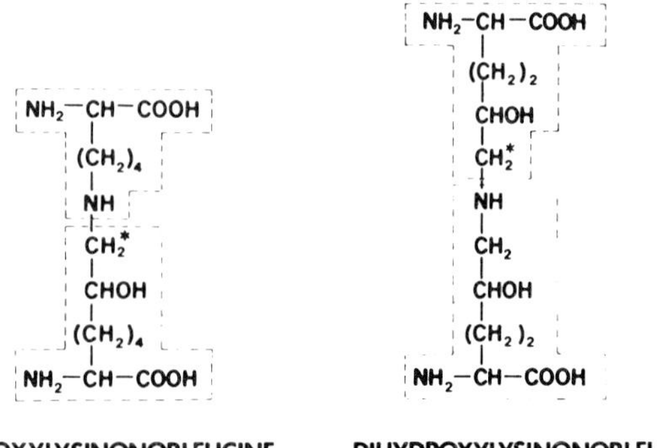

Fig. 11-19. Structures of most abundant cross-links in ligament after reduction with $NaBH_4$. Asterisks indicate sites of tritium labeling with radioactive isotope reduction. Basic amino acid skeletons contributing to cross-links are enclosed by dotted lines.

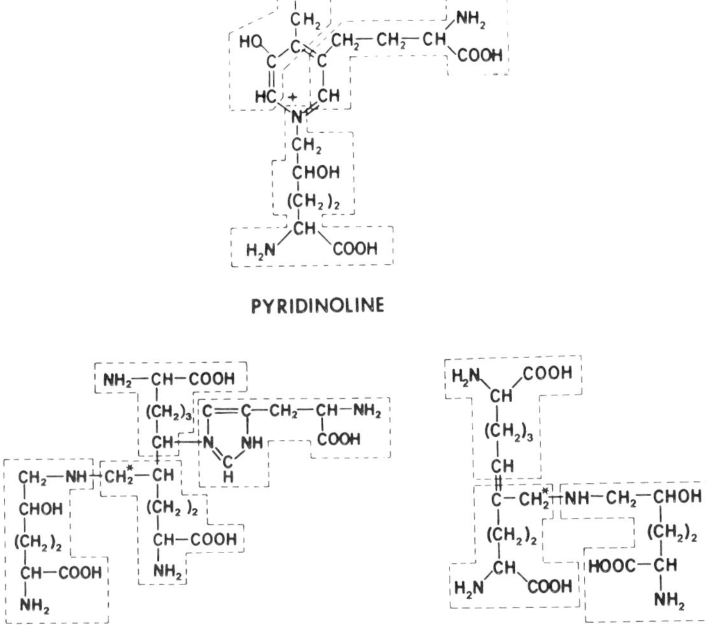

Fig. 11-20. Cross-links found in various proportions in collagen from different tissues. Individual amino acids (mostly lysine and lysine-derived aldehydes and histidine) are identified in dotted areas.

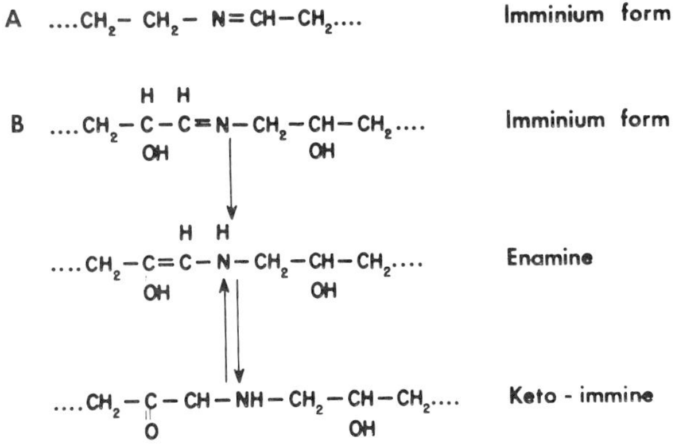

Fig. 11-21. Two types of cross-links are illustrated. **A,** Cross-link between lysine from one collagen polypeptide and lysine-derived aldehyde from another. Schiff base formed is in imminium configuration, and double bond is susceptible to cleavage by acids. **B,** Cross-link formed between hydroxylysine derived from one molecule and hydroxylysine-derived aldehyde from another molecule. This cross-link is prevalent in bone and in collagens rich in hydroxylysine. Initial imminium form contains hydroxy group conjugated with $N = C$ bond. This can form enamine, which readily tautomerizes to ketoimine.

are crucial to the gliding function at intercept points where fibers cross in the tissue matrices. As noted previously, gliding is an essential physical property of ligaments and other periarticular connective tissues. The water and proteoglycans also confer viscoelastic properties to ligaments. The movement of water in the system is inhibited by its entrapment between the large, highly charged molecules of proteoglycans. At high strain rates therefore the water cannot displace completely in the brief time of force application, resulting in strain properties that are different from those at slow rates. In the latter case water displacement is greater, because force is applied more slowly therefore allowing greater ligament strain.

Proteoglycans are relatively uniform chemically in the different periarticular connective tissues. The proteoglycan subunit consists of a core protein with protein-linked glycosaminoglycan side chains. Hyaluronic acid, chondroitin-4 sulfate, and chondroitin-6 sulfate, and dermatan sulfate represent the majority of the glycosaminoglycans (GAGs) present. Except for hyaluronic acid, the GAGs are covalently linked to proteins to create aggregate molecules of massive molecular weight. They are highly negatively charged and possess a large number of hydroxyl groups. These fixed charges confer predictable properties on the connective tissue through physical-chemical properties, as previously mentioned. Hydroxyl groups attract water through hydrogen binding and contribute important features to the collagen fiber–ground substance interaction.

RELATIONSHIP OF STRUCTURE AND FUNCTION

Ligaments are well-suited structurally, mechanically, and biomechanically to the physiologic functions they perform.

Recruitment of collagen fibers from their resting state (crimp) can provide increasing joint stability in anatomically determined positions of bony congruence as motion and joint displacement occur. Neural feedback mechanisms protect static stabilizers by adding dynamic control and prevent displacement that would exceed their mechanical limits. Multiple ligaments serve a single joint, providing a mechanism for the maintenance of static protection through wide ranges of movement where dynamic stabilization may be inadequate.

Since ligaments are predominantly (but not entirely) a backup mechanism of joint stabilization to the dynamic mode, they must be able to respond quickly when primary systems fail. Histologic laxity is minimal, and the parallel fiber arrangement allows for early tensile resistance once the crimp pattern is straightened. Their viscoelastic nature, which is a combination of component properties and interactions, is similarly adapted to resisting sudden loads. The chemical structure and inter-molecular cross-linking of the collagen, its interaction with the ground substance, and the water-binding capacity of the protein polysaccharides and collagen are all mechanically significant characteristics. Collectively they serve to maintain fiber orientation and distance in an organized meshwork for optimal load distribution and response. As fast loading rates cause increases in ultimate failure and ligament stiffness, joints are maximally protected during rapid movements. Ligaments, however, are still the *weak link* of the bone-ligament-bone apparatus in extremely fast loading situations. At slow loading rates when dynamic supports are less likely to be exceeded, the ligaments are relatively extensible and allow minimal mechanical impediment to normal ranges of motion.

Ligament insertions are functionally adapted to force dissipation by passing through fibrocartilage to bone and are less susceptible to disruption in the transition area than the extremes on either side (bone or peri-insertional ligament substance). Through a careful history of load and loading rate the mechanism and site of failure (bone versus ligament) should be more predictable. Fast loading should produce midsubstance injury if physiologic limits are broken. Slower loading should produce avulsion injury. As with all dynamic physiologic systems there are functional adaptations to age, temperature, and sex, even though collagen turnover in ligaments may be slow. Extrapolations from animal work suggest that maximal tensile resistance of ligaments is reached at skeletal maturity, which is the time of maximum probable need. Epiphyseal plate closure (the weak link in the skeletally immature) and peak physical activity potential at maturity coincide with this event. The mechanism of adaptation may well involve changes in content and organization of ligament substance secondary to any number of extraligamentous parameters (e.g., growth, sex, hormones, or activity).

The fact that ligaments are in fact dynamic structures requires particular emphasis. Both stress and stress deprivation have been shown to have considerable impact on the structure-function relationship and will be considered in the following section. This in turn will form the background for a discussion of ligament healing with and without stress application.

STRESS AND MOTION EFFECTS ON LIGAMENT

Every change in the form and function of a bone, or of its function alone is followed by certain definite changes in its internal architecture and equally definite secondary alterations in its mathematical laws.[113]

It is our view that *Wolff's law* should not be restricted to bone but should be extended to include a more generalized statement of connective tissue adaptation to applied stresses. Wilhelm Roux,[91] a German anatomist and embryologist, may have recognized this deficiency when he published his "law of functional adaptation" stating that "an organ will adapt itself structurally to an alteration, quantitative or qualitative, of function". Unfortunately, his work did not receive widespread recognition in orthopaedic literature. Wolff and Roux would probably not be surprised to learn that ligaments are morphologically, biomechanically, and biochemically sensitive to both stress enhancement and stress deprivation. This sensitivity appears to fall in a spectrum spanning stress-deprived (immobilized) through normal (arbitrarily defined as activities of daily living) to stress-enhanced (exercised) conditions.

Stress deprivation (immobilization)

Morphology. The effects of stress deprivation on synovial joints are profound. Intraarticular changes include time-dependent proliferation of fibro-fatty synovial connective tissue in a manner reminiscent of pannus to the point of obliterating the joint space. If the process is allowed to continue for many months,[92,96] cartilage necrosis is seen from pressure effects in contact areas,[92,106] breech of the subchondral plate takes place by ingrowth of mesenchymal marrow tissue,[36,37] cartilage erosion and ulceration happen in noncontact areas,[37] and adhesions occur with tears of articular cartilage at the point of adhesion attachment.[36,37,51]

Intraarticular and extraarticular ligaments and periarticular connective tissues are also profoundly affected by immobilization. Gross inspection reveals them to be less glistening in gross appearance and more *woody* on palpation or dissection. Histologically there is a pattern of increased randomness of fibers and cells compared with longitudinal sections of controls stained with hematoxylin and eosin. Partial loss of parallelism of collagen fibers in cruciate ligaments has been observed in an animal model after 9 weeks of immobilization[4] (Fig. 11-22) with distortion of the pattern of cellular alignment and presentation of more random matrix organization. Others

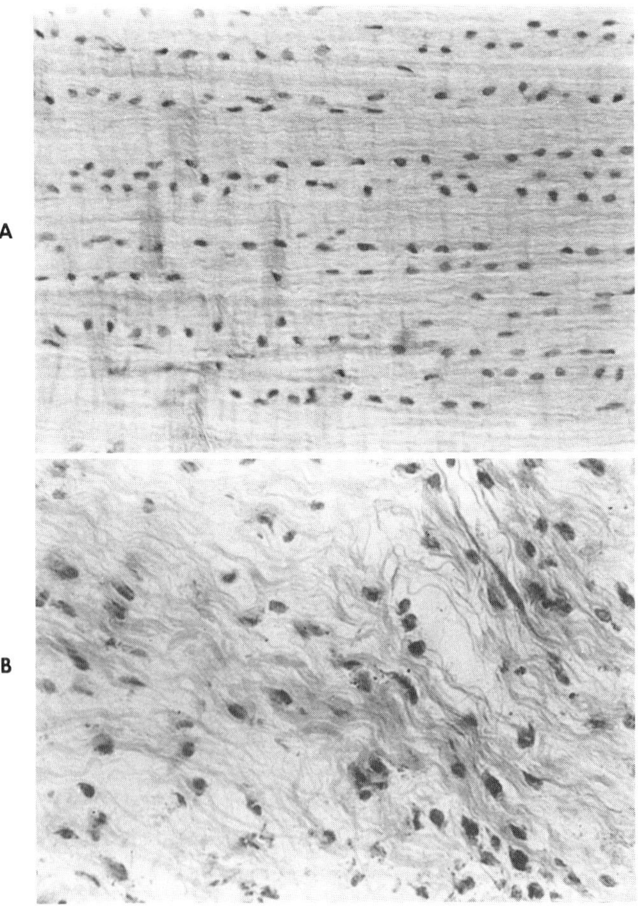

Fig. 11-22. A, Anterior cruciate ligament from cage activity rabbit knee ($\times$310). **B,** Anterior cruciate ligament from 9-week immobilized rabbit knee showing matrix disorganization ($\times$310). (From Akeson, W.H., and others: Biorheology **17**:95, 1980.)

reported that *intercellular collagen fiber bundles* may be decreased in thickness and number secondary to immobilization[97] (i.e., atrophy of collagen).

Electron microscopy has confirmed increased cellularity in capsular structures that are stress deprived.[9] This increased population of cells contains increased cytoplasm and prominent secretory endoplasmic reticulum, which are consistent with an increased metabolic state (Fig. 11-23). A metamorphosis of these proliferative cells to *myofibroblasts*[43] (active in the contractile function of granulation tissue) is, however, apparently not a factor in this hypermetabolic contracture process of joints.

Biomechanics. Increased knee joint stiffness after immobilization has been demonstrated using an *arthrograph*[116] (Fig. 11-24). This apparatus measures the severity of contracture formation in the form of a torque–angular deformation diagram. The amount of torque required to initially extend the knee to a specific joint angle and the area of hysteresis (measuring the energy requirements) during cycling are quantitative indexes[79] (Fig. 11-25) that have been used.

Increases in knee joint stiffness demonstrated by this method have been attributed to a number of changes already described in the joint tissues (adhesions, pannus, and decreased lubricity) and probably include restricted extensibility of loose periarticular collagen weave by fixed contact at strategic sites (Fig. 11-26). Newly produced random collagen formation is hypothesized to form these interfibrillar contacts and would be expected to restrict normal fiber sliding and motion in extensible

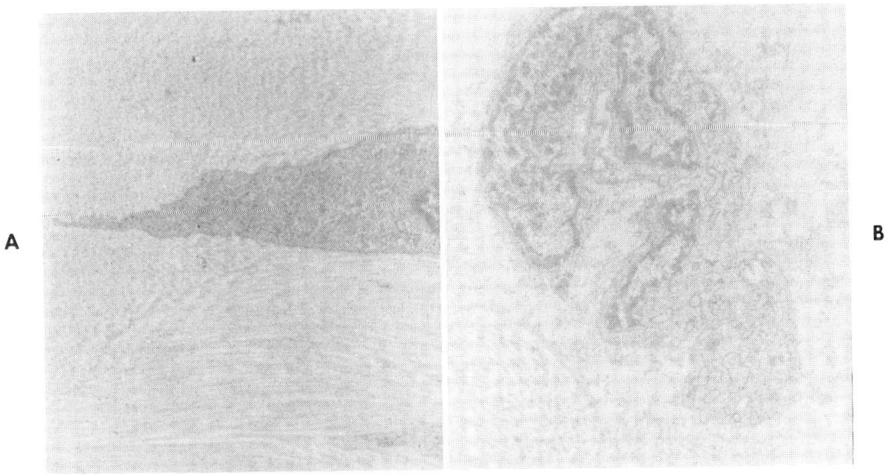

Fig. 11-23. A, Electron micrograph of fibroblast from posterior capsule of cage activity rabbit knee. Nucleus of this cell is relatively inactive, showing smooth margins and minimal secretory apparatus. **B,** Electron micrograph of fibroblast from posterior capsule of rabbit knee joint that has been immobilized, showing invagination of nucleus and considerably increased rough endoplasmic reticulum and Golgi apparatus (metabolically active). (From Amiel, D., and others: A biochemical and morphological comparison of connective tissue from Dupuytren's palmar fasciitis and immobilized joint contracture. In American Academy of Orthopaedic Surgeons: Symposium on heritable disorders of connective tissue, St. Louis, 1982, The C.V. Mosby Co.)

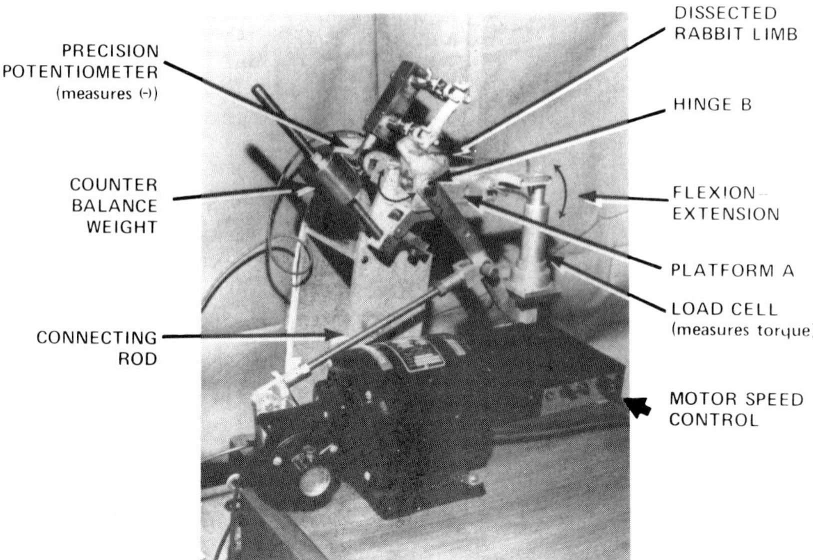

Fig. 11-24. Previously described arthrograph system for measurement of joint stiffness. (From Woo, S. L.-Y., and others: Arthritis Rheum. **18:**257, 1975.)

structures such as capsule of the shoulder or posterior aspect of the knee (Fig. 11-27).

Ligament substance, however, is uniquely affected by immobility. Rather than becoming relatively more stiff in tension, as may be postulated from increased joint stiffness (contracture), ligaments become less stiff after several weeks of stress deprivation,[73,120] with the ultimate load, linear stiffness, and energy-absorbing capacity of a bone–medial collateral ligament–bone preparation being reduced to about one third of normal[12] (Fig. 11-28).

To differentiate between whether such quantitative reductions are a result of cross-sectional atrophy[98] or alteration in tissue mechanical properties, a specialized video dimensional analyzer system was used to obtain a stress-strain relationship of normal and immobilized lateral collateral ligaments (Fig. 11-29). The diminished slope of the stress-strain curve seen in the immobilized ligaments suggests some compromise in the mechanical properties of the ligament substance. Despite the possibility of intercept point-binding (stiffening) in more randomly distributed and newly produced collagen, qualitative softening of the ligament substance predominates (Fig. 11-30).

In addition to these changes in ligament substance compliance, immobilization significantly decreases the strength of the bone-ligament-bone apparatus.* This decrease in strength is a result of change in ligament substance itself and in its bony insertion sites. After 8 weeks of immobilization in the primate, for example, Noyes[73,76]

---

*References 73, 76, 98, 100-103, 116, 120.

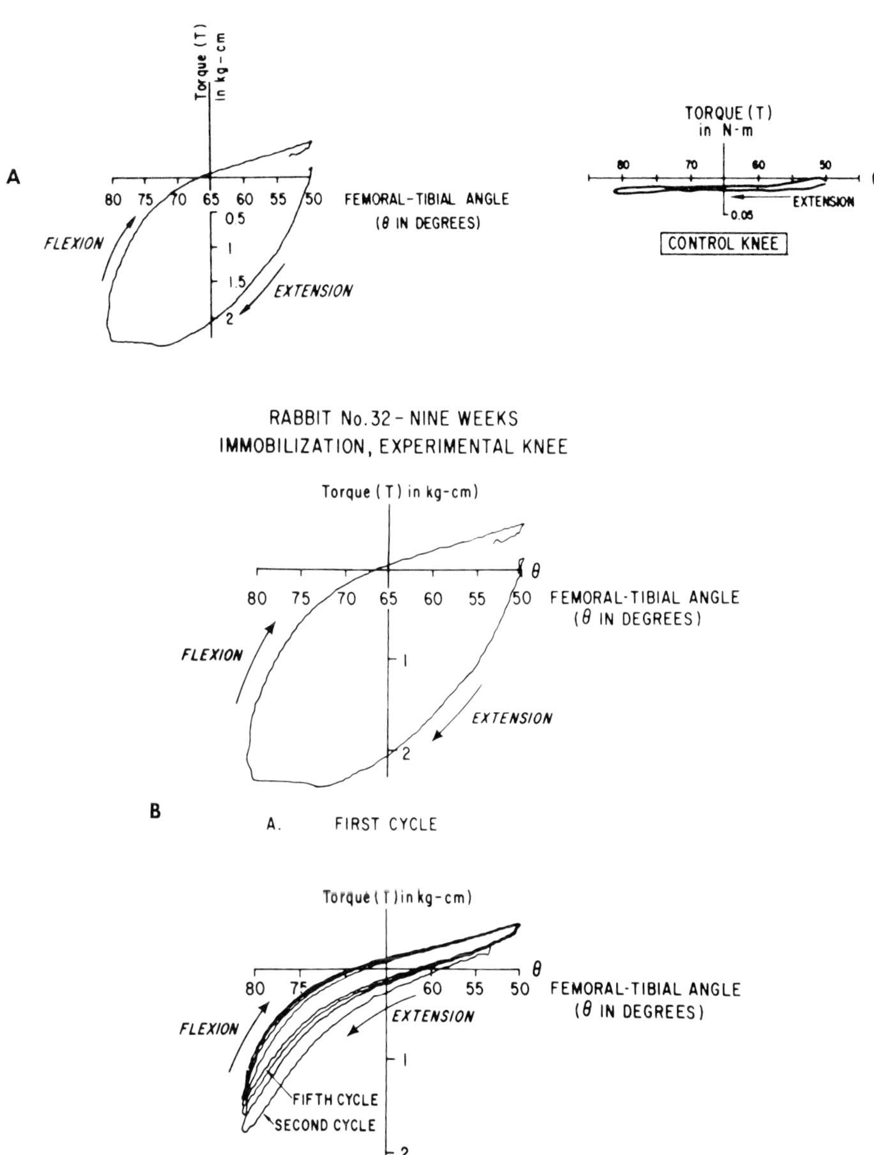

Fig. 11-25. A, Diagram comparing typical torque-angular deformation diagram of first cycle of extension-flexion of rabbit knees with 9 weeks of immobilization *(left)* versus contralateral nonimmobilized control *(right).* The area of each test represents energy required to bend joint (immobilized joint showing contracture formation). **B,** Recording on x = and y = axes of torque-angular deformation diagram of experimental contracture rabbit knee showing differences between first and successive cycles (energy of bending decreases successively). (From Woo, S. L.-Y., and others: Arthritis Rheum. **18**[3]:257, 1975.)

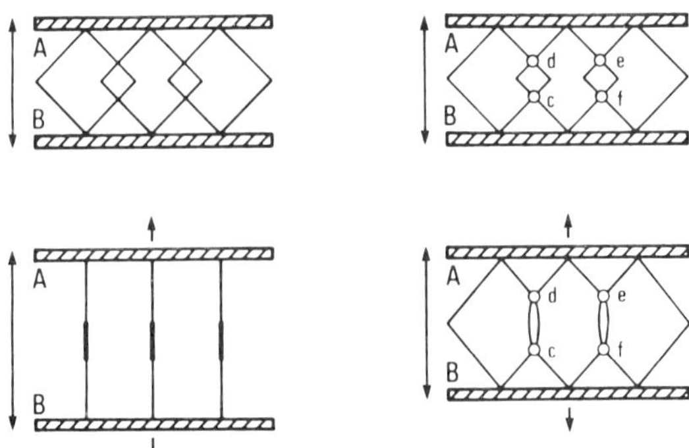

Fig. 11-26. Schematic representation of idealized collagen weave. Fixed contact at strategic points (e.g., *d* and *e*) can severely restrict extension of this collagen weave. (From Woo, S. L.-Y., and others: Arthritis Rheum. 18[3]:257, 1975.)

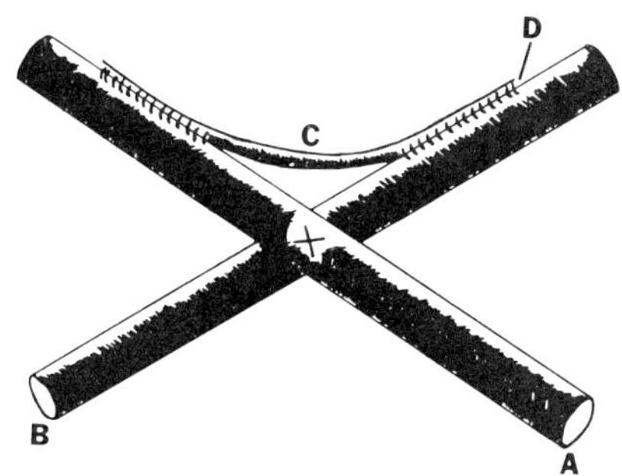

Fig. 11-27. Possible mechanism of intercept binding of two crossing collagen fibrils (*A* and *B*) by newly synthesized fibril *C*, which is cross-linked at contact points *D*. (From Akeson, W.H., and others: Biorheology 17:95, 1980.)

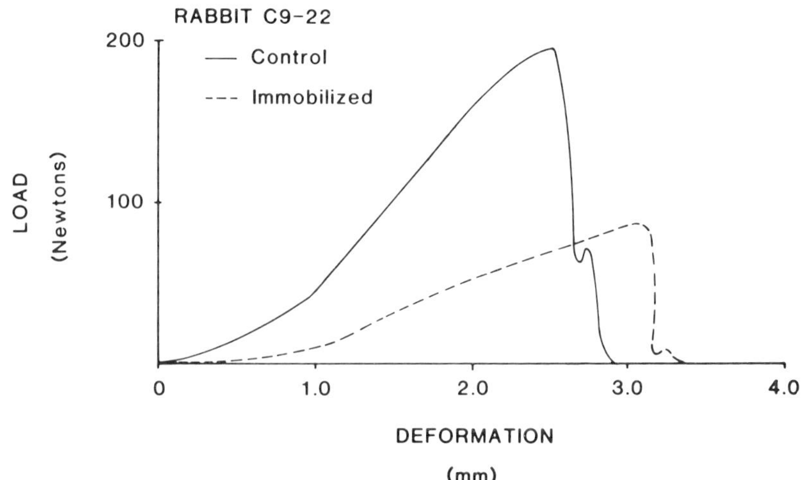

Fig. 11-28. Typical load-deformation curves of lateral collateral ligaments of normal and immobilized knees of same rabbit. (From Amiel, D., and others: Acta Orthop. Scand. 53:325, 1982.)

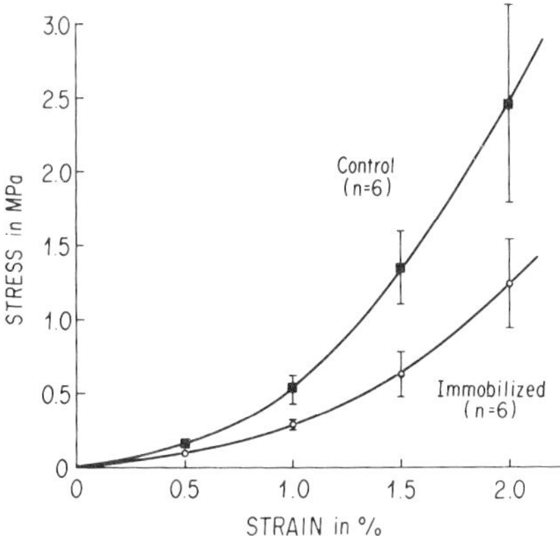

Fig. 11-29. Stress-strain relationship of normal and immobilized rabbit lateral-collateral ligaments. (From Amiel, D., and others: Acta Orthop. Scand. **53:**325, 1982.)

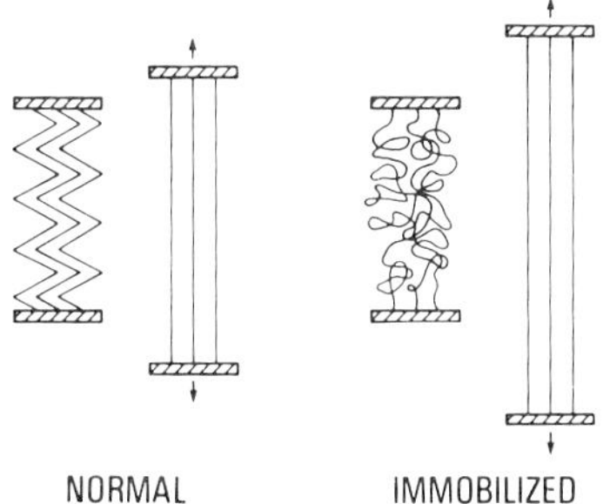

Fig. 11-30. Schematic representation of qualitative changes in ligament weave that allow increased extensibility despite intercept binding.

demonstrated a 39% decrease in maximum failure load of the anterior cruciate ligament complex and attributed a portion of these losses to insertional cortical atrophy with resulting avulsion. Laros and Tipton[64] documented osteoclastic periosteal resorption around ligament insertion sites and noted that it was anatomically specific (more tibiofibular insertions than femoral). They speculated that periosteal proximity to insertion sites may partially determine the site specificity of resorption around the ligaments. (The broad tibial insertion of the collateral ligaments is contiguous with periosteum but the femoral is not.) They also showed that even partial immobilization (restricted activity) had similar deleterious effects on insertion sites, which raised serious doubt about the validity of using cage activity *controls* in animal model testing.

Biochemistry. There are a number of significant biochemical changes in periarticular connective tissue as a consequence of stress deprivation. These include decreased water content,[102,103] decreased total glycosaminoglycans,[2,5] increased collagen turnover,[3,23,83] and parallel increases in certain types of collagen cross-linking associated with increased synthesis.[3,10]

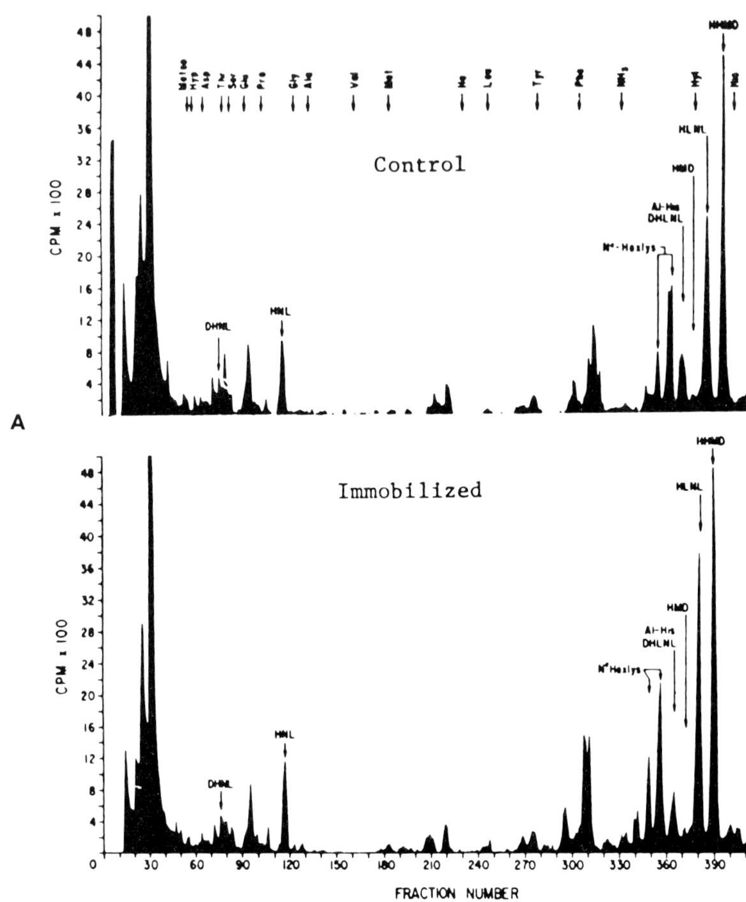

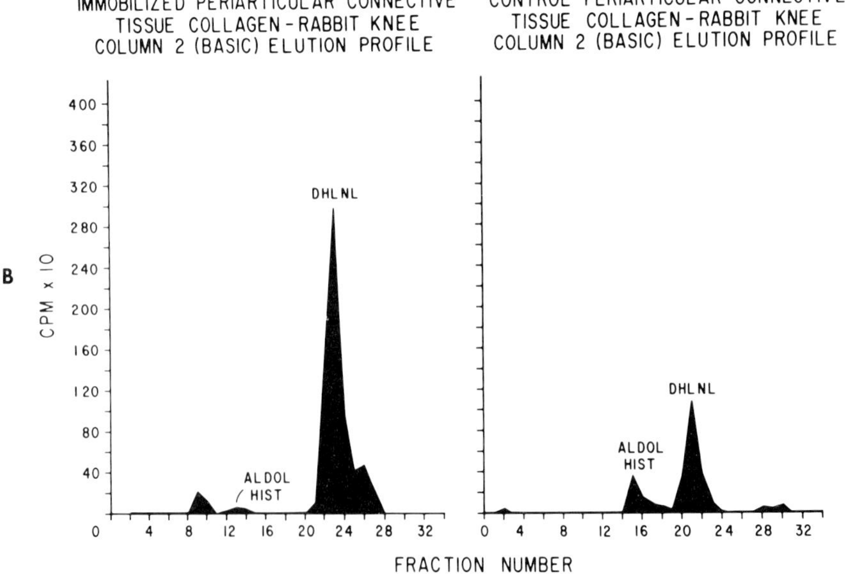

Fig. 11-31. For legend see opposite page.

Fig. 11-31. A, Radioactive elution profile of a 3N *p*-toluene sulfonic acid hydrolysate of [³H]NaBH₄ reduced collagen from control and immobilized periarticular connective tissue from rabbit knee. Abbreviations for radioactive compounds are *DHNL*, dihydroxynorleucine; *HNL*, hydroxynorleucine; *Nᵋ-hexolys*, Nᵋ-hexosyllsine; *Al-His*, aldol-histidine; *DHLNL*, dihydroxylysinonorleucine; *HMD*, hydroxymerodesmosine; *HLNL*, hydroxylsinonorleucine; *HHMD*, histidinohydroxymerodesmosine. **B,** Elution profiles of aldol-histidine-dihydroxylysinonorleucine peak from control and immobilized periarticular connective tissue collagen rechromatographed on extended basic column. (From Akeson, W.H., and others: Connect. Tissue Res. **5**:15, 1977.)

Table 11-1. Mean values in changes in reducible cross-links in normal and immobilized periarticular connective tissue from 8 rabbit knees*

Reduced cross-links	E − C/C × 100 (%)	Paired T-test
HLNL	+49	$p < .005$
DHLNL	+116	$p < .005$
HHMD	+29	$p < .05$

From Akeson, W.H., and others: Connect. Tissue Res. **5**:15, 1977.
*Changes expressed as percent change from control.

There is only a small alteration in the total collagen content and no change in the collagen type present in the immobilized tissues.[10,61,98] A qualitative change of collagen is indicated, however, by the dramatic alteration in collagen cross-links, which is consistent with the reduced stiffness observed mechanically. These cross-link changes include significant increases in the reducible intermolecular cross-links DHLNL, HLNL and HHMD[3] (Fig. 11-31 and Table 11-1).

Long-term labeling studies have addressed the question of collagen metabolism in stress-deprived connective tissues more specifically in order to resolve previous debates on the subject.[12,56,61,62] It now appears that immobility causes significantly increased metabolic turnover of collagen with increased synthesis and degradation.[12] Slightly more degradation combined with losses of water and glycosaminoglycans probably contribute to the decrease in weight-length ratios of the ligaments and to a net decrease in mass.[12,102] These changes may well be specific to ligaments, and it has been suggested that cruciate ligaments are particularly susceptible to these changes.

Duration of immobilization is a significant factor in the magnitude of some of these changes. For example, one model has shown no change in ground substance at 6 weeks[97] whereas significant decreases were noted at 9 weeks in another.[2,5] This may also be a reflection of species variation in response, position of the limb, or rigidity of fixation. It appears that at least 12 weeks of immobility is necessary before the just noted reduction in ligament mass is detectable.[12] Metabolic changes and cross-link alterations probably occur relatively early, but require time to become detectable with available techniques.

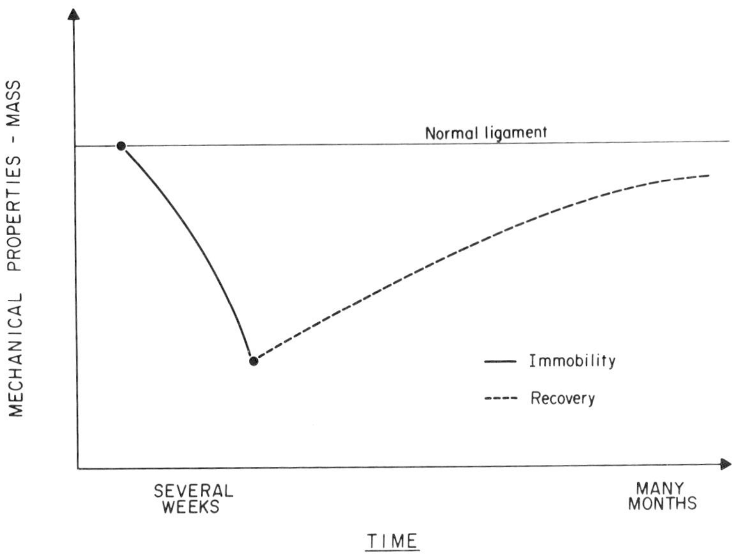

Fig. 11-32. Schematic representation of early degradation in properties of immobilized ligament complex, requiring many months of recovery toward normal values.

Recovery. It is also important to note that recovery of these mechanical alterations after immobilization is a slow process. It may take more than 5 months to regain normal compliance and more than 1 year for a ligament complex to regain normal tensile strength after being immobilized for only 8 weeks.[76] Insertion site recovery may be the slowest consistent with the long-term processes of bone metabolism (Fig. 11-32). More detailed experimental data are required on the recovery process, since the concept has obvious implications in rehabilitation programs and should be placed on a firm scientific foundation.

Discussion and summary. Diarthrodial joints are profoundly affected by stress deprivation. Although there is variation in tissue response, all tissues of the joint are affected. The ligament complex (bone-ligament-bone) undergoes morphologic, biomechanical, and biochemical changes. Recovery from these changes is slow and presumably dependent on a number of factors other than reinstitution of exercise. These factors include species, age, sex, specific ligament hormones, and periosteal proximity. Stress deprivation causes both qualitative and quantitative alterations in ligament substance that appears to progress exponentially through the first 12 weeks of immobility, resulting in rapid and severe deterioration in mechanical properties. Recovery from some of these effects is linear rather than mirroring the geometric onset. Based on limited data the recovery process requires many months or possibly years. Stress-deprivation effects on structural properties of ligaments remain evident for over a year after the reinstitution of function.

Ligaments demonstrate a unique response in the process of joint contracture. Although restrictive properties of the contracture itself and certain biochemical parameters of the loose periarticular connective tissues recover in only a few weeks,[6] ligaments are much more chronically affected. Joint reconditioning and overall rehabilitation must obviously be planned with these ligament changes in mind.

Stress effects (exercise)

The effect of exercise on ligaments has only recently been investigated with confusing and contradictory results.* Reasons for discrepancies may include the use of various animal models, inadequate intergroup matching of important variables, different experimental procedures, and inconsistent definition of controls and *exercised* animals. Despite these drawbacks, which include inconsistent physiologic proof of exercise effectiveness in other systems (such as organ weights, heart rates, serum cholesterol levels, adipocyte diameters, enzyme activities, and muscle weights[98,107]), a comparative review of results will be presented to summarize the current controversies and to ideally provide adequate background for further investigation.

Morphology. Exercise does not cause persistent gross changes in the appearance of ligament substance itself. There is a suggestion of decreased water content with a duller appearance and a slight loss of fiber waviness immediately after exercise.[111] Increases in ligament mass may occur with certain long-term exercise programs, and increases in cross-sectional area and weight have been reported.[98] Microscopically, this increased mass has been suggested as secondary to fiber bundle hypertrophy (with increased collagen matrix between cell bodies) as opposed to cellular hyperplasia.[97,98]

As noted previously, insertions of ligaments are particularly stress sensitive, and morphologic reversal of stress deprivation changes in subperiosteal insertions secondary to exercise have been recognized.[64,76] Although these changes are difficult to quantitate and may be specific to individual ligaments, a spectrum of effects paralleling the spectrum of activity from immobilized through normal to exercised can probably be found. The use of cage activity animals as normal controls has been questioned,[64,98] particularly in a comparative study with exercise, and must be carefully considered when evaluating previous results.

Biomechanics. According to a number of investigators, several properties of bone-ligament complexes are affected by exercise. These changes must be qualified as either transitory (viscoelastic) or persistent, with the latter of primary concern for possible lasting improvement of qualities for clinical purposes. Although not definitely established, it would appear that persistent changes in ligament complexes do occur secondary to exercise. Since the mechanisms of these changes are unknown, either direct stress application to substance or insertions or secondary hormonal and nutritional differences[28,98,103] may be responsible.

As noted previously, the majority of mechanical tests to failure have been conducted on bone-ligament-bone preparations. Failure strengths therefore are usually an index of the weakest link in that system, and at low loading rates most commonly

---

*References 1, 28, 88, 98, 107, 115, 121, 122.

involve the insertions. The absolute separation force[122] of these complexes in various models is usually increased by exercise[1,28,97,98,121] (Fig. 11-33).

Such results are obtained for medial collateral,[100,120] lateral collateral,[122] and anterior cruciate knee preparations.[73,76] Most researchers have attributed this improvement to pure insertional change rather than differences in ligament substance. It may be a combined effect, however, as evidence for midsubstance effects of exercise also exists.[28]

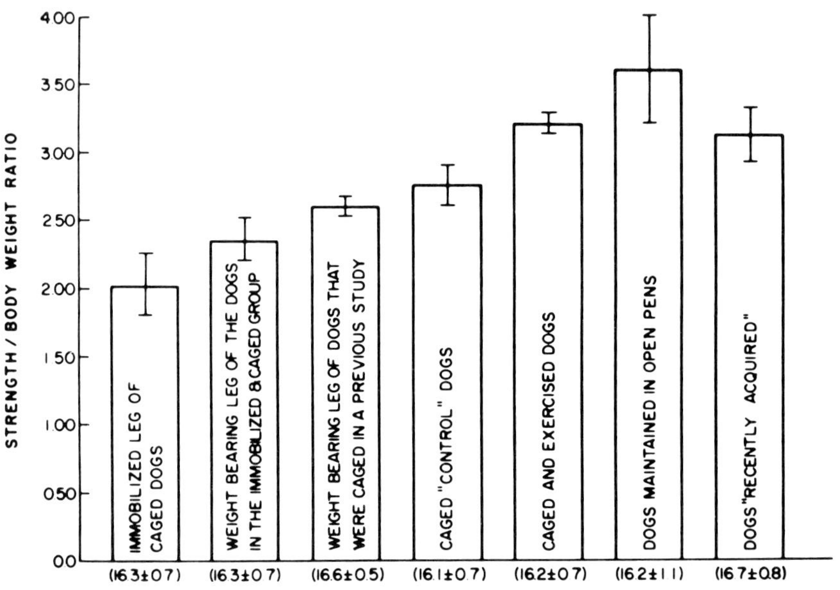

Fig. 11-33. Junction strength/body weight ratios of male mongrel dogs assigned to different activity groups. (From Tipton, C.M., and others: Med. Sci. Sports Exerc. 7[3]:165, 1975.)

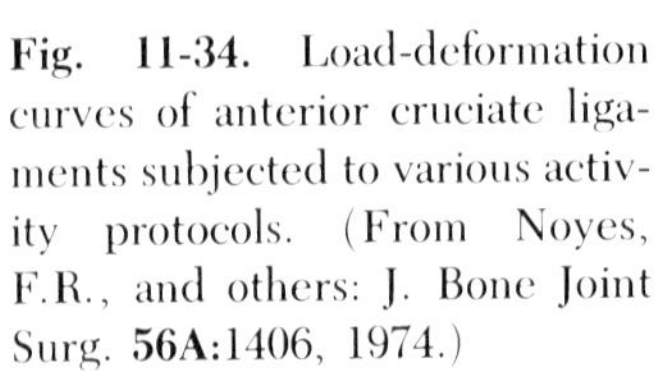

Fig. 11-34. Load-deformation curves of anterior cruciate ligaments subjected to various activity protocols. (From Noyes, F.R., and others: J. Bone Joint Surg. 56A:1406, 1974.)

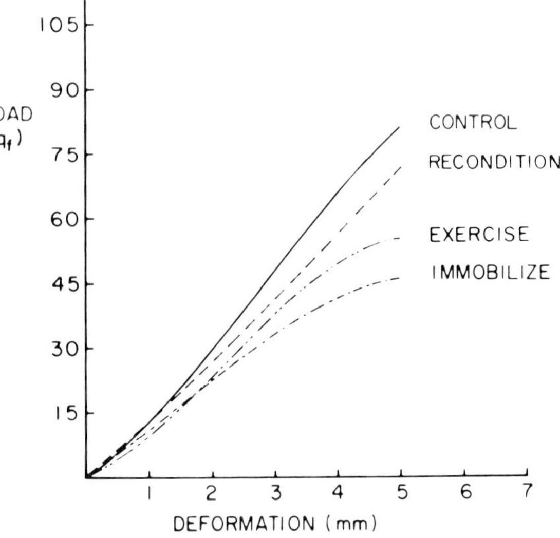

Although some have reported elastic stiffness of ligaments to be either significantly increased[25,100] or slightly increased[120] secondary to exercise, others have noted the opposite, that is, ligaments demonstrating chronically decreased stiffness after exercise (increased compliance)[76,97] (Fig. 11-34).

Still others have reported no significant change in stiffness in response to exercise.[21,88] These discrepancies are probably multifactorial and may include evidence that male animals may be more affected than females and certain species may be more affected than others. Another cause for these discrepancies may be that training protocols are varied.[25,98,107]

Exercise recovery from immobilization (reconditioning) must be regarded as a slightly different situation. Exercise effects may be more pronounced and therefore less controversial in aiding the return toward normal of biomechanical properties.[76]

While immobilization effects (predominantly degradative) may be dramatic and exponential with time, exercise effects appear to be more gradual in onset and effectiveness in conditioning and reconditioning situations. Immobilization and exercise effects once established, however, are probably long lasting in an animal that maintains normal activity because of relatively slow normal ligament turnover. However, more data are required to describe the minimum exercise needed to maintain the benefit of intensive exercise training on ligaments.

Biochemistry. The biochemical changes of ligaments in response to exercise have not been completely elucidated. Collagen content (per unit mass) may be increased[97]; however, this has not been a consistent finding. Other studies have noted no changes in collagen, water, or glycosaminoglycan content as a result of exercise.[120]

To our knowledge other biochemical parameters, such as collagen cross-links and collagen metabolism, have not yet been studied in exercised ligaments. Collagen turnover in exercised tendons is apparently increased,[56] and a similar effect may be expected in ligament, but has not been demonstrated.

Systemic biochemical mediation of changing ligament properties has been suggested, with exogenous testosterone and thyroxine in some way increasing ligament complex strength.[98] Although these effects may be insertional (on bone), the possibility of synergistic action of movement and hormonal influence on ligament substance must be considered.[103]

Summary of effects. Ligament complexes seem to be influenced both qualitatively and quantitatively by exercise through mechanisms that are as yet undefined. Changes are subtle and demonstrate minimal gross alteration.

Ligaments increase slightly in mass by fiber bundle hypertrophy, which may be caused by increased collagen production. When compared with normal ligaments, those that have undergone training have not shown any other biochemical changes. Recovery from immobilization, however, demonstrates improvement more quickly than recovery without exercise. At best the recovery is extremely slow in comparison to the rapid onset of stress-deprivation effects. Data available indicate ligament complexes from joints immobilized a few weeks require more than 1 year to recover.

Exercise apparently alters several mechanical properties of bone-ligament-bone complexes through action on both bony insertions and ligament substance. These

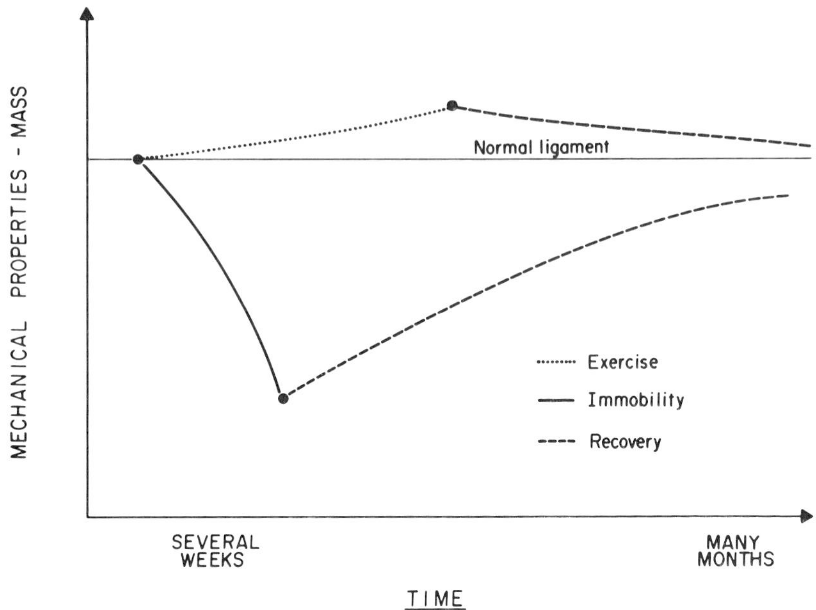

Fig. 11-35. Schematic representation of exercise and immobilization effects and recovery on ligament complex properties. Note general patterns of deviation from normal (generalization of this formulation remains largely speculative).

alterations are once again more dramatic in postimmobilization recovery of properties than in exercise of normal subjects.

Exercise effects on ligament may vary depending on age, sex, species, nutrition, hormones, type of exercise, and perhaps the specific ligament involved. Further elucidation of these and other variables that may mediate exercise phenomena is certainly indicated. If plotted on a time line, the trend of stress-related and motion-related soft tissue homeostasis is probably not a mirror image of that for immobility (Fig. 11-35).

The time necessary for exercise to demonstrate an effect on normal ligaments is more prolonged than that for immobility. The time for recovery from both is long and the end points are uncertain, but it would appear that exercise is beneficial in accelerating the reconditioning of ligaments after immobility.

LIGAMENT HEALING
Wound healing

In simplest terms, hemorrhage and inflammation usually dominate for the first 1 to 7 days after an injury (biomechanical *productive phase*).[24] A *proliferative phase* when connective tissue cells proliferate usually follows and reaches a peak 2 to 3 weeks after injury. Then the prolonged maturation of the *remodeling phase* begins. The variability of duration of each phase from these guidelines depends on a number of systemic factors (age, nutrition, or hormones) and local factors (tissue type, blood supply, infection, mechanical stresses, temperature, or chemical environment).

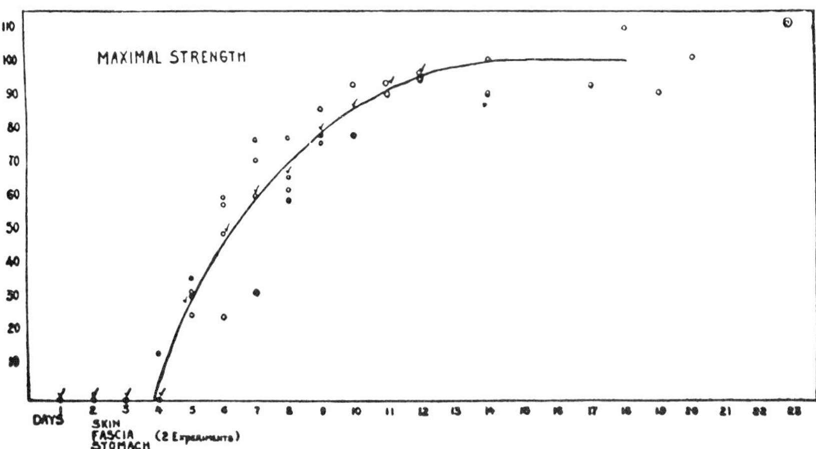

Fig. 11-36. Recovery of tensile strength in healing wounds. (From Howes, E.L., and others: JAMA **92**:42, 1929.)

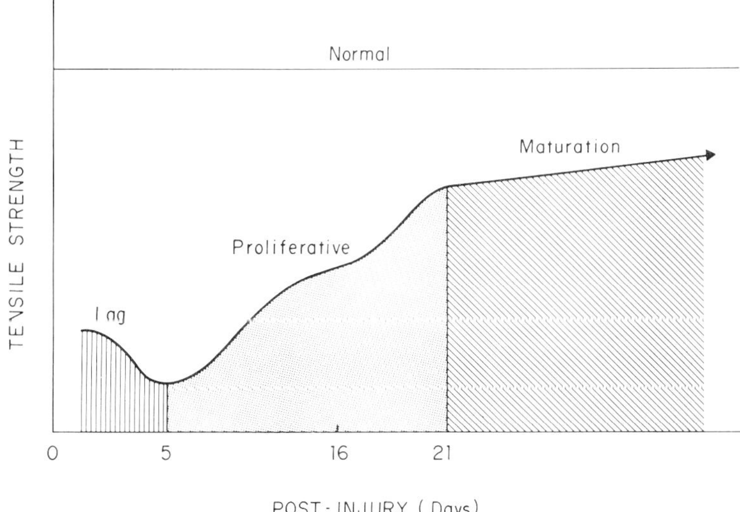

Fig. 11-37. Stages of mechanical recovery in healing tendons. (From Mason, M.L., and Allen, H.S.: Ann. Surg. **113**[3]:424, 1941.)

The first attempt to supplement the histologic phases of wound healing with correlative biomechanical strength versus time studies was by Howes and others[57] (Fig. 11-36). Their curve of the early return of skin wound healing strength has remained a standard in terms of experimental wound study. Probably, however, the true maturation phase of healing was not addressed in this study or in the many studies that followed.

Mason and Shearon[66] applied tensile testing to tendon healing, and Mason and Allen[65] subsequently concluded that the return of tensile strength in tendons is similar to that for other tissues (and presumably ligaments) (Fig. 11-37).

In addition to correlating histologic phases with tensile strength, attention was focused on the third phase of healing (maturation or remodeling) as being particularly important in changing viscoelastic properties of the wound on the basis of ongoing matrix reorganization.[52]

The biochemical study of wound healing began with previously described assays of normal tissue components and mediators of inflammation.[24] Dunphy and Udupa[34] correlated biochemical observations with biomechanical observations and demonstrated a direct relationship between collagen content and wound strength in tension in the early days of recovery. Although the rate of collagen synthesis and deposition reaches a maximum at approximately the fourteenth day (in skin), it remains slightly elevated for many weeks after injury. Its correlation with increasing tensile load to failure persists through that period. However, tensile load to failure continues to increase for at least 60 days after the collagen content plateaus. This increase is probably on the basis of specific collagen reorganization and maturation, collagen cross-linking, and other matrix interaction processes.

The importance of ground substance–collagen interaction can be illustrated by the observation that the collagen-mucopolysaccharide ratio is reportedly a better determinant of wound failure load in tension than collagen alone.[25] The duration of increased metabolic activity (synthesis, degradation, and remodeling) in the scar is variable, but is probably prolonged.[58]

Ligament healing and treatment

Morphology. The first histologic description of the states of ligament healing in an animal model appeared in the work of Miltner[68,69] in 1932, and subsequently a series of specific and multidisciplinary studies of these processes have been published.* In general these studies can be divided into two groups.

Nonrepaired ligaments. Depending on degree of injury the joint of the involved ligament and the gap created by separation of soft tissue fibers usually fill rapidly with blood. In complete disruptions, free ligament ends usually recoil with the tortuous appearance of the relaxed ligament bodies and are connected only by the forming hematoma.[59] Ligament stumps may be relatively shredded in a diffuse manner, taking the characterstics *mop ends* appearance of failure. Within hours an inflammatory reaction begins, with a progressive edematous infiltrate that renders the ligament substance increasingly friable.[68] The area of damage and subsequent reaction is often much larger than expected from external examination and therefore proprotionately slower to resolve.[81] Gross evidence of vascular *granulation tissue* begins in the first few days and proliferates through hemorrhagic tissues to fill potential spaces and obliterate normal tissue planes in the area. Inflammation and granulation predominate for 2 to 3 weeks as progressive fibrosis occurs. The tenuous attachment of ligament ends via the fibrin clot is strengthened by the increasing collagen matrix.

---

*References 30, 31, 59, 77-79, 97, 100, 102, 103.

At about 1 month resorption of joint fluid and edema reveals a considerable extent of underlying *scar formation* and maturation begins. Contraction and remodeling of this scar in the animal model is sufficiently advanced at 6 weeks for some to note "complete healing" has occurred.[68,69] However, months or years may be required to even approach normality.[38,77] *Old ligament* is often identifiable in the scar as a result of its relative density for many months after injury, bridged by a relatively loose and disorganized scar. Histologically, the healing response of the nonrepaired ligament is similar to that of other connective tissues. Hemorrhage, fluid, and inflammatory cells predominate for the first week after injury.[68] An increasing fibroblastic response occurs in the second and third weeks, with deposition of increasing amounts of collagen. Ligament cells notably contribute to this fibroplasia to the extent that hypercellularity is evident from one end to the other.[38,59] At 4 weeks the fibroblastic response diminshes, inflammatory cells and edema decrease, and matrix alignment begins. Progressive remodeling of swirls of scar fibers in the defect takes place, and cellularity decreases slowly. Occasional metaplasia to cartilage cells occurs, depending on local and systemic factors. Old ligament (usually near the insertions if the injury was midsubstance) becomes recognizable and separable from scar formation because of its return toward normal cellularity after a few months. Eighteen months after injury the bridging scar has become relatively hypocellular, is still slightly disorganized, and has a different staining quality than normal.[38] The histologic endpoint of the process may have been reached, but this requires confirmation.

Repaired ligaments. With repair, there may be certain qualitative and quantitative alterations in the processes just described. In a canine model of collateral ligament transection, Clayton and Wier[30,31] noted diminution of separation in ligament ends and therefore significantly decreased scar formation with repair. Suturing of sharply divided ligaments in fact led to what might be called *primary ligament healing* with no visual break in the continuity of the original tissue at the suture line. Unsutured ligaments always healed with a gap and slightly more scar tissue. O'Donoghue,[79] using a similar model, noted more orderly healing in the early stages as a result of repair rather than by relatively diffuse extensive scar formation. Repairs appeared "more taut" and had increased collagenization with shorter stages of inflammation and proliferation.[79] Healing was therefore apparently hastened, at least during the first few weeks after injury. Repair was shown to be particularly important in the cruciate ligaments, since without suture apposition of ends they had no mechanical potential for healing.[77,78] Even the primary anterior cruciate ligament repair is challenged by many clinicians on the basis of failure of healing caused by the *hostile* environment of the synovial space. The importance of ligament integrity in preventing arthritis was also demonstrated in long-term follow-up of failures of variations in cruciate healing.[77] Types of suture material and applied tension were also suggested as important factors in determining cruciate healing in these studies through their effects on potential necrosis and duration of inflammation. Details of the influence of vascularity on the anterior cruciate repair in the unfavorable intrasynovial environment are described in detail in other chapters of this book.

Biomechanics

Nonrepaired ligaments. Reports of tensile tests of healing ligaments have been infrequent, and most have employed relatively slow strain rates. These studies, however, suggest that the return to normal strength and elastic stiffness in ligaments is slower than that in skin and tendon, but its general pattern of recovery is similar.[39] The importance of the remodeling phase of ligament healing in this recovery cannot be overemphasized; it is analogous to fracture healing (Fig. 11-38). The rate of return of the ligament's structural and mechanical properties is probably dependent on stress, however, and may therefore be controlled to some extent by physical means.[28,30,107]

Repaired ligaments. There is evidence of an early advantage in strength properties of repaired ligaments over those that are nonrepaired.[31,79] This advantage, however, may not be sustained. Clayton and Weir[31] demonstrated an earlier return of tensile load to failure in those repaired, but this advantage was not clearly maintained in animals of longer term follow-up. Sutured and unsutured ligaments had nearly equal failure strength when both had been subjected to exercise.[30] O'Donoghue[78] was also unable to conclude that repair had a lasting tensile advantage over nonrepair except in the cruciate, where all nonrepairs failed to heal. A significant number of repaired cruciates, however, also failed to heal.[77,78] Ligament lengthening during healing is critically important to functional results. To our knowledge the only published report of an experimental test of this parameter was Clayton and others,[30] who found that

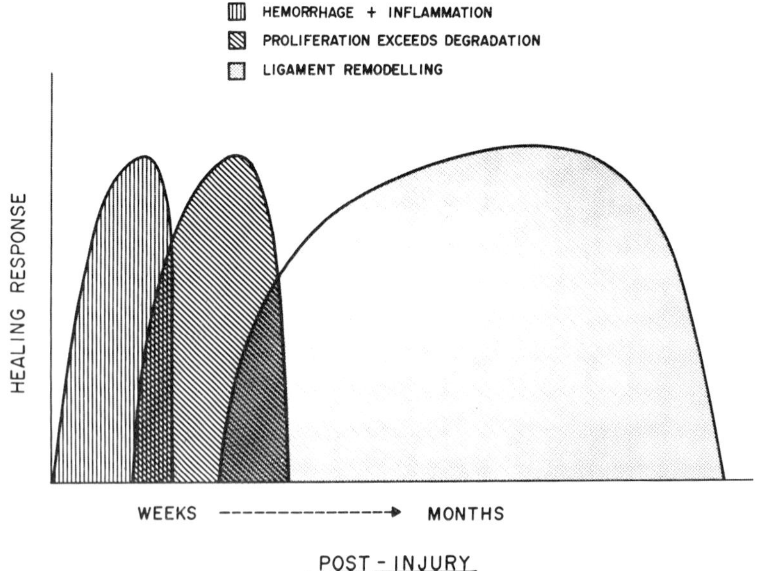

Fig. 11-38. Theoretical representation of phases of ligament healing showing relative durations and overlap of stages. Treatment is aimed at optimizing proliferation and remodeling in as short a time as possible.

sutured and unsutured ligaments heal with equal length when measured at rest, but as a result of a possible increased elasticity of the scar, the nonrepaired may be more distensible when stressed. O'Donoghue's observation[79] that repair combined with immobilizatoin resulted in the "most taut" collateral ligament was not confirmed biomechanically and therefore remains experimentally inconclusive.

Biochemistry. The biochemistry of ligament healing has received little attention to date, Indications are that collagen content parallels the slow increase of tensile strength and return of elastic stiffness in the early phase of healing.[39]

Preliminary data suggest that collagen content of the healing ligament may contain up to 30% to 40% Type III collagen in the early months after injury (typical of granulation tissue) and possibly decrease slowly with time. Remodeling of ligament scar in collagen cross-link changes has been shown to be an equally prolonged process[39] that requires further elucidation. Biochemically therefore ligament healing is probably not particularly unique except perhaps for the extremely slow-attempted reconstitution of its original highly organized structure.

Stress effect on healing. There can be little doubt that stress application or deprivation alters normal ligaments. Healing tendons are stress sensitive during the early and maturation phases of their healing when guarded movement produces increases in ultimate strength.[65,117] There is evidence to suggest that the biochemical composition of healing ligaments is similarly responsive to stress application.

Experimental animal models with identically injured and repaired ligaments treated by immobilization, cage activity, or active exercise showed that immobilized ligaments were weakest, cage activity ligaments were stronger, and actively exercised ligaments were strongest.[97,98,107] This led Tipton[98] to conclude that the strength of repaired ligaments is at least temporarily increased with exercise training and decreased with immobilization. Although the endpoint of this exercise effect is uncertain, Tipton and co-workers[98,107] have suggested that the rate of return to normal strength of ligament substance may be significantly reduced with an exercise program.

In investigations of short healing periods of only a few weeks' duration, stress appeared to have minimal effects on the compliance of healing ligaments.[120] The effects of exercise and early motion on other parameters of healing[50] (in particular, laxity[56]) and possible mechanisms of stress action in these situations require further study in the areas, for example, of blood supply[90] and hormones.[98]

Discussion. Midsubstance ligament injury and healing constitute a diffuse process. The *one wound–one scar* concept of healing creates problems of equal significance for ligaments and tendons. Furthermore, anatomically isolated ligaments (e.g., anterior cruciate) may lack the healing benefit of surrounding connective tissues in the hostile intraarticular environment.[50] It has been said that the physical injury of ligaments is typically more severe than for tendons.[90] Certainly there is a proportionally greater need for intrinsic healing potential in the case of the anterior cruciate, and there may be difficulty with its nutrition. Certain ligaments apparently contribute to their own healing process. But most ligaments probably depend heavily on the surrounding tissues for provision of vascular neogenesis, fibroplasia, mechanical support, and additional nutrition through their prolonged recovery. The cruciates may, however, be unique in their ability to use nutrients in synovial fluid in addition to those in the blood. During remodeling ligaments are no doubt more sensitive to all the conditions that normally affect them (i.e., stress, immobilization, and hormones) on the basis of their relatively increased metabolic rates (or cellularity). Ligament repair unquestionably alters several parameters of healing in the early stages, but it is of unproven lasting benefit in all cases.

It is difficult to equate tendon healing, where scar formation must be minimized to promote function, with ligament healing, in which scar formation may actually be beneficial. It is equally difficult to reconcile the applicability of a tendon-type injury model with sharp laceration and repair to the typical catastrophic *mop-end* rupture of severe joint sprains. Relevance may be sacrificed for experimental reproducibility, which is a definite problem in the development of models for ligament healing and repair.

Stress effects are particularly significant to this discussion, since they can potentially alter some of the most important ligament characteristics. Remodeling and orientation of the randomly cross-linked collagen matrix are crucial to complete recovery from either injury or immobilization. Movement may modify the milieu of fiber production or degradation either directly or through some indirect vascular or metabolic pathways. Lack of movement permits relative randomization and probably produces the potential for macromolecular cross-bridges to interfere with normal tissue gliding, which is of more functional consequence in loose connective tissues where fiber crossing is a normal feature.

Injury represents certain surprising parallels to stress deprivation in terms of biologic response. Randomness of structure in a hypermetabolic ligament is a clear similarity. Recovery is slow from both processes, and both are sensitive to many systemic and local factors.

CLINICAL RELEVANCE

Ligament disorders may be more important to clinical practice than is commonly appreciated. They are involved in congenital disorders, for example, congenital dysplasia of the hip, Ehlers-Danlos syndrome, talipes equinovarus, and arthrogryposis, and a number of acquired conditions. They can be affected either primarily or secondarily in many of these conditions, including the connective tissue disorders (rheumatoid arthritis, ankylosing spondylitis, gout, Marfan's syndrome, and ochronosis), degenerative joint diseases (osteoarthritis, hemophiliac arthritis), infection (septic joints or bursae), neoplasms (bony or soft tissue), neurologic conditions (Charcot's joint), toxins (lathyrism), and trauma.

Trauma is the best recognized cause of ligament pathology. Although the significance of catastrophic ligament failures at the knee, ankle, or shoulder are well known, so-called sprains (likely the majority of injuries) are often diagnosed and treated with relative ease. Perhaps the most common entities in orthopaedic practice are injuries of the back and neck, and these probably often involve ligament injuries.

Commonly used clinical modalities including immobilization, traction, and physiotherapy clearly have a positive and negative influence on ligaments. Preoperative correction of joint deformity often relies on ligament softening and stretching by using combinations of these techniques.

The historic perspective of ligament injury biology therefore is somewhat surprising considering its prevalence and significance. Persistent confusion and grouping of connective tissue injuries into clinical treatment categories has retarded its scientific study along the way. The vast majority of ligament conditions for example, minor ankle sprains, probably do return to functional limits with minimal attention and further perpetuate the lack of incentive for specific ligament research.

The understanding of normal ligament physiology is an important prerequisite for the study of ligament healing. Correlations of morphology, biochemistry, and biomechanics of normal ligaments provide an appreciation of their complexity and functional abilities. Normal ligaments are not inert structures. Although limited by metabolic activity and blood supply, they are, however, able to respond to changes in their environment.

Commonly used orthopaedic modalities, such as rest and exercise, have dramatic effects on ligament properties. These effects should be considered in treatment planning that will affect the joints. Recovery of strength in injured ligaments is exceedingly slow as a result of their physiologic processes, and they must be treated accordingly.

Ligament healing is a complex process that has been inadequately studied. It remains to be demonstrated whether all ligaments heal by identical mechanisms and if these mechanisms are similar to tendons. The anterior cruciate ligament, because of its location, apparently has the greatest biologic disadvantage for healing potential. Of practical importance are the factors that accelerate healing, such as suturing and exercise. Prolonged immobilization in these situations is apparently contraindicated. It must be added, however, that many experimental models have been challenged because follow-up time has often been short and experimental design has been flawed. Important questions regarding ligament elongation during the prolonged healing process remain unresolved, with or without repair, and with various degrees of stress application. Regimens of repair and activity are far from being defined for the clinical setting and may eventually be shown to be injury and joint or ligament specific.

The biologic story of ligaments is far from complete. Only through a better understanding of the processes of ligament physiology (morphology, chemistry, and mechanics) will healing be understood, and treatment of all conditions involving ligaments optimized.

REFERENCES

1. Adams, A.: Effect of exercise upon ligament strength, Res. Q. Exerc. Sport, 1966.
2. Akeson, W.H., Amiel, D., and LaViolette, D.: The connective tissue response to immobility; a study of chondroitin-4 and -6 sulfate and dermatan sulfate changes in periarticular connective tissue of control and immobilized knees of dogs, Clin. Orthop. **51**:183, 1967.
3. Akeson, W.H., and others: Collagen cross-linking alterations in joint contractures;: changes in the reducible cross-links in periarticular connective tissue collagen after nine weeks of immobilization, Connect. Tissue Res. **5**:15, 1977.

4. Akeson, W.H., Amiel, D., and Woo, S. L.-Y.: Immobility effects on synovial joints: the pathmechanics of joint contracture, Biorheology **17**:95, 1980.
5. Akeson, W.H., and others: The connective tissue response to immobility: biochemical changes in periarticular connective tissue of the immobilized rabbit knee, Clin. Orthop. **93**:356, 1973.
6. Akeson, W.H., and others: Rapid recovery from contracture in rabbit hindlimb, Clin. Orthop. **122**:359, 1977.
7. Akeson, W., and others: The biology of ligaments. In Funk, J., editor: Basic principles of knee rehabilitation, St. Louis, 1983, The C.V. Mosby Co.
8. Alm, A., and others: The anterior cruciate ligament: a clinical and experimental study on tensile strength, morphology and replacement by patellar ligament, Acta Chir. Scand. Suppl. **445**:15, 1974.
9. Amiel, D., and others: A biochemical and morphological comparison of connective tissue from Dupuytren's palmar fasciitis and immobilized joint contracture. In Akeson, W.H., Bronstein, P., and Glimcher, M.J., editors: American Academy of Orthopaedic Surgeons: Symposium on heritable disorders of connective tissue, St. Louis, 1982, The C.V. Mosby Co.
10. Amiel, D., and others: Effect of nine week immobilization on the types of collagen synthesized in periarticular connective tissue from rabbit knees, Connect. Tissue Res. **8**:27, 1980.
11. Amiel, D., and others: Tendons and ligaments: a morphological and biochemical comparison, J. Orthop. Res.**1**:257, 1984.
12. Amiel, D., and others: The effect of immobilization on collagen turnover in connective tissue: a biochemical-biomechanical correlation, Acta Orthop. Scand. **53**:325, 1982.
13. Arnoczky, S.P., Rubin, R.M., and Marshall, J.L.: Microvasculature of the cruciate ligaments and its response to injury, J. Bone Joint Surg. **61A**:1221, 1979.
14. Asboe-Hansen, G., editor: Connective tissue in health and disease, Copenhagen, 1954, Munksgaard.
15. Baer, E.: The multicomposite structure of tendon collagen: relationships between ultrastructure and mechanical properties, Proceedings of the third international congress of biorheology, La Jolla, Calif., 1978.
16. Bailey, A.J.: In Florkin, M., and Stotz, E., editors: Comprehensive biochemistry, 297-423, Amsterdam, 1968, Elsevier/North Holland.
17. Bailey, A.J., Robins, S.P., and Balian, G.: Biological significance of the intermolecular cross-links of collagen, Nature **251**:105, 1974.
18. Barr, M.L.: The human nervous system: an anatomical viewpoint, New York, 1972, Harper & Row, Publishers.
19. Bayles, T.A.: The biology of connective tissue cells, no. 7, New York, 1982, Arthritis and Rheumatism Foundaiton Conference Series.
20. Bloom, W., and Fawcett, D.W.: A textbook of histology, ed. 10, Philadelphia, 1975, W.B. Saunders Co.
21. Booth, F., and Tipton, C.M.: Ligamentous strength measurements in prepubescent and pubescent rats, Growth **34**:177, 1970.
22. Bronstein, P., Kang, A.H., and Piez, K.A.: The limited cleavage of native collagen with chymotrypsin, trypsin and cyanogen bromide, Biochemistry **5**(12):3803, 1966.
23. Brooke, J.S., and Slack, H.G.B.: Metabolism of connective tissue in limb atrophy in the rabbit, Ann. Rheum. Dis. **18**:129, 1959.
24. Brookis, J.G.: The scientific fundamentals of surgery, New York, 1972, Appleton-Century-Crofts, p. 186.
25. Bryant, W.M., and Weeks, P.M.: Secondary wound tensile strength gain: a function of collagen and mucopolysaccharide interaction, Plast. Reconstr. Surg. **39**:84, 1967.
26. Bull, H.B.: Protein structure and elasticity. In Remington, J.W., editor: Tissue elasticity, Washington, 1957, American Physiologic Society.
27. Burleigh, P.M.C., and Poole, A.R.: Dynamics of connective tissue macromolecules, New York, 1975, American Elsevier Publishing Co., Inc.
28. Cabaud, H.E., and others: Exercise effects on the strength of the rat anterior cruciate ligaments, Am. J. Sports Med. **8**:79, 1980.
29. Clark, L.: The tissues of the body, ed. 6, Oxford, 1971, Oxford University Press.
30. Clayton, M.L., Miles, J.S., and Abdulla, M.: Experimental investigations of ligamentous healing, Clin. Orthop. **61**:146, 1968.
31. Clayton, M.L., and Weir, G.J.: Experimental investigations of ligamentous healing, Am. J. Surg. **98**:373, 1959.

32. Cooper, R.R., and Misol, S.: Tendon and ligament insertion, J. Bone Joint Surg. **52A**:1, 1970.
33. Crowninshield, R.D., and Pope, M.P.: The strength and failure characteristics of rat medial collateral ligaments, J. Trauma **16**:99, 1976.
34. Dunphy, J.E., and Udupa, K.N.: Chemical and histochemical sequences in the normal healing of wounds, N. Engl. J. Med. **253**:847, 1955.
35. Engel, A., and Larsson, T.: Aging of connective and skeletal tissue, Symposium 1 to 3, 1969, Nordiska Bokhandelns Forlay.
36. Enneking, W.F., and Horowitz, M.: The intraarticular effects of immobilization on the human knee, J. Bone Joint Surg. **54A**:973, 1972.
37. Evans, E.B., and others: Experimental immobilization and remobilization of rat knee joints, J. Bone Joint Surg. **42A**:757, 1960.
38. Frank, C., Schachar, N., and Dittrich, D.: The natural history of healing in the repaired medial collateral ligament: a morphological assessment in rabbits, J. Orthop. Res. **1**:179, 1983.
39. Frank, C., and others: Medial collateral ligament healing: a multidisciplinary assessment in rabbits, Am. J. Sports Med., **11**:379, 1983.
40. Frisen, M., Magi, M., Sonnerup, L., and Viidik, A.: Rheological analysis of soft collagenous tissue. I. Theoretical considerations, J. Biomech. **2**:13, 1969.
41. Fung, Y.C.B.: Elasticity of soft tissues in simple elongation, Am. J. Physiol. **213**(6):1532, 1967.
42. Fung, Y.C.B.: Biorheology of soft tissues, Biorheology **10**:139, 1973.
43. Gabbiani, G., and others: Granulation tissue as a contractile organ, J. Exp. Med. **135**:719, 1972.
44. Gallop, P.M., and others: Isolation and identification of α amino aldehydes in collagen, Biochemistry **7**:2409, 1968.
45. Gallop, P.M., Blumenfeld, O.O., and Seifter, S.: Structure and metabolism of connective tissue proteins, Annu. Rev. Biochem. **41**:617, 1972.
46. Gardner, E.D.: Physiology of movable joints, Physiol. Rev. **30**:127, 1950.
47. Gelman, R.A., and Blackwell, J.: An analysis of fibrous long spacing forms of collagen, Connect. Tissue Res. **2**:31, 1973.
48. Gove, P.B., editor: Webster's new collegiate dictionary, Springfield, Mass., 1977, G. & C. Merriam Co.
49. Grant, M.E., and Prockop, D.J.: The biosynthesis of collagen. I., N. Engl. J. Med. **286**:194, 1972.
50. Gustavson, K.H.: The chemistry and reactivity of collagen, New York, 1956, Academic Press, Inc.
51. Hall, M.C.: Cartilage changes after experimental immobilization of the knee joint of the young rat, J. Bone Joint Surg. **45A**:36, 1963.
52. Hamilton, R., Apesos, J., and Korostaff, E.: Viscoelastic properties of healing wounds, Plast. Reconstr. Surg. **45**:274, 1970.
53. Harkness, R.D.: Biological functions of collagen, Biol. Rev. **36**:399, 1961.
54. Harris, E.F., an McCroskery, P.A.: The influence of temperature and fibril stability on degradation of cartilage collagen by rheumatoid synovial collagenase, N. Engl. J. Med. **290**:1, 1974.
55. Hascall, V.C., and Sajdera, S.W.: Protein polysaccaride complex from bovine nasal cartilage, J. Biol. Chem. **244**:2384, 1969.
56. Heikkinen, E., and Vuori, I.: Effect of physical activity on the metabolism of collagen in aged mice, Acta Physiol. Scand. **84**:543, 1972.
57. Howes, E.L., Sooy, J.W., and Harvey, S.C.: The healing of wounds as determined by their tensile strength, JAMA **92**:42, 1929.
58. Hunt, T.K., and Dunphy, J.E.: Fundamentals of wound management, New York, 1979, Appleton-Century-Crofts, p. 30.
59. Jack, E.A.: Experimental rupture of the medial collateral ligament of the knee, J. Bone Joint Surg. **32B**:396, 1950.
60. Kennedy, J.C., and others: Tension studies of human knee ligaments, J. Bone Joint Surg. **58A**:350, 1976.
61. Klein, L., Dawson, M.H., and Heiple, K.G.: Turnover of collagen in the adult rat after denervation, J. Bone Joint Surg. **59A**:1065, 1977.
62. Klein, L., Player, J.S., and Heiple, K.G.: Isotopic evidence for resorption of soft tissues and bone in immobilized dogs, J. Bone Joint Surg. **64A**:225, 1982.
63. Kuei, S.C., and others: The viscoelastic, thermoelastic and time dependent properties of the knee ligaments, Trans. Orthop. Res. Soc. San Francisco **4**:25, 1979.
64. Laros, G.S., Tipton, C.M., and Cooper, R.R.: Influence of physical activity on ligament insertions in the knees of dogs, J. Bone Joint Surg. **53A**:275, 1971.

65. Mason, M.L., and Allen, H.S.: The rate of healing of tendons, Ann. Surg. **113**(3):425, 1941.
66. Mason, M.L., and Shearon, C.A.: The process of tendon repair, Arch.Surg. **25**:615, 1932.
67. Mechanic, L.G.: An automated scintillation counting system for continuous analysis: cross-links of [³H]NaBH₄ reduced collagen, Anal. Biochem. **62**:349, 1974.
68. Miltner, L.J., and Hu, C.H.: Experimental reproduction of joint sprains, Proc. Soc. Exp. Biol. Med. **30**:883, 1932-33.
69. Miltner, L.J., Hu, C.H., and Fang, H.C.: Experimental joint sprain: a pathologic study, Arch. Surg. **35**:234, 1937.
70. Muir, H.: Biochemistry. In Freeman, M.A.R., editor: Adult articular cartilage, Kent, England, 1979, Pitman Medical Publishing Co., Ltd.
71. Neuberger, A., and Slack, H.G.B.: The metabolism of collagen from liver, bones, skin, and tendon in the normal rat, Biochem. J. **53**:47, 1953.
72. Nimni, M.E.: Collagen: its structure and function in normal and pathological connective tissues, Semin. Arthritis Rheum. **4**:95, 1974.
73. Noyes, F.R., DeLucas, J.L., and Torvik, P.J.: Biomechanics of anterior cruciate ligament failure: an analysis of strain rate sensitivity and mechanisms of failure in primates, J. Bone Joint Surg. **56A**:236, 1974.
74. Noyes, F.R., and others: Clinical biomechanics of the knee: ligament restraints and functional stability. In American Academy of Orthopaedic Surgeons: Symposium on the athlete's knee: surgical repair and reconstruction, St. Louis, 1980, The C.V. Mosby Co.
75. Noyes, F.R., and others: Effect of intraarticular corticosteroids in ligament properties, Clin. Orthop. **123**:197, 1977.
76. Noyes, F.R., and others: Biomechanics of ligament failure. II. An analysis of immobilization, exercise, and reconditioning effects in primates, J. Bone Joint Surg. **56A**:1406, 1974.
77. O'Donoghue, D.H., and others: Repair and reconstruction of the anterior cruciate ligament in dogs: factors influencing long term results, J. Bone Joint Surg. **53A**:710, 1971.
78. O'Donoghue, D.H., and others: Repair of the anterior cruciate ligament in dogs. II. J. Bone Joint Surg. **48A**:503, 1966.
79. O'Donoghue, D.H., Rockwood, C., and Zarecznyj, B.: Repair of knee ligaments in dogs. I. The lateral collateral ligament, J. Bone Joint Surg. **43A**:1167, 1961.
80. Ogata, K., Whiteside, L.A., and Andersen, D.A.: The intra-articular effect of various postoperative managements following knee ligament repair: an experimental study in dogs, Clin. Orthop. **150**:271-276, 1980.
81. Palmer, I.: On injuries to the ligaments of the knee joint, Acta Chir. Scand. Suppl. **53**:1, 1938.
82. Paz, M.A., and others: α Amino alcohols as products of a reductive side reaction of denatured collagen with sodium borohydride, Biochemistry **9**:2123, 1970.
83. Peacock, E.E.: Comparison of collagenous tissue surrounding normal and immobilized joints, Surg. Forum **14**:440, 1963.
84. Petruska, J.A., and Hodge, A.J.: A subunit model for the tropocollagen macromolecule, Proc. Natl. Acad. Sci. USA **51**:871, 1964.
85. Piez, K.A., Eigner, E.A., and Lewis, M.S.: The chromatographic separation and amino acid composition of the subunits of several collagens, Biochemistry **2**:58, 1963.
86. Piper, T.L., and Whiteside, L.A.: Early mobilization after knee ligament repair in dogs: an experimental study, Clin. Orthop. **150**:277, 1980.
87. Ramachandran, G.N., and Gould, B.S.: Treatise on collagen, New York, 1968, Academic Press, Inc.
88. Rasch, P.J., and others: Effect of exercise, immobilization and intermittent stretching of knee ligaments of albino rats, J. Appl. Physiol. **15**:289, 1960.
89. Rosenburg, L.: Cartilage proteoglycans, Fed. Proc. **32**:1467, 1973.
90. Rothman, R.H., and Slogoff, S.: The effect of immobilization on the vascular bed of tendon, Surg. Gynecol. Obstet. **124**:1064, 1967.
91. Roux, W.: Die Entwicklungsmechanic, Leipzig, 1905.
92. Salter, R.B., and Field, P.: The effects of continuous compression on living articular cartilage: an experimental investigation, J. Bone Joint Surg. **42A**:31, 1960.
93. Scapinelli, R.: Studies on the vasculature of the human knee joint, Acta Anat. **70**:305, 1968.
94. Sjoerdsma, A., and others: Hydroxyproline and collagen metabolism, Ann. Intern. Med. **63**:672, 1965.

95. Tanzer, M.L.: Crosslinking of collagen, Science **180**:561, 1973.

96. Thaxter, T.H., Mann, R.A., and Anderson, C.E.: Degeneration of immobilized knee joints in rats: histological and angiographic study, J. Bone Joint Surg. **47A**:567, 1965.

97. Tipton, C.M., and others: Influence of exercise on the strength of the medial collateral ligaments of dogs, Am. J. Physiol. **218**:894, 1970.

98. Tipton, C.M., and others: The influence of physical activity on ligaments and tendons, Med. Sci. Sports Exerc. **7**(3):165, 1975.

99. Tipton, C.M., Matthes, R.D., and Martin, R.R.: Influence of age and sex on the strength of bone-ligament junctions in knee joints of rats, J. Bone Joint Surg. **60A**:230, 1978.

100. Tipton, C.M., Matthes, R.D., and Sondage, D.S.: In situ measurement of junction strength and ligament elongation in rats, J. Appl. Phys. **37**(5):758, 1974.

101. Tipton, C.M., Schild, R.J., and Flatt, A.E.: Measurement of ligamentous strength in rat knees, J. Bone Joint Surg. **49A**:63, 1967.

102. Tipton, C.M., Schild, R.J., and Tomanek, R.J.: Influence of physical activity on the strength of knee ligaments in rats, Am. J. Physiol. **212**:783, 1967.

103. Tipton, C.M., Tcheng, T-K, and Mergner, W.: Ligamentous strength measurements from hypophysectomized rats, Am. J. Physiol. **221**:1144, 1971.

104. Torp, S., and others: Structure property relationships in tendon as a function of age, Proceedings of Colston Conference, Bristol, England, 1974, University of Bristol.

105. Traub, W., and Piez, K.A.: The chemistry and structure of collagen, Adv. Protein Chem. **25**:243, 1971.

106. Trias, A.: Effect of persistent pressure on the articular cartilage: an experimental study, J. Bone Joint Surg. **43B**:376, 1961.

107. Vailas, A.C., and others: Physical activity and its influence on the repair process of medial collateral ligaments, Connect. Tissue Res. **9**:25, 1981.

108. Viidik, A.: Elasticity and tensile strength of the ACL in rabbits as influenced by training, Acta Physiol. Scand. **74**:373, 1968.

109. Vogel, H.G.: Influence of maturation and age on mechanical and biochemical parameters of connective tissue of various organs in the rat, Connect. Tissue Res. **6**:161, 1978.

110. Warwick, R., and Williams, P.L., editors: Gray's anatomy, ed. 35, Philadelphia, 1973, W.B. Saunders Co.

111. Weisman, G., Pope, M.H., and Johnson, R.J.: The effect of cyclic loading on knee ligaments, Trans. Orthop. Res. Soc. San Francisco, **4**:24, 1979.

112. Whiteside, L.A., and Sweeney, R.E., Jr.: Nutrient pathways of the cruciate ligaments, J. Bone Joint Surg. **62A**:1176, 1980.

113. Wolff, J.: Das Gesetz der Transformation der Knochan, Berlin, 1892.

114. Woo, S. L.-Y.: Mechanical properties of tendons and ligaments. I. Quasistatic and nonlinear viscoelastic properties, Biorheology **19**:385, 1982.

115. Woo, S. L.-Y.: Mechanical properties of tendons and ligaments. II. The relationship of immobilization and exercise on tissue remodeling, Biorheology **19**:397, 1982.

116. Woo, S. L.-Y., and others: The connective tissue response to immobility: a correlative study of the biomechanical and biochemical measurements of the normal and immobilized rabbit knee, Arthritis Rheum. **18**:257, 1975.

117. Woo, S. L.-Y., and others: The importance of controlled passive motion on flexor tendon healing: a biomechanical study, Acta Orthop. Scand. **52**:615, 1982.

118. Woo, S. L.-Y., Gomez, M.H., and Akeson, W.H.: The time and history dependent viscoelastic properties of medial collateral ligaments, J. Biomech. Eng. **103**:293, 1981.

119. Woo, S. L.-Y., and others: On the measurement of mechanical properties of ligament substance from a bone-ligament-bone preparation, J. Orthop. Res. **1**:22, 1983.

120. Woo, S. L.-Y., and others: Effect of immobilization and exercise on strength characteristics of bone-medial collateral ligament-bone complex. Am. Soc. Mech. Eng. **32**:62, 1979.

121. Zuckerman, J., and Stull, G.A.: Effects of exercise on knee ligament separation force in rats, J. Appl. Physiol. **26**:716, 1969.

122. Zuckerman, J., and Stull, G.A.: Ligamentous separation force in rats as influenced by training, detraining, and cage restriction, Med. Sci. Sports Exerc. **5**(1):44, 1973.

12. Biomechanical function of knee ligaments

Jack L. Lewis
William D. Lew
George T. Shybut
Murali Jasty
James A. Hill

The majority of research in knee biomechanics has been guided by the needs of clinical diagnosis. The classic work of Brantigan and Voshell[1] served as a model for the study of the knee for many years. Their goal was to show the relationship between ligamentous structures and changes in knee joint displacement during clinical laxity tests when these ligaments were transected. This test methodology has been helpful in interpreting clinical diagnostic tests. However, many questions regarding ligament function remain unanswered, which is partly a result of the inherent limitations of this test method. The results of this technique depend on the order of ligament cutting, and the applied external loads are those that will cause the greatest clinically observable difference in displacement from normal for a given ligamentous deficit, which is not necessarily a functional situation.

An alternate approach was introduced by Noyes and others.[6] Their test methodology involved determining the relative restraint provided by knee ligaments during controlled input displacements that occur in clinical laxity tests with the goal of sharpening the diagnostic value of the laxity test. This has proved to be a fruitful approach, but also leaves many questions unanswered, since it is directed toward diagnosis instead of actual ligament function.

Since the question of the function of ligaments is unanswered, it will remain an area of research for some time. However, this research takes on a greater urgency as a result of the increased interest in the surgical reconstruction of knees with ligament deficiencies. Methods and criteria for evaluating surgical ligamentous reconstructions are needed, but are not available partly because previous work has

☐ Supported by grant no. G008300070 from the National Institute of Handicapped Research, Department of Education, Washington, D.C.

concentrated on the analysis of clinical diagnostic tests rather than on defining the required function of knee ligaments.

We propose a different approach, one that would initially establish the mechanical function of ligaments. After mechanical ligament function is clarified, evaluation of surgical substitutes should become more evident and generally provide a more solid basis on which to approach problems of the knee. In spite of the long history of knee ligament research, there is little known about the detailed functioning of ligaments. For example, do ligaments help stabilize all external joint loads or only traumatic loads? The answer is unknown. Determining the functional significance of ligaments is obviously a long-term project, and definitive statements cannot be provided in this chapter. However, two projects will be described that approach the knee from the point of clarifying the functional significance of ligamentous tissue.

In the first project, ligament force transducers were installed on the four major cruciate and collateral ligament bands of fresh knee specimens, and the in vitro ligament forces were measured for a wide range of external load directions. The thesis was that any given ligament carries load (or functions) over a wide range of external load directions and that these external loads are often different from and occur in addition to external loads applied during clinical laxity testing. The goal of this project was to catalogue ligament forces during these external load conditions.

In the second project, the same ligament force transducers were surgically installed on the in vivo collateral ligaments in the stifle (knee) joints of living dogs, and ligament forces were measured during functional activities. These tests demonstrate the close interaction between muscles and ligaments that occurs during in vivo function.

HYPOTHESIS OF LIGAMENT FUNCTION

The goal of this type of project is to establish and support a hypothesis on ligament function that can be tested by further experimentation. The hypothesis suggested by the projects to be described is as follows.

Ligaments serve a high and low load function. The high load function is to stabilize the joint against external loads that act too rapidly for the muscles to equilibrate or are too large to be stabilized by the muscles. Ligament strength is important to this function. The low load function is to maintain proper joint kinematics to allow adequate joint lubrication and muscle function to occur. Ligament geometry (i.e., origin and insertion location) and ligament load–deflection characteristics at low loads are also important to this function. Most ligament function is the low load type, and only occasional high load function occurs during traumatic situations. Intermediate load function can occur, especially in the pathologic joint. Each ligamentous band functions over a wide range of external joint load directions.

This hypothesis is not original, since parts of it have been suggested by other researchers[5,7] throughout the years. However, the proposition and testing of a hypothesis is a logical approach to a better understanding of ligament function. It is offered as a testable hypothesis to be revised as experiments proceed.

IN VITRO HUMAN STUDY

In the first project, ligament force buckle transducers were used to directly measure forces in all or portions of the cruciate and collateral ligaments of seven fresh knee specimens that were subjected to a wide variety of low level external loads. The objective was to catalogue external load directions that will load particular ligaments, that is, to better define the functional load ranges of the knee ligaments. Although these cadaver tests do not include the effect of musculature, the ligament force data generated provide useful functional information.

Methods and materials

Buckle transducers (Fig. 12-1) are small devices that, when force calibrated, are capable of directly measuring the tension in flexible biologic structures. The transducers were introduced by Salmons[5] and were applied by Lewis and others[3] to the measurement of knee ligament forces in vitro[2] and in vivo.[4] The transducers consist of a rectangular stainless steel frame on which strain gages are bonded and a removable crossbar that is seated on the frame. The transducer is installed by manipulating the ligament through the inner portion of the frame so that the crossbar is seated on the frame yet under the ligament (Fig. 12-2). The ligamentous fibers are slightly deflected from their normal configuration. Tension in the ligament causes it to straighten itself by pushing against the crossbar and thus deforming the crossbar and frame. The strain gages on the frame sense this deformation and give an output proportional to the ligament force.

Seven fresh cadaver knee specimens were obtained from above-the-knee amputations. The specimens were without contractures, abnormal ligamentous laxity, or significant degenerative arthritic changes. The specimens were kept moist throughout testing with saline solution. The tibia, fibula, and femur were transected approximately 15 cm proximal and distal to the joint space (Fig. 12-3). All soft tissues

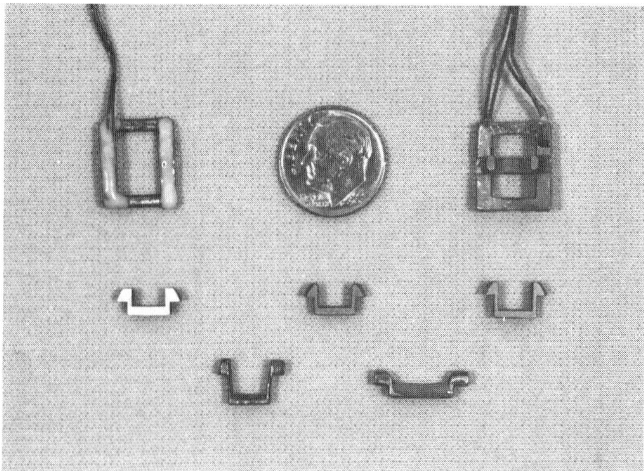

Fig. 12-1. Representative buckle transducer designs used in project.

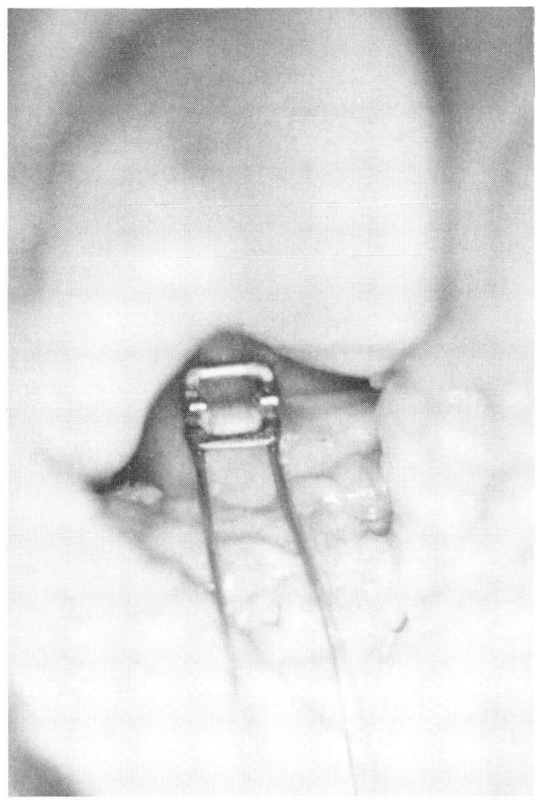

Fig. 12-2. Buckle transducer installed on anterior half of in vitro anterior cruciate ligament.

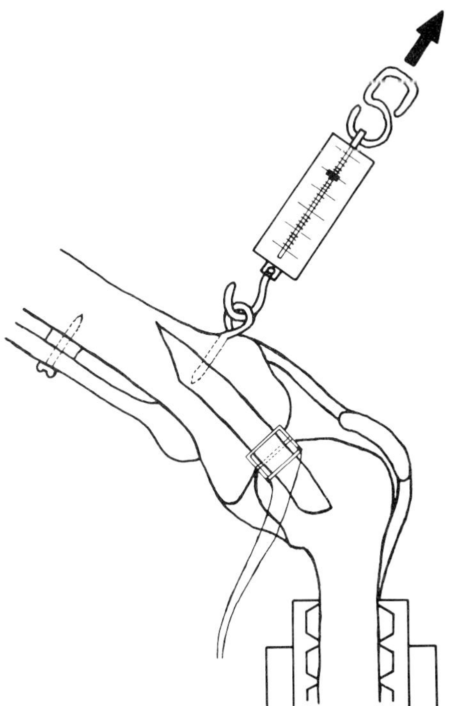

Fig. 12-3. Sketch of in vitro experimental setup.

were removed except the ligaments, capsular structures, and patellar complex. The fibula was secured to the tibia with a bone screw. Seven eyebolts were attached to the tibia so that calibrated spring scales could be used to manually apply a variety of external loads through the eyebolts to the knee specimen. The eyebolts were placed in specific locations on each of the seven tibias relative to bony landmarks so that external load magnitudes were known and were the same from specimen to specimen.

Buckle transducers were installed on the following ligament bands: (1) the anteromedial band of the anterior cruciate ligament, (2) the posterior half of the posterior cruciate ligament, (3) the anterior portion of the superficial band of the medial collateral ligament, and (4) the entire lateral collateral ligament. Buckles were not installed on an entire cruciate ligament because of space limitations in the intercondylar region. Current buckle designs could not accommodate an entire cruciate cross section, although buckle transducers could be designed to do so. Even though each entire cruciate ligament was not instrumented, measurement of forces in ligamentous bands provides important implications regarding the function of the entire ligament.

The femur of each specimen was securely clamped in a vise, and the tibia was allowed to flex freely and extend over the femur (Fig. 12-3). Buckle transducer output was fed into a four-channel Beckman strip chart recorder (Model R611). Impingement of the buckle transducers with bone or soft tissue that could potentially lead to a false output was checked for and eliminated before actual testing by a detection technique.[3] The effect of ligament shortening on the distribution of ligament forces around the knee as a result of the presence of the buckle transducers was also routinely detected by a technique described by Lewis and others[3] and was minimized by the proper relation of buckle crossbar depth and the amount of tissue contained in the transducer. A slight amount of shortening is unavoidable, since the operation of a buckle depends on a loaded ligament straightening itself and deforming the crossbar and frame. However, it has been shown that the shortening effect can be quantified and minimized and that it does not significantly alter knee ligament mechanics around the joint. Each buckle transducer–ligament complex was force calibrated in situ several times throughout the test procedure, using a method previously described by Lewis and others.[3]

After these preliminary preparations a variety of low level external load conditions was manually applied to each specimen by one or more calibrated spring scales acting through appropriate tibial eyebolts at 0, 20, 45, and 90 degrees of flexion. When given the location of the eyebolts and the fact that all spring scales were loaded to 44.5 N (10 pounds of force), the approximate magnitude of the basic load states at each of the flexion angles was (1) anterior- and posterior-directed force, 44.5 N; (2) internal and external rotation, 3.7 Nm; (3) varus, 3.9 Nm; (4) valgus, 4.2 Nm; (5) hyperextension, 4.5 Nm; and (6) passive unloaded flexion. All possible combinations of two of the basic load states were also applied at each of the flexion angles, for example, posterior force + valgus and hyperextension + internal rotation. The load directions (orientation of the spring scales) and specimen flexion angles were visually estimated. As a result of this manual load application technique, buckle ligament forces were found to be repeatable within an average of 10%.

Results

Selected results from this project are summarized in Fig. 12-4 to 12-8. The solid bars in these figures represent the mean ligament forces as a result of the application of the indicated basic external load directions to the series of specimens. Only mean ligament forces significantly different from zero force are presented as determined by a 90% confidence interval. The following observations can be made from this and other data not included in the figures:

1. Ligaments were not significantly loaded during passive unloaded flexion.

2. Each ligament band responded to a wide variety of external load directions.

3. The anteromedial band of the anterior cruciate ligament was highly loaded during several load conditions near extension—anterior force, varus, and internal rotation.

4. The posterior half of the posterior cruciate ligament was highly loaded for various external load directions near 90 degrees of flexion—posterior force, varus-valgus, and internal-external rotation.

5. The medial collateral ligament was highly loaded during internal-external rotation and valgus throughout the flexion range.

6. The lateral collateral ligament was highly loaded during varus and external rotation throughout the flexion range.

7. The anteromedial half of the anterior cruciate ligament and both collateral ligaments were highly loaded during hyperextension.

8. Combinations of the basic external load directions changed respective ligament forces in an additive but nonlinear manner. If a ligament was highly loaded during two basic load conditions applied separately, a combination of those load directions also produced a high force in the ligament (Fig. 12-8).

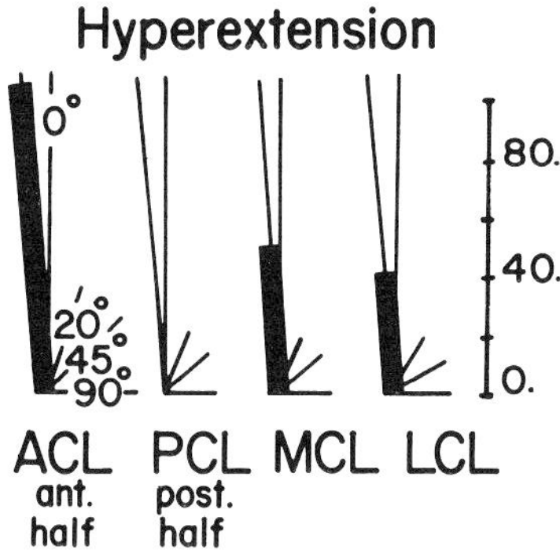

Fig. 12-4. Mean ligament forces (in newtons) from seven specimens subjected to hyperextension load condition.

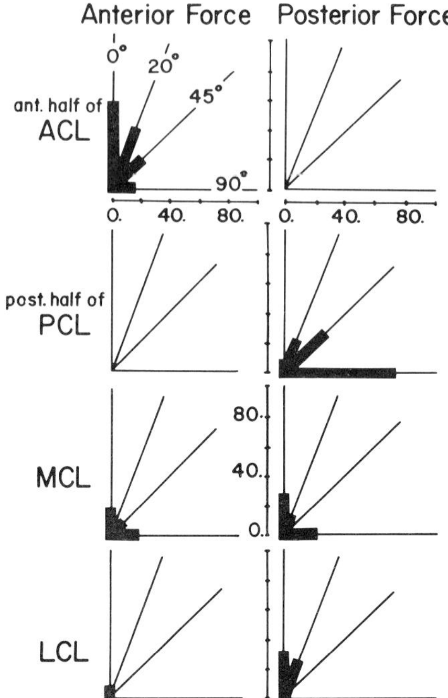

Fig. 12-5. Mean ligament forces (in newtons) from specimens to which anterior (seven knees) and posterior (six knees) directed force load states were applied.

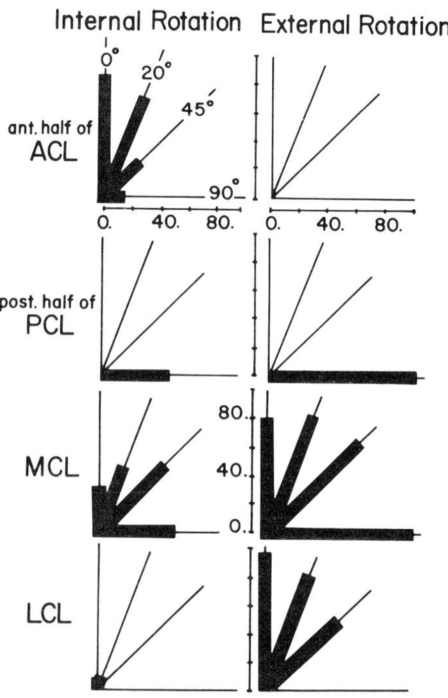

Fig. 12-6. Mean ligament forces (in newtons) from knees subjected to internal (seven specimens) and external (six specimens) rotation load conditions.

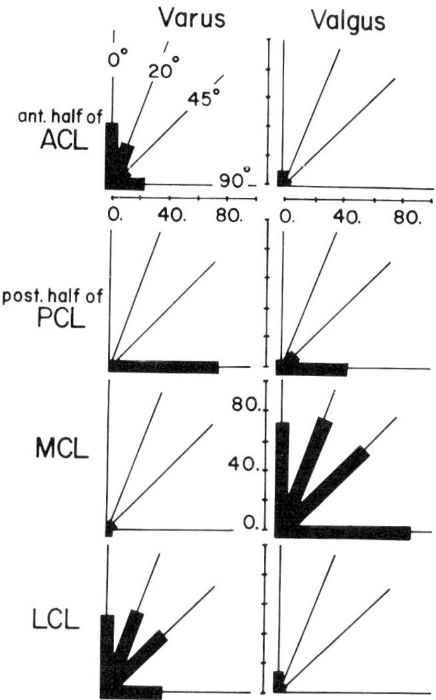

Fig. 12-7. Mean ligament forces (in newtons) from specimens subjected to varus (seven knees) and valgus (six knees) load states.

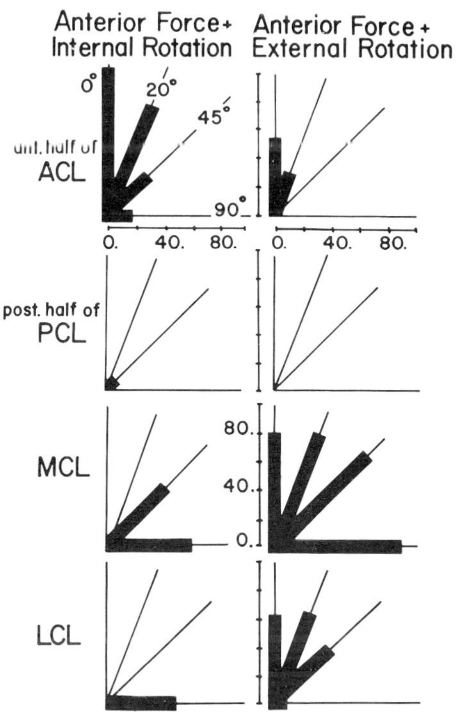

Fig. 12-8. A typical result of the combination of basic load states showing mean ligament forces (in newtons) during anterior force + internal rotation and anterior force + external rotation.

9. A large amount of scatter in ligament force data exists among the seven specimens for given load conditions. The mean percent error (standard deviation) for each instrumented ligament-ligament band during load cases in which the ligament was significantly loaded is as follows: anteromedial half of the anterior cruciate, 60%; posterior half of the posterior cruciate, 98%; medial collateral, 66%; and lateral collateral, 61%. The contribution of experimental errors to this scatter, such as bony impingement, ligament shortening, in situ calibration, repeatability of manual load application, inability to position eyebolts in precisely the same locations in each of the specimens, and inability to instrument precisely the same ligamentous bands in each of the specimens, were quantified, and it was estimated that they accounted for approximately one half of the ligament force scatter. It was therefore concluded that the remaining half of the scatter was caused by the biologic or anatomic variability among the specimens, that is, differences in bony geometry and soft tissue attachment. It is suggested that anatomic differences among the knees of individuals have a substantial effect on ligament function.

10. The proposed ligament force data correlate with mechanisms of ligamentous injury; that is, ligament bands that were highly loaded during the in vitro test situation are frequently found to be injured or torn (as is the entire ligament) as the result of a functional in vivo injury mechanism with a similar external load direction yet of higher magnitude. For example, the posterior half of the posterior cruciate ligament was found to be highly loaded during application of posterior force at 90 degrees of flexion (Fig. 12-5). The entire posterior cruciate ligament is often torn as a result of a direct blow to the anterior aspect of the tibia with the knee in flexion as occurs in a classic dashboard injury. Figs. 12-4 and 12-6 indicate that the anteromedial band of the anterior cruciate ligament is highly loaded in hyperextension and internal rotation at extension. An athlete who is running and attempts a cutting maneuver in which he suddenly turns toward his planted foot and subjects the tibia to internal rotation at extension sometimes sustains an isolated anterior cruciate injury in which the entire ligament is torn. Thus the experimental results are supported by clinical observations. The results show that any given ligamentous band resists external joint loads for a wide range of directions, not only those used in diagnostic testing.

IN VIVO CANINE STUDY

The second project was directed at understanding the in vivo function of ligaments and how they interact with muscle function. In vitro specimen studies as just described provide an indication of ligament function during the absence of muscular activity, which might be expected to occur during a traumatic mechanism of injury when the external load occurs too rapidly for muscles to equilibrate, with the ligaments providing the only constraint. However, in vivo studies must also be conducted to directly assess the effect of muscular activity on ligament function. In this project, buckle ligament force transducers were installed on the collateral ligaments of canine stifle (knee) joints with ligament forces being monitored during clinical laxity tests and several functional states. Since these tests are difficult to perform and data were taken on only two dogs postoperatively, the conclusions must be considered preliminary. These conclusions are presented because they are the only data we are aware of that measure in vivo ligament forces during functional activities.

Methods and materials

The buckle transducers were surgically installed on the collateral ligaments of the knees of two dogs. Each dog weighed approximately 20 kg. The lateral collateral ligament of the right knee of animal A and both medial collateral ligaments of animal B gave usable data. Data were collected from animal A 10 days after transducer implantation surgery and from animal B 1 day after surgery. Leads from the strain gages were passed subcutaneously up the hind leg to the back of each animal and were made accessible through an exit wound that was allowed to heal with lead wires in place. During testing the animals appeared to function normally for approximately one-half hour, which suggests the surgery had minimal effect on the joint mechanics, since the buckles were extracapsular. However, after the half-hour test the dogs seemed to favor the leg that underwent operation.

The strain gages on the buckle of animal A were foil gages, Micromeasurements EA-06-031DE-120, and those on the buckles in animal B were semiconductor gages, BLH SPB1-12-12. The strain gage outputs were recorded on a Beckman Dynograph Model R611 strip chart recorder.

The first procedure was to perform clinical laxity tests on each instrumented canine joint, such as is done when assessing ligamentous integrity during diagnostic examination of the human knee. This consisted of manually applying selected external loads to the joint, especially those that were thought to load the collateral ligaments, such as internal-external rotation at extension and varus-valgus at extension. Passive flexion-extension and hyperextension were also applied. The transducer output was recorded during these external clinical laxity loads. During human clinical laxity tests the patient is asked to relax the muscles, and it is assumed that the ligaments carry all the applied external load. In the dog such cooperation is not assured. However, the muscle bundles (especially the hamstrings) appeared to be lax, which was determined by palpation during the test procedure, and it was felt that the ligaments were providing the only constraints. The objective of these tests was to intentionally load the instrumented ligament to provide a comparison with functional external loads. Not all transducers were calibrated for force so these tests provided a necessary standard. In humans, joint loads used in clinical laxity tests are approximately 10% of the loads necessary to cause ligamentous injury.[5] It is assumed the clinical laxity test loads for the animals were the same.

In the second set of tests, buckle outputs were recorded during the following functional activities: (1) walking and turning on level ground, (2) trotting on level ground, (3) dropping from approximately 30 cm and landing on all four feet, (4) static loading of approximately 100 N over the back legs with minimal position change from standing, (5) stepping over a 25 cm barrier, and (6) a sudden unexpected valgus load applied to the joint by a rope tied to the canine limb.

It was planned to force calibrate the buckles after performing the above tests; however, all but one transducer failed before removal so only one buckle was calibrated. This was done by directly loading a nylon strap of approximately the same cross section as the canine ligament as it passed through the buckle transducer in question.

Results

In vivo canine ligament–buckle transducer responses during the clinical laxity external loads are shown in Fig. 12-9 for the lateral collateral ligament of animal A and the right medial collateral ligament of animal B. Buckle responses for the same ligaments during the functional tests are shown in Fig. 12-10. The traces are uncalibrated for force. The gains of the transducers were identical for the laxity tests and the functional tests so the amplitudes of the traces in the two figures for each ligament are directly comparable. Buckle transducer responses for each of two ligaments were normalized relative to their maximum values as shown in Fig. 12-11.

The collateral ligaments of the canine knee would be expected to behave similarly to those in the human knee, although there will likely be some significant differences. The response to the clinical laxity tests was therefore about as expected. That is, the lateral collateral was loaded in varus and external rotation at extension, and the medial collateral was loaded in valgus and internal-external rotation at extension. There is a small but measurable ligament load in unloaded flexion-extension, but the magnitude varies from negligible in subject A to 20% of the maximum in the right medial collateral ligament of subject B. This variability may be indicative of ligament shortening caused by the presence of the buckle in subject B. This is certainly a small effect, but represents an upper bound on the error caused by shortening. If shortening is the cause of this ligament force, it implies that the lengths of the ligaments and bony geometry are such that low ligament forces result from normal unloaded flexion-extension joint motion.

The variability in precisely duplicating the clinical laxity tests with regard to repeatably loading the ligaments is shown in several of the traces in Fig. 12-9, for example, internal rotation and valgus for the right medial collateral ligament of subject B. The repeatability is less than perfect partly because of the inability to manually repeat the external force magnitude and its direction.

When these observations are taken into account, several conclusions become apparent from the in vivo clinical and functional data:

1. In level walking there was minimal ligament force, although there was increased ligament force during turning, particularly in the lateral collateral.

2. Ligament force during trotting was slightly greater than during level walking (approximately 20%).

3. Ligament force from dropping the dog from 30 cm was slightly greater than that during level walking. The dog seemed to be ready for the resulting external load and absorbed all of it with muscle activity.

4. Increased joint contact force does not necessarily increase ligament force for

CLINICAL LAXITY LOADS

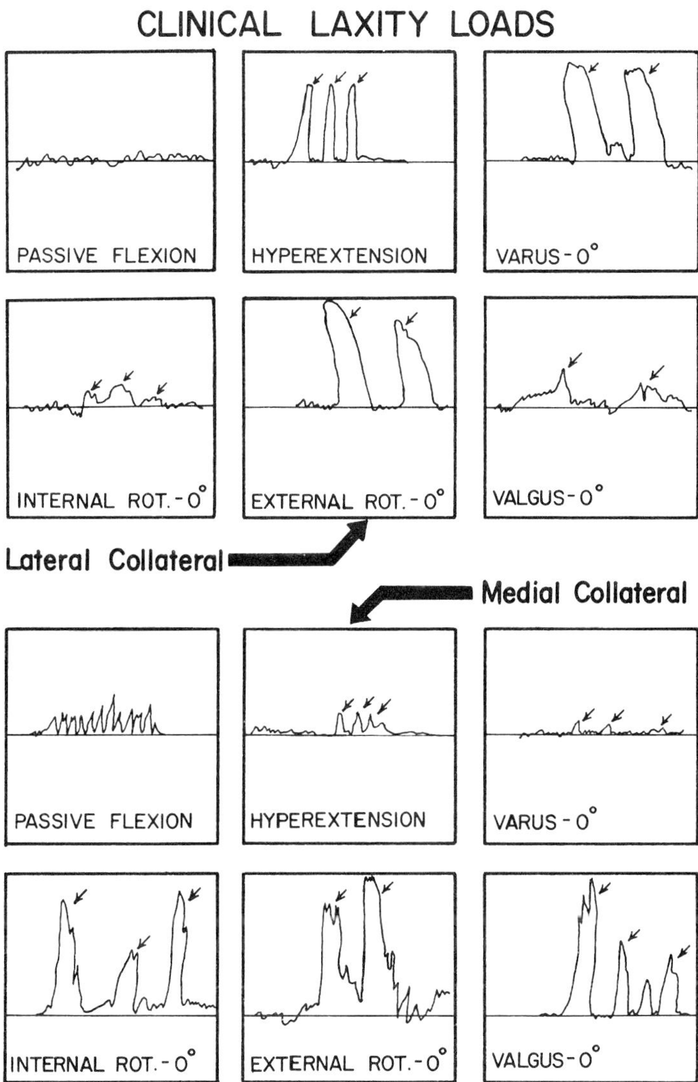

Fig. 12-9. Traces representing in vivo canine ligament forces during passive flexion-extension and other clinical laxity loads applied at extension for instrumented lateral collateral ligament of animal A and right medial collateral ligament of animal B.

a controlled position. In fact, for the static load case tested (constant vertical load on the hind legs) ligament loads were the smallest functional forces recorded, which implies the external load was stabilized by increased joint contact forces and by the muscles in isometric contraction.

5. While stepping over a stool, ligament forces were slightly higher than during level walking (approximately 25%).

6. Application of the sudden valgus load or "clip" to the knee produced one of

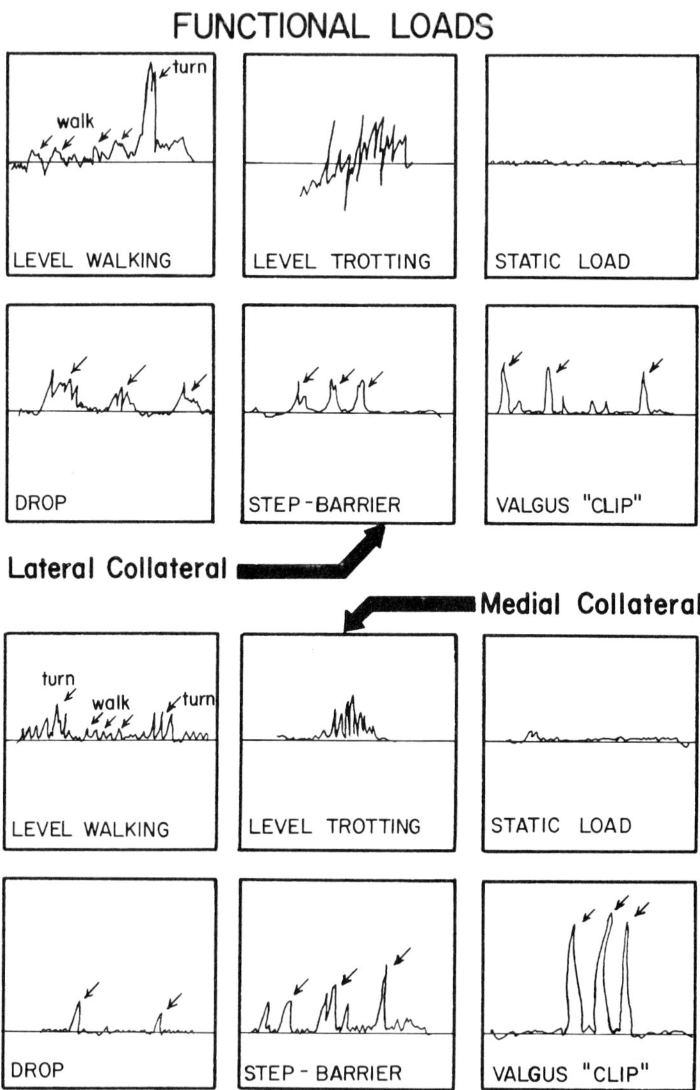

Fig. 12-10. Traces representing in vivo canine ligament loads during indicated functional activities for lateral collateral ligament of animal A and right medial collateral ligament of animal B.

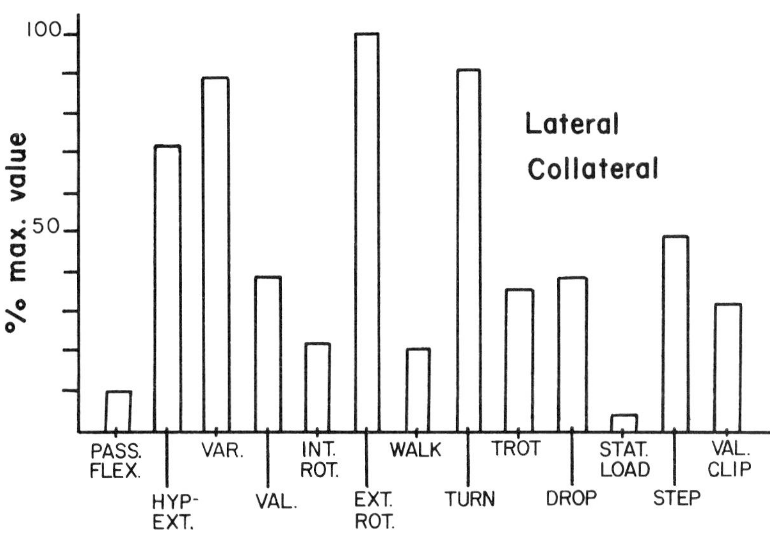

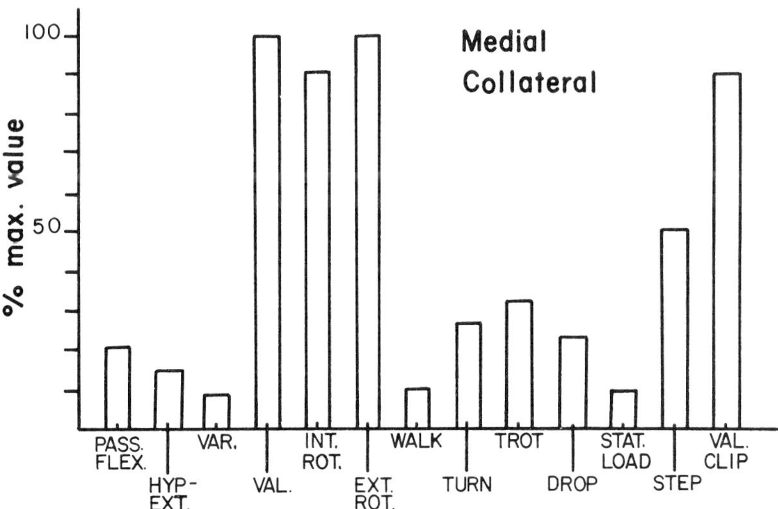

Fig. 12-11. Buckle transducer voltage responses in traces of Fig. 12-9 and 12-10 are normalized with respect to their maximum value for each ligament.

the largest functional responses (in the medial collateral) comparable in magnitude to the clinical laxity responses. The animals did not anticipate the application of the external load, and their ligaments provided the restraint, since the musculature could not react quickly enough.

7. For all three ligament measurements the largest ligament forces occurred during the clinical laxity tests. Except for the sudden valgus load when the animal was not able to react quickly enough, the ligament forces measured during the more "voluntary" dynamic functions were small but not negligible and were substantially higher during turning (in the lateral collateral). For the one calibrated transducer the largest force measured was approximately 18 N. With the exception of the lateral collateral during turning and the medial collateral during the valgus clip the functional ligament loads recorded were all less than 38% of the maximum clinical laxity test load for animal A and less than 50% and 25% of the maximum clinical laxity test loads of the two ligaments for animal B. Since the clinical laxity test ligament forces are far below failure loads for the ligaments, the functional ligament forces must be negligible in relation to the failure loads. This conclusion is also suppported by error sources that would tend to exaggerate smaller forces and have less effect on higher forces.

DISCUSSION

The in vitro project demonstrates that each ligament or ligamentous band becomes loaded during a wide range of external joint load conditions (directions). Ligament forces as a result of these experimentally applied low magnitude external loads reflect actual ligament function during high level mechanisms of injury when ligaments provide the major knee restraint, since the traumatic load occurs too rapidly for musculature to equilibrate. This is substantiated by the correlation of the proposed forces in the ligaments-ligament bands with mechanisms of injury of similar load directions in which the entire ligament is torn or injured. Neither high nor low level functional ligament forces must be confused with the ligament response in clinical laxity tests, since the functional situations are considerably more complex. Clinical diagnostic external loads are not necessarily functional, since they are chosen to visibly yield the greatest change in joint displacement because of the absence of a particular ligament. This project also demonstrates the effect of anatomic variability among individuals, particularly with regard to bony geometry and ligament attachment locations, on the mechanics of knee ligaments.

The in vivo canine project demonstrates the profound influence of muscle activity on ligament function and suggests that high level ligament function is relatively rare, occurring only during traumatic situations with the majority of knee ligament function of the low level type. During the functional activities when the animals were aware of the external loading situation, in vivo ligament forces were minimal compared to forces produced by clinical laxity loads (except for the lateral collateral during turning), which suggests that muscular activity and joint contact forces provide the major joint restraint during common low level functional activities. The hypothesis is also substantiated by the results of the sudden application of the valgus clip to the animals' knees. Ligament forces in this case were among the largest of the functional activities, since the animals were not aware of the situation and did not have time to voluntarily stabilize the traumatic external load with muscular activity. All ligament forces obtained during the in vivo study in both functional and diagnostic load situations were far below ligament failure levels.

Limitations

Several limitations exist with the experimentation used in the two projects. In the canine study, it was difficult to keep the buckle transducers operational in the in vivo surroundings. The major problem was buckle failure as a result of breakage in the strain gage lead wires caused by the constant motion of the animals and the presence of the in vivo fluids. The buckles inherently mask low level ligament force data and make it difficult to look at the details of the proposed low level functional region. This is because of noise that results from tension on the strain gage lead wires and from the unavoidable effect of the overlying layers of soft tissue covering the surgically implanted buckles. The in vivo study also did not address the basic question of how muscle forces are transferred to the ligaments in the pathologic knee. One specific problem with the proposed in vivo data is that ligament forces for animal B were recorded only 1 day postoperatively to make sure that data could be acquired before the buckle failed. It is not clear what effect this short recovery time had on the function of the animal, although the animal did not appear to be guarding the affected limb.

The in vitro project had many potential sources of error, but all were quantified and their contribution to the scatter in the proposed ligament force data was estimated. One limitation of this project is that current buckle designs could not accommodate the entire cross section of a cruciate ligament. Thus forces were measured for only specific cruciate bands. Because of the correlation between ligament band–force data and mechanisms of injury in which the entire ligament is frequently found to be torn, we feel that forces in a ligament band reflect the approximate function of the entire ligament, although there are probably significant differences. Experimental errors in this in vitro project could be reduced with improved buckle designs capable of accommodating a larger ligament and with an improved external load application technique.

Future directions

Both projects presented support the proposed hypothesis, although more extensive experimental verification is needed. Improvements with the design and use of the buckle transducers, particularly in the in vivo application, will be very helpful. One of the most important conclusions implied by the projects and the hypothesis is that little is known about the detailed functioning of ligamentous tissue. There is still much to be learned. We believe that improved treatment of knee ligament injuries will result from a better understanding of knee ligament function.

REFERENCES

1. Brantigan, O.C., and Voshell, A.F.: The mechanics of the ligaments and menisci of the knee joint, J. Bone Joint Surg. **23A**:45, 1941.
2. Lew, W.D., and Lewis, J.L.: The effect of knee-prosthesis geometry on cruciate ligament mechanics during flexion, J. Bone Joint Surg. **64A**:734, 1982.
3. Lewis, J.L., Lew, W.D., and Schmidt, J.: A note on the application and evaluation of the buckle transducer for knee ligament force measurement, J. Biomech. Eng. **104**:125, 1982.
4. Lewis, J.L., and Shybut, G.T.: In vivo forces in the collateral ligaments of canine knees, Trans. Orthop. Res. Soc. Las Vegas **6**:4, 1981.
5. Markolf, K.L., Graff-Radford, A., and Amstutz, H.C.: In vivo knee stability, J. Bone Joint Surg. **60A**:664, 1978.
6. Noyes, F.R., and others: Clinical biomechanics of the knee: ligament restraints and functional stability, In American Academy of Orthopaedic Surgeons: Symposium on the athlete's knee, St. Louis, 1980, The C.V. Mosby Co.
7. Pope, M.H., and others: The role of musculature in injuries to the medial collateral ligament, J. Bone Joint Surg. **61A**:398, 1979.
8. Salmons, S.: Meeting report: the Eighth International Conference on Medical and Biological Engineering, J. Biomed. Eng. **4**:467, 1969.

13. Models of ligament repairs and grafts

Edward S. Grood
David L. Butler
Frank R. Noyes

STAGES OF HEALING

It is common for the events that occur during healing of wounds to be classified into sequential time intervals or phases. Although the nomenclature used and the time intervals assigned by various researchers vary,[17,33,42,54] four phases are typically described: exudation, inflammation, proliferation, and maturation. The initial or exudation phase includes bleeding from the ruptured blood vessels, formation of a fibrin clot, and entrapment of blood cell elements. The inflammatory response following the initial bleeding phase involves the infiltration of many types of cells, including macrophages, polymorphonuclear cells, and other blood cell elements that aggregate around the injury site. Over the first few days a proliferation of fibroblasts occurs that is responsible for the subsequent synthesis of collagen and ground substance and may also be involved in the resorption of the structurally damaged collagen framework at the injury site.

In the early stages of healing the blood vessels show an increased permeability with exudation and associated swelling of the surrounding tissue. To support the increased metabolic demands of the resorption and reparative processes that occur after injury a capillary budding arises followed by a prolific vascular invasion that facilitates the transport of cells, nutrients, and metabolic waste products. The structural changes in the vasculature that occur have been studied using microangiographic techniques.* The vascular proliferation is often initially disorganized, but undergoes subsequent alignment with the direction of force transmission and tissue deformation.[20,21] Later in the healing process, during the maturation phase, the number of cells and the number of vessels will decrease toward the preinjury levels.

The cellular and vascular changes that occur are part of the response necessary to remove debris and fill defects, as well as an attempt to reestablish the extracellular

□ Supported in part by grant no. AM21172 and grant no. AM27517 from the National Institute of Arthritis, Diabetes, Digestive and Kidney Diseases.
* References 3, 5-8, 20, 30, 41, 42.

composition and microstructure of the ligament or tendon. The extent to which the preinjury microstructure is reestablished and the factors affecting this restructuring are still not worked out.

The early fibroblastic proliferation that occurs following injury supports the need for increased collagen and glycosoaminoglycan synthesis. What is known about the detailed sequence of events involved in collagen synthesis (i.e., transcription, translation, and hydroxylation), the secretion of tropocollagen molecules from the cell, and their assembly into an organized extracellular structure has recently been reviewed by Prockop and others.[43] Like the vascular invasion the early rebuilding of the collagen framework may be highly disorganized, requiring subsequent realignment of fibers with the load transmission axis and fiber maturation involving cross-linking in and between molecules to obtain strength. The initial disorganization of newly synthesized collagen, its uniting of opposing ends of the injury, and subsequent alignment are illustrated in Potenza's reports[46,47] on the healing of full-thickness wounds in canine flexor tendons. In addition, there is an increase over time in the diameter of the collagen fibrils. Studies on the healing of partial defects in the rabbit achilles tendon by Postacchini and Demartino[45] demonstrate the increase in the diameter of the collagen fibrils that occurs during the maturation phase. The increase in fibril diameter does not automatically occur and was notably absent in Postacchini's earlier study[44] of full-thickness defects where the opposing ends of a cut tendon were allowed to retract. Postacchini believed that the primary difference between their partial- and full-thickness models, which accounted for the observed difference in growth of fibril diameter, was the forces applied to the healing region. He argued that retraction of the ends of the full-thickness defect model shortened the muscle and put it in a less favorable position on its length-tension curve, which reduced the forces the muscle could produce and lowered the forces applied to the healing region. However, no forces were measured for either model, and the opposite argument could be made where the partial defect model was stress protected by the adjacent normal tendon while the full-thickness defect was required to transmit whatever reduced forces the shortened muscle applied to the tendon. Thus the stimuli that are responsible for fiber maturation and, specifically, the increase in collagen fibril diameter are not yet fully understood.

An elevated rate of collagen synthesis has been reported to persist for some time after the extracellular structure is apparently reconstituted.[31] It is unlikely that this continued synthesis represents excess collagen; rather it probably reflects continued structural development or the higher metabolic turnover of young collagen that has not cross-linked sufficiently to reduce its solubility and increase its inertness to the local biochemical-biomechanical environment.

FACTORS ALTERING HEALING

Many factors affect the processes that occur during healing. A clear understanding of the major factors is important when trying to interpret the literature or when comparing results from two or more studies. These factors include the animal species used, the age of the animals employed and their past level of activity, the tissue model selected, the method of injury and repair, and the postoperative treatment employed. The conclusions reached from the study will also depend on the evaluation methods employed and the time periods selected for evaluation.

Species choice

The most common species used are the dog* and rabbit,† although studies have been conducted in the rat,[31,52,53] cat,[29] and primates.[10,14] The differences in ligament healing between species have not been specifically studied, but it is reasonable to expect that tissue size and metabolic rate have strong influences on the rate of soft tissue healing just as they do on hard tissue healing. This is an important consideration when trying to extrapolate the results of experimental studies in animals to their application in the treatment of human patients, particularly with regard to specifying the time periods when a repair is sufficiently strong to allow resumption of certain activities.

Age and activity levels

Even in a species there may be significant differences between animals. Two major factors to be considered are previous activity levels of the animal and its age. Most experimental animals have been bred for laboratory use. This creates two problems. First, animal activity is limited by cage confinement, which produces an artificial disuse state. While it is not known if this alters the healing process, it does affect measurement of repair strength by increasing the incidence of bone avulsion fractures in normal control ligaments. One example of this is our unpublished study in purebred beagles. Since we were concerned with the effects of postoperative cage confinement, we arranged for care on a farm where the dogs could have ad lib activity in a larged fenced area. Late in the study we became concerned because mechanical testing of control bone-ligament-bone preparations yielded a high incidence of bone avulsion fractures. On further checking with the breeders we learned that the animals were raised in wire cages held above the ground to allow easy cleaning of the facilities. Only on a limited basis did the animals have a chance for activity. Although we cannot be certain, the limited activity of the animals may have resulted in increased bone porosity which led to the high incidence of bone avulsion fractures that occurred.

One approach to overcoming the problem of disuse is the use of wild captured animals. Wild captured primates are available, but increasing numbers are being raised in confined conditions for laboratory use. The mongrel from a dog pound may represent another wild captured animal with more normal levels of past activity. The problems in using wild captured animals include the unknown level of past activity, unknown past diseases, and unknown current age. Further, animal-to-animal vari-

---

* References 2, 4, 9, 12, 13, 15, 20, 21, 28, 33, 39, 40, 47-49.
† References 18, 22, 27, 44, 45, 50, 55.

ations are expected to be larger than if a genetically homogeneous purebred line is used. This is not a serious problem if conclusions can be based in intraanimal differences (e.g., right-left comparisons) or if a large number of animals are used.

The second major factor relates to the age of the experimental animal. Rabbits and purebred dogs are normally sold before closure of growth plates. The results of studies using such animals[18,19] must be carefully interpreted, keeping in mind the effect of growth hormones on the healing process. Unfortunately, it is common for researchers to report the use of adult animals without indicating how their age was verified. In rabbits the judgment of age is often based on animal weight, which may be an unreliable indicator.

Tissue model

Once the animal species is specified, including age and past history of the study group, a tissue model must be selected. Important differences exist between tendons, intraarticular ligaments, and extraarticular ligaments with regard to mechanical environment, biologic environment, and healing response. The healing response and biologic environment will be considered first while discussion of the difference in mechanical environment is deferred until later. The healing response in tendons appears to be fairly localized around the injury site, whereas the response in ligaments appears to be more diffuse and incorporates a much larger fraction of the tissue. Specifically Potenza's studies[46,47] show a local invasion of granulation tissue that fills the gap between the two ends of a divided flexor tendon. Arnoczky's studies[5] on revascularization of the anterior cruciate ligament following a partial-defect injury show a profuse vascular invasion through the entire body of the ligament. This extensive vascular proliferation seems to indicate a significant remodeling in uninjured tissue. However, it is not yet possible to exclude the traumatic effect of the surgery as the cause of the vascular response.

In contrast with the tendency to resorption in the injured and repaired anterior cruciate ligament,[5,38,39] the reparative process in tendons often produces a fibrous callus surrounding the injured area. Walker and others[55] found large increases in cross-sectional area at 5 months after repair of the achilles tendon. We noted that a similar callus developed following sharp surgical transection and repair of the patellar tendon in beagles. The development of a callus is not limited exclusively to tendons. Frank and others[19] reported an increase in cross-sectional area following injury to the medial collateral ligament. This suggests that the lack of callus development in the anterior cruciate ligament may be a result of its intraarticular location.

It has been suggested that the poor healing response of the anterior cruciate ligament is caused by deleterious effects of the synovial fluid. We remain unconvinced that normal synovial fluid has an adverse effect, because tendons are exposed to a similar fluid in their sheath, particularly in regions where they change direction and are exposed to lateral compressive loads.[22] We are not aware of any evidence that tendon healing is inhibited when injury occurs in these areas. When considering the effect of synovial fluid on ligament healing it is necessary to distinguish the influence of pathologic synovial fluid that occurs with osteoarthritis and other degenerative diseases of the knee separately from the influence of normal synovial fluid.

The major difference between the healing of intraarticular ligaments and extraarticular ligaments may be that the tissue surrounding the extraarticular ligaments offers an abundance of extrinsic blood vessels and nutrients that aid in initiating and maintaining the repair process. The intraarticular ligaments do not have a readily available blood supply surrounding them on all sides. Perhaps of greater importance is the tissue adjacent to extraarticular ligaments that provides a scaffold for the development of a callus. This is not available to the cruciate ligaments. Mankin[32] has suggested that the inability of partial-thickness defects in cartilage to heal may be caused by synovial fluid preventing adherence of a fibrin clot (available as a result of intraarticular bleeding), thereby depriving the cartilage of a necessary stimuli or the scaffold required to fill defects. A similar mechanism where clot adherence is prevented on the surface of the cruciate ligaments as a result of the presence of the synovial fluid and the intraarticular movement of the ligament is worth further investigation.

Method of injury and repair

The most common type of injury studied is a sharp scalpel division that produces a local disruption. A more diffuse traumatic injury has been simulated by only a few researchers,[18] typically by passing a suture or wire underneath the tissue and rapidly applying a force until rupture occurs. To our knowledge no researcher has done histologic studies to evaluate the extent or reproducibility of injuries generated by this technique, or how the injuries compare to in vivo trauma. Clearly the surgery required to expose the tissue being studied is important, since it will affect the local blood supply in adjacent tissue and in the tissue model being studied.

Once injury is produced it is important to consider the nature of the repair, including the types of sutures used and the specific surgical techniques employed. If no repair is performed, the tissue ends at the injury site retract. The influence of the gap produced on the initial repair and subsequent remodeling processes is not fully understood. However, any loss of continuity of the ligament or tendon ends has been reported to have a significant deleterious effect.[30,38-40] If a repair is performed, the type of suture material used, as well as the stitch employed, will affect the initial repair strength[30] and subsequent return in strength.[27] Significant reductions in tensile strength and stiffness have been reported as a result of simply suturing undivided tendon.[27] This effect was not just a result of mechanical trauma and interruption of blood supply, but was also influenced by the type of suture material used.

Mechanical environment

Postoperative care. Once the wound is closed the postoperative care given must be considered, since it partly determines the mechanical environment (force and motion) and dictates whether appropriate or excessive tension is provided to the healing tissue. The level of forces placed on ligaments in the postoperative period after repair or reconstruction is highly variable and difficult to control. This is true in experimental animals as well as in humans, where a number of factors, such as use of cast braces, splints, and crutches, affect the forces applied to the repaired tissues.

The influence of force and motion on both normal and healing tissues is of interest, particularly because of recent advocation of early and continuous passive-motion programs. The application of early motion after ligament repair or reconstruction raises two important questions. First, what are the forces imposed on the repair-reconstruction, and second, are effects beneficial or are the forces produced so large that disruption or stretching of weak tissues occurs? These questions need to be answered if early motion programs are to be successfully used following ligament repair or reconstruction. Studies indicate that forces applied to the anterior cruciate ligament during active knee extension are greatest from 30 degrees of flexion to full extension.[24,51] This suggests that active terminal extension exercises with weights should be avoided early after repair, particularly if the surgeon feels the tissues are weak. It is often possible, however, to maintain early knee motion after certain ligament repairs or reconstructions. The surgeon must employ the use of certain suture techniques and high strength grafts providing sufficient initial strength to allow immediate passive or active-assisted knee motion. In addition to range of movement, the attachment location, the initial tension placed on the repair, and the flexion angle of the knee at the time of repair-implantation will also determine the magnitude of in vivo forces imposed.[25] The effect of these parameters is a result of their influence on the changes in tissue length that occur with knee motion.[26]

Given an appropriately installed graft and a proper program of passive motion, the question still remains if there are any benefits to the graft caused by the motion. Preliminary studies[10,11] indicate that 3 weeks of intermittent passive motion (16 hr/day, 7 days a week) in a primate does not affect the strength of either free or vascularized patellar tendon graft replacements of the anterior cruciate ligament. We believe early passive motion may be highly beneficial in lessening articular cartilage disuse changes. However, its effect on ligament healing remains speculative.

Internal forces. The mechanical environment is not completely determined by external forces, such as the weights used during rehabilitation exercises. In addition, the internal forces resulting from muscle contraction must be considered. In this regard there are significant differences between tendons and ligaments. Tendons attach muscle to bone so that some force is transmitted through all full-thickness injuries even in the presence of significant retraction at the cut or ruptured ends. Thus the healing region is seldom totally unloaded unless the involved joint can be placed in a position that shortens the muscle sufficiently to make it completely ineffective.

In contrast, ligaments are attached to bone at both ends, and forces can only be induced when these ends separate sufficiently to strain the repair site. If the ligament retracts after it is ruptured and the gap fills with new tissue, the length of the ligament is effectively increased. This longer structure will remain slack unless large, abnormal bone motions occur that are sufficient to induce a strain. Although contraction of skin wounds is a well-known mechanism for closing defects, there is only limited evidence[19] that this phenomenon is capable of restoring a ruptured ligament to its original length and returning joint laxity to normal. This suggests that the in vivo forces that are applied to the injury-repair site may be significantly different for tendons and ligaments.

LIGAMENT REPAIR MODELS
Anterior cruciate ligament

Healing has been studied in a number of knee ligament repair models including the anterior cruciate ligaments,[5,10,38,39] the lateral collateral ligaments,[16,40] and the medial collateral ligaments.[18,19,29,52] O'Donoghue and others[38] reported the largest return of strength of all the anterior cruciate repair models. After a 3½-year period, strength was 40% of control. The reported return in strength is an overestimate of the true return, since O'Donoghue was unable to determine the strength of the normal anterior cruciate ligament. This is because the tibia fractured where it was gripped before the ligament ruptured. Studies by Cabaud and others[12] on healing of anterior cruciate ligaments in the rhesus monkey and the dog are consistent with O'Donoghue's findings and the reported inability of the body to fill partial defects created in the ligament.[5] Overall the results from animal studies suggest a long period of low strength following primary repair of the anterior cruciate ligament.

Lateral collateral ligament

Healing of primary repairs in the lateral collateral ligament was investigated by O'Donoghue and others[40] in dogs. Both histologic and mechanical changes were measured. Our unpublished data on the healing of traumatically induced lateral collateral ligament injuries in purebred beagles are consistent with O'Donoghue's results and demonstrate just under a 50% return in strength at 6 months. In contrast, a patellar tendon repair model in the same animal returned to 100% of normal strength by 6 months, illustrating the differences in response between ligament and tendons.

Medial collateral ligament

The medial collateral ligament is an unusual healing model in that several investigators have reported a complete return in strength in time periods that are short in terms of what is known about soft tissue healing. Studies by Clayton and Weir[15] and Vailas and others[52] show recovery to normal control strength between 6 and 8 weeks. The agreement of these studies makes it difficult to disregard their results. However, we believe there are several explanations for the rapid return of strength found in the medial collateral by these researchers. First, the strength of the control ligaments may be low, since failure of the medial collateral most often occurs at its tibial attachment. Thus failure tests may measure the strength of the attachment of the ligament and not the strength of the ligament itself. Our studies on wild captured rhesus monkeys demonstrated that the medial collateral ligament failed at a maximum stress of 70 megapascals (MPa),[23] a value not too dissimilar from the values we found for the anterior cruciate (66 MPa) in the rhesus.[34] However, from the data presented by Vailas and others[52] on the strength of the medial collateral in rats, we have estimated a failure stress of less than 20 MPa. This suggests significant disuse effects may be acting in the rat model they used.

A second problem with the medial collateral ligament repair model, which we noted in the beagle, was that the ligament appeared to be under considerable tension. When the ligament was divided, the ends retracted and made it difficult to obtain a good surgical approximation. Ultimately we abandoned the medial collateral in favor of the lateral collateral because of these problems.

The most recent studies on healing of the medial collateral ligament were conducted in immature rabbits by Frank and co-workers.[18,19] Using a comprehensive battery of evaluation methods including histologic, biochemical, and biomechanical analyses, they found that ruptured and unrepaired medial collateral ligaments returned to 63% of control strength by 14 weeks. From 14 to 40 weeks the strength changed little even though significant changes occurred in measured biochemistry, indicating a return toward normal control values. This dissociation of biochemical and biomechanical changes in the maturation phase of healing may be explained by the characteristics of these two analysis methods along with the observed heterogeneity of the tissue from histologic evaluation. Since it is necessary to have adequate amounts of material for biochemical assay, tissue samples normally include not only the repair site but also adjacent more normal tissue. Subsequent homogenization before analysis results in values representative of the average behavior in the tissue. Mechanical testing, however, yields values representative of the weakest link in the tissue. Thus even if the majority of the tissue heals normally, strength may remain low because of small local areas of weakness that have little influence on biochemical measurements.

GRAFT MODELS

The healing of ligament grafts is more complicated than the healing of primary repairs. One characteristic that distinguishes ligament grafts from ligament repairs is the healing of the attachment of the graft. This may involve healing at the soft tissue–to–soft tissue, soft tissue–to–cancellous bone, or bone-to-bone interfaces, depending on the graft tissue employed and the method of attachment. The necessity for healing of the attachment of the graft offers an additional opportunity for failure that primary ligament repair avoids. Furthermore, the location of the attachment and the composition (structure) of the graft will affect both the length of the fibers in the graft and the strain the fiber bundles experience during various activities and joint motions. In addition, a variety of different tissues have been used for grafts, including the iliotibial band,[28,38] central and medial portions of the patellar tendon,*

---

* References 1, 4, 6, 9, 10, 14, 28, 36.

and the semitendinosus tendon.[50] Significant differences exist among these tissues with regard to initial strength[37] and likely with regard to healing potential.

In spite of these differences there are many similarities between the healing of primary repairs and the biologic changes that occur in the substance of the graft tissue. O'Donoghue,[38] using standard histologic techniques, reported that iliotibial band graft replacements of the anterior cruciate ligament undergo a revascularization process. Alm and co-workers,[1,3,4] Arnoczky and others,[6] Clancy and others,[14] and our group[10,11] made similar observations using the central and medial thirds of patellar tendon as graft materials, whereas Roth and Kennedy[50] reported revascularization of the semitendinosus anterior cruciate ligament replacement.

The occurrence of revascularization along with the observed histologic changes demonstrates that an active remodeling process occurs in the substance of the graft. This raises a question about the ultimate fate of the collagen in the graft at the time of its implantation. Using radioactive labeling techniques, Klein and others[31] reported that achilles tendon allografts undergo a one-for-one replacement of old mature collagen with weaker immature collagen. Based on histologic evidence a similar replacement of collagen in autografts most likely occurs, though not necessarily on a one-for-one basis. This suggests that significant decreases must occur in the strength of the graft substance after transplantation.

The changes in graft strength over time have been measured for many of the tissues employed. Ryan and Drompp[49] reported less than 20% of control strength at 26 weeks using the central third of the patellar tendon. O'Donoghue and others[38] reported less than 35% of control strength at 3½ years with strength on the decline when the iliotibial band was used to replace the anterior cruciate in dogs. The largest values of graft strength were reported by Clancy and others,[14] who measured recovery to 50% of control strength at 1 year using patellar tendon grafts. Roth and Kennedy[50] found less than 15% control strength after 26 weeks employing the semitendinosus tendon. Our preliminary results indicate 27% of control strength for a vascularized patellar tendon graft (medial third) after 26 weeks in cynomolgus monkeys. Hulse and others[28] and Butler and others[9] combined the iliotibial band with the lateral portion of the patellar tendon and found only a 28% return of strength in 26 weeks.

The reporting of graft strength as a percentage of control has several difficulties that need to be recognized when interpreting results. First, there is the problem of correctly measuring control values that may be affected by the previous activity levels of the animal model used[35] and by the test method. Related variables, such as rate[34] and method of tissue alignment during testing, also affect the uniformity of loading and the resulting ultimate tensile strength. Activity level is important because disuse like that induced by confinement in small cages produces bone loss resulting in increased incidence of bone avulsion fractures that occur at lower strains and loads.[34] As noted earlier we found that a high level of bone avulsion failures occurred when we measured the strength of control tissues in purebred beagles raised for laboratory research. This was one of the major reasons we have used wild captured cynomolgus monkeys in our recent studies. As expected, the incidence of bone avulsion was reduced to a relatively low incidence consistent with our previous studies in rhesus monkeys.[34]

To reduce the test-related problem of nonuniform loading, we now use cast grips fabricated by driving a pin through the long axis of the anterior cruciate ligament in a control knee and casting the entire preparation in plaster of Paris. The plaster was formed to the desired grip shape and used to prepare a sand mold for casting. The resulting cast grips were machined so that the mounting surfaces were perpendicular to the pin that had been passed through the anterior cruciate ligament. These grips hold the tibia and femur at odd angles that result in a vertical orientation of the anterior cruciate ligament and an anatomic orientation of the bone ends.

We have not directly compared ligament strength values measured using these grips with strength values measured using more conventional grips in the same bone-ligament-bone model. We have measured failure stresses in femur–anterior cruciate ligament–tibia units in cynomolgus monkeys that are significantly higher than the values we previously measured in the rhesus monkey using more conventional grips.

The importance of this is that higher values of control strength result in lower reported strength in repair and graft tissue when the results are expressed on a percentage basis. The opposite is also true, and inadequate testing methods that produce low values of strength in control tissues result in apparently better healing of the repair or graft model. The classic examples are O'Donoghue's study[38,39] on the anterior cruciate ligament in the dog. O'Donoghue was unable to measure the tensile strength of normal anterior cruciate ligament, because the tibia always fractured through a hole placed in it for gripping purposes.

Another important factor in interpreting results is whether the reported control values reflect the strength of the original graft tissue or the strength of the ligament being replaced. The former indicates how the tissue changed as a result of transplantation, and the latter indicates the extent to which the graft replaces the functional capacity of the normal ligament.

Besides the difficulty in correctly measuring the control values there are other important variables not often reported in the literature. Abnormal hypertrophy of the tissue and tissue adhesions are factors that might contribute to increased strength, but do not necessarily reflect a return to normal properties of the ligament or its effect on joint function. The function of a ligament results from the individual action of its component bundles, which have differing lengths, attachment locations, and, presumably, functions. The role of these bundles in controlling joint kinematics and the contact conditions (area, location, and stress) occur under force conditions well below the ligament's ultimate tensile strength. Thus we need to evaluate healing by using the traditional methods of measuring mechanical properties of the ligament and by using newer approaches to quantitating the changes that occur in joint kinematics.

SUMMARY

The healing of ligaments and tendons and the remodeling of the graft replacements are complex processes affected by many variables. We have reviewed a number of these variables that can be controlled in experimental studies, including three that can be controlled by the surgeon: placement, initial tension, and knee flexion angle. Better reporting and more careful control of these variables are needed in future experimental and clinical studies. Further information is needed on the relative importance of each individual variable. Experimental studies need to be designed and carried out that will permit this analysis. Improvements are also needed in the methods used to evaluate the healing response. Currently, microangiographic and light histologic evaluations are subjective, and quantitative stereologic methods need to be applied. Improved correlation of these results with biochemical and mechanical measurements is also needed. The problem of correlating biochemical measurements in average tissue properties with biomechanical measurements of the weakest link must also be overcome. One approach would be to develop biochemical methods that are sensitive enough to be used on small samples taken only from the repair region.

Many studies of ligament repair, including our studies, examine the return in strength over time. In using strength as one measure of the extent of healing it is useful to recognize that the body does not have the ability to directly monitor tissue failure limits. It does have the ability, however, to monitor the stiffness of the tissue because stiffness affects neuromuscular control characteristics. In reviewing our data and that in the literature, we have noticed that stiffness appears to return to normal much earlier than strength. In fact, only a few researchers have reported full return in strength. In Hirsch's study[27] on the achilles tendon, stiffness returned to control values after about 8 weeks while strength required 24 weeks to return. Our unpublished studies on the lateral collateral tendon indicate that stiffness returns to control value when strength is only 60% of normal. Similar results have also been reported by Gelberman and co-workers[20,21] in canine flexor tendons. Thus perhaps the most interesting issue for future study is determination of the predominate functional objectives of healing beyond the obvious ones of filling gaps and restoring continuity and a determination of the precise internal stimuli that control the extent of healing.

REFERENCES

1. Alm, A.: Survival of part of patellar tendon transposed for reconstruction of anterior cruciate ligament, Acta Chir. Scand. **139:**443, 1973.
2. Alm, A., Ekstrom, H., and Stromberg, D.: Tensile strength of the anterior cruciate ligament in the dog, Acta Chir. Scand. Suppl. **445:**15, 1974.
3. Alm, G., and Stromberg, B.: Vascular anatomy of the patellar ligaments, Acta Chir. Scand. Suppl. **445:**25, 1974.
4. Alm, A., and Stromberg, B.: Transposed medial third of patellar ligament in reconstruction of the anterior cruciate ligament surgical and morphological study in dogs, Acta Chir. Scand. Suppl. **445:**37, 1974.
5. Arnoczky, S.P., Rubin, R.M., and Marshall, J.L.: Microvasculature of the cruciate ligaments and its response to injury, J. Bone Joint Surg. **61A:**1221, 1979.
6. Arnoczky, S.P., Tarvin, G.B., and Marshall, J.L.: Anterior cruciate ligament replacement using patellar tendon: an evaluation of graft revascularization in the dog, J. Bone Joint Surg. **64(2):**217, 1982.
7. Arnoczky, S.P., and others: The over-the-top procedure: a technique for anterior cruciate ligament substitution in the dog, J. Am. Animal Hosp. Assoc. **15:**283, 1979.
8. Braithwaite, F., and Brockis, J.G.: The vascularization of a tendon graft, Br. J. Plast. Surg. **4:**130, 1950.

9. Butler, D.L., and others: Biomechanics of cranial cruciate ligament reconstruction in the dog, Vet. Surg. **12**(3):113, 1983.

10. Butler, D.L., and others: The effects of vascularity on the mechanical properties of primate anterior cruciate ligament replacements, Trans. Orthop. Res. Soc. Anaheim **8**:93, 1983.

11. Butler, D.L., and others: The importance of vascularity and continuous motion in biological ligament substitution, Paper presented at the meeting of the American Society of Biomechanics, Rochester, Minn., Sept. 1983.

12. Cabaud, H.E., Rodkey, W.G., and Feagin, J.A.: Experimental studies of acute anterior cruciate ligament injury and repair, Am. J. Sports Med. **7**:18, 1979.

13. Chiroff, R.T.: Experimental replacement of the anterior cruciate ligament, J. Bone Joint Surg. **57A**:1124, 1975.

14. Clancy, W.G., and others: Anterior and posterior cruciate ligament reconstruction in rhesus monkeys, J. Bone Joint Surg. **63A**:1270, 1981.

15. Clayton, M.L., Miles, J.S., and Abdulla, M.: Experimental investigations of ligamentous healing, Clin. Orthop. **61**:146, 1968.

16. Clayton, M.L., and Weir, G.J.: Experimental investigations of ligamentous healing, Am. J. Surg. **98**:373, 1959.

17. DeVito, R.V.: Healing of wounds, Surg. Clin. North Am. **45**:441, 1965.

18. Frank, C., Schachar, N., and Dittrich, D.: The natural history of healing in the repaired medial collateral ligament, J. Orthop. Res. **1**:79, 1983.

19. Frank, C., and others: Medial collateral ligament healing: a multidisciplinary assessment in rabbits, Am. J. Sports Med. **11**:379, 1983.

20. Gelberman, R., Menon, J., Gonsalves, M., and Akeson, W.: The effects of mobilization on the vascularization of healing flexor tendons in dogs, Clin. Orthop. **153**:283, 1980.

21. Gelberman, R.H., and others: The effects of mobilization on the tensile strength, excursion, and revascularization of healing flexor tendons, Trans. Orthop. Res. Soc. Atlanta **5**:16, 1980.

22. Gillard, G.C., and others: The influence of mechanical forces on the glycosaminoglycans content of the rabbit flexor digitorum profunders tendon, Connect. Tissue Res. **7**:37, 1979.

23. Grood, E.S., Noyes, F.R., and Miller, E.H.: Comparative mechanical properties of the medial collateral and capsular structure of the knee, Trans. Orthop. Res. Soc. **1**:223, 1977.

24. Grood, E.S., and others: Biomechanics of the knee extension exercise: effect of sectioning the anterior cruciate ligament, J. Bone Joint Surg. **66A**:725, 1984.

25. Grood, E.S., and others: On the placement and the initial tension of anterior cruciate ligament substitutes, Trans. Orthop. Res. Soc. Anaheim, **8**:92, 1983.

26. Grood, E.S., and Hefzy, M.S.: Sensitivity of insertion location on deformation of the anterior cruciate ligament, Paper presented at the Symposium on Biomechanics of the American Society of Mechanical Engineers, Houston, June 20-22, 1983.

27. Hirsch, G.: Tensile properties during tendon healing, Acta Orthop. Scand. Suppl. **153**:7, 1974.

28. Hulse, D.A., and others: Biomechanics of cranial cruciate ligament reconstruction in the dog, Vet. Surg. **12**(3):109, 1983.

29. Jack, E.A.: Experimental rupture of the medial collateral ligament of the knee, J. Bone Joint Surg. **32B**:396, 1950.

30. Ketchum, L.D., Martin, N.L., and Kappel, D.A.: Experimental evaluation of factors affecting the strength of tendon repairs, Plast. Reconstr. Surg. **59**:708, 1977.

31. Klein, L., and Lewis, J.A.: Simultaneous quantification of ^{3}H-collagen replacement during healing of rat tendon grafts, J. Bone Joint Surg. **54A**:137, 1972.

32. Mankin, H.J.: Current concepts review: the response of articular cartilage to mechanical injury, J. Bone Joint Surg. **64A**:460, 1982.

33. Mason, M.L., and Allen, H.S.: The rate of healing of tendons: an experimental study of tensile strength, Ann. Surg. **113**:424, 1941.

34. Noyes, F.R., DeLucas, J.L., and Torvik, P.J.: Biomechanics of anterior cruciate ligament failure: an analysis of strain-rate sensitivity and mechanisms of failure in primates, J. Bone Joint Surg. **56A**:236, 1974.

35. Noyes, F.R., and others: Biomechanics of ligament failure. II. An analysis of immobilization, exercise, and reconditioning effect on primates, J. Bone Joint Surg. **56A**:1406, 1974.

36. Noyes, F.R., and others: Intraarticular cruciate reconstruction. I. Perspectives on graft strength, vascularization, and immediate motion after replacement, Clin. Orthop. **172:**71, 1983.
37. Noyes, F.R., and others: Anterior cruciate ligament reconstruction: mechanical properties of human ligament grafts, J. Bone Joint Surg. **66A:**344, 1984.
38. O'Donoghue, D.H., and others: Repair and reconstruction of the anterior cruciate ligament in dogs, J. Bone Joint Surg. **53A:**710, 1971.
39. O'Donoghue, D.H., and others: Repair of the anterior cruciate ligament in dogs, J. Bone Joint Surg. **48A:**503, 1966.
40. O'Donoghue, D.H., and others: Repair of knee ligaments in dogs, J. Bone Joint Surg. **43A:**1167, 1961.
41. Peacock, E.E., Jr.: A study of the circulation in normal tendons and healing grafts, Ann. Surg. **149:**415, 1958.
42. Peacock, E.E., Jr.: Biological principles of the healing of long tendons, Surg. Clin. North Am. **45:**461, 1965.
43. Prockop, D.J., and others: The biosynthesis of collagen and its disorders. I. N. Engl. J. Med. **301**(1):13, 1979.
44. Postacchini, F., and others: Regeneration of rabbit calcaneal tendon: a morphological and immuno-chemical study, Cell Tissue Res. **195:**81, 1978.
45. Postacchini, F., and Demartino, C.: Regeneration of rabbit calcaneal tendon: maturation of collagen and elastic fibers following partial tenotomy, Connect. Tissue Res. **8**(1):41, 1980.
46. Potenza, A.D.: Critical evaluation of flexor tendon healing and adhesion formation within artificial digital sheaths, J. Bone Joint Surg. **45A:**1217, 1963.
47. Potenza, A.D.: Tendon Healing within the flexor digital sheath in the dog, J. Bone Joint Surg. **44A:**49, 1962.
48. Preston, E.T.: Tendon healing in dogs with emphasis on tensile strength and cellular patterns, South. Med. J. **66:**1364, 1973.
49. Ryan, J.R., and Drompp, B.W.: Evaluation of tensile strength of reconstructions of the anterior cruciate ligament using the patellar tendon in dogs, South. Med. J. **59:**129, 1966.
50. Roth, J.H., and Kennedy, J.C.: Intra-articular reconstructions of the anterior cruciate ligament in rabbits, Trans. Orthop. Res. Soc. Atlanta **5:**109, 1980.
51. Suntay, W., and others: Biomechanics of the knee extension exercise, Proceedings of the sixth annual meeting of the American Society of Biomechanics, Seattle, Wash., Oct. 1982.
52. Vailas, A.C., and others: Physical activity and its influence on the repair process of the medial collateral ligaments, Connect. Tissue Res. **9:**25, 1981.
53. Viidik, A., Holm-Pedersen, P., and Rudgren, A.: Some observations on the distant collagen response to wound healing in young and old rats, Scand. J. Plast. Reconstr. Surg. **6:**114, 1972.
54. Viljanto, J.: Biochemical basis of tensile strength in wound healing, Acta Chir. Scand. Suppl. **333:**6, 1964.
55. Walker, P., Amstutz, H.C., and Rubinfeld, M.: Canine tendon studies. II. Biomechanical evaluation of normal and regrown canine tendons, J. Biomed. Mater. Res. **10:**61, 1976.

PART TWO

Treatment

14. Evaluation of acute knee injuries

William G. Clancy, Jr.

KNEE INJURIES

Knee injuries can be broken down into two main classifications: traumatic and nontraumatic. Traumatic injuries are those in which one specific traumatic event occurred that precipitated the knee problem. The pain, swelling, or other manifestations may have been significant at the time of injury or may have later developed into a significant problem. Therefore the injury can be classified as either acute traumatic or chronic traumatic. The nontraumatic injury is one in which the athlete cannot recall any specific instance of a knee injury or any particular traumatizing event that could be associated with the present knee problem.

Acute knee injuries can be initially divided into a number of categories:

1. Ligament sprain
   a. Medial collateral ligament
   b. Anterior cruciate ligament
   c. Lateral collateral ligament
   d. Posterior cruciate ligament
   e. Combination of the above
2. Meniscal tears
3. Extensor mechanism injuries
   a. Patellar dislocation
   b. Patellar subluxation
4. Epiphyseal fractures
   a. Distal femoral epiphyseal injury
   b. Proximal tibial epiphyseal injury
5. Articular cartilage traumatic injuries
   a. Patellar articular fracture
   b. Femoral condyle articular fracture
   c. Tibial plateau osteochondral fractures
6. Extraarticular soft tissue injury
   a. Peripatellar traumatic bursitis
   b. Sympathetic knee effusion secondary to a grade II or grade III quadriceps contusion

ACUTE KNEE INJURIES
History

The mechanism of the injury is one of the most important aids in making a diagnosis. An open mind must be kept when evaluating the patient after hearing a description of the mechanism of injury. The knowledge of the mechanism can cause the examiner to focus on a particular diagnosis, miss a second injury, or misinterpret the clinical finding.

For example, the patient may say that he saw his right patella sitting out laterally after he fell down, and it went back into place when he straightened his knee out. Further questioning by another examiner, however, revealed that the patient was dribbling a basketball downcourt when he stopped suddenly, cut to his left, felt a pop, and his knee gave out. He went to his physician the next day with a large tense effusion. On physical examination, which was limited as a result of pain, there was pain just proximal to the adductor tubercle. There was also pain along the medial collateral ligament with some moderate increased medial laxity with valgus testing at 30 degrees of knee flexion, but no laxity to valgus testing at full extension. However, the Lachman test was definitely positive. Therefore this patient had a complete tear of his anterior cruciate ligament, a second degree tear of his medial collateral ligament, and a patellar dislocation. This patient has had a serious knee injury, and only a careful history and complete examination yielded the full diagnosis. An incomplete history and physicial examination would have left the examiner with the diagnosis of only a patellar dislocation.

Over the past few years many new concepts and diagnostic tests have been developed that have improved the clinical examination, which should yield an accuracy of over 90% of the primary diagnosis without the aid of arthrography or arthroscopy.

Mechanism of injury

I. Contact injury
    A. Valgus or varus stress
        1. Without rotation suspect:
            a. Collateral ligament injury
            b. Epiphyseal fracture
            c. Patellar dislocation or subluxation
        2. With rotation suspect:
            a. Collateral ligament and cruciate injury
            b. Collateral ligament and patellar dislocation or subluxation
    B. Fall on a flexed knee:
        a. With the foot in dorsiflexion the blow is sustained on patellofemoral joint—suspect patellar articular injury
        b. With the foot in plantar flexion the blow is taken on tibial tubercle—suspect a posterior cruciate ligament injury

    C. Anterior blow to tibia causing knee hyperextension suspect:
        a. Anterior cruciate ligament injury
        b. Anterior and posterior cruciate ligament injury
   II. Noncontact injury
    A. Hyperextension suspect—anterior cruciate ligament injury
    B. Deceleration suspect:
        a. Anterior cruciate ligament injury
    C. Deceleration and tibial internal rotation or femoral external rotation on a fixed tibia suspect:
        a. Anterior cruciate ligament injury
    D. Lateral cut with tibia in external rotation suspect:
        a. Patellar dislocation or subluxation
    E. Twisting injury with valgus or varus loading suspect:
        a. Meniscus tear

Pain

The localization of the pain by the patient may not be as helpful as expected, since the patient may focus on the location of the greatest amount of pain and not relate other sites of pain.

Medial pain. A medial collateral ligament injury may produce pain at one or a combination of the following locations: medial femoral epicondyle, medial joint line, or proximal tibia. This pain could be located only at the medial joint line, but this is not common except perhaps in first-degree sprains.

Patellar dislocations will usually result in anterior medial parapatellar pain and medial parapatellar pain. However, on examination there is almost always significant pain to palpation just proximal to the adductor tubercle where the vastus medialis tears from the intermuscular septum. This sign remains positive for 5 to 7 days and is almost pathognomonic of a patellar dislocation or subluxation.

Medial meniscal injury frequently results in posterior medial joint line pain and mild medial joint line pain. There is seldom any anterior medial pain unless there is a displaced bucket-handle tear in which the anterior part of the bucket has not fully extended itself and is held tight around the medial femoral condyle. Isolated anterior horn tears represent less than 1% of meniscus tears. Thus isolated anterior medial pain is usually not a sign of a meniscal tear.

Lateral joint line pain. In lateral collateral ligament injuries, isolated tears are usually localized to the midlateral joint line and fibular head. If the pain is also posterolateral, then a complex lateral ligament injury or lateral meniscus injury must be suspected. Lateral meniscus injuries are seen more frequently with midlateral pain than with posterolateral pain.

Posterolateral pain. Posterolateral pain represents either a lateral meniscal injury or, more frequently in my experience, an avulsion of the anterior cruciate ligament from the lateral femoral condyle.

Posterior pain. In acute knee injuries, posterior pain is associated with either a mild strain of one of the gastrocnemius muscles, a mild sprain of the posterior capsule, or a posterior cruciate ligament tear.

Effusion

An acute knee injury with a history of no previous injury seen 24 hours after the injury will have no effusion, a mild effusion, or a large effusion.

Large tense effusion (no previous history of injury). If there is a large tense effusion, it will almost always represent a hemarthrosis. The two diagnoses that represent over 80% of the causes of an acute tense hemarthrosis are an acute anterior cruciate ligament tear or a patellar dislocation or significant subluxation.[2,6] In the adolescent a third diagnosis of epiphyseal fracture must be considered. A complete isolated tear of the medial or lateral collateral ligaments will seldom lead to a large tense hemarthrosis, because the knee capsule is torn and most of the blood leaks out of the capsule down into the leg. A meniscal tear will seldom lead to a large bloody hemarthrosis, because most tears are in the body of the meniscus, which has no blood supply.

Mild effusion. Usually the fluid, if aspirated, is either serosanguinous or serous. If so, a meniscus tear or an isolated partial or complete tear of either the medial or lateral collateral ligaments should be suspected. An isolated tear of either collateral ligament is seldom associated with an interbody tear of a meniscus. When these two entities are present there must be some injury to one of the cruciate ligaments.

If the mild effusion is grossly bloody, then the examiner must look for a medial or lateral collateral ligament tear and an associated tear of either cruciate ligament or an isolated tear of the posterior cruciate ligament, which for unknown reasons seldom leads to a gross hemarthrosis as does its counterpart the anterior cruciate ligament.[1]

PHYSICAL EXAMINATION
Range of motion

The range of motion of the injured knee should always be compared to the uninjured knee. The patient should first be in the supine position with both heels on the examining tables, since this will allow the examiner to know what the neutral position is when examining for hyperextension. Most people have a few degrees of hyperextension when examined in this position. Loss of hyperextension when compared to the opposite knee is frequently a sign of a completely displaced bucket-handle tear. If the knee goes into hyperextension and there is posteromedial or posterolateral pain, a posterior horn tear of either meniscus is indicated.

Inability to fully flex the knee may be a result of the acute injury or a large effusion. Inability to fully extend the knee may be because of a displaced meniscus tear or a result of partial collateral ligament injury. The collateral ligament is most relaxed at 30 degrees of flexion and under maximum stretch at full extension. It may appear to be locked at 30 degrees, but this is pseudolocking resulting from pain.

Effusion

The inexperienced examiner may confuse a traumatic peripatellar bursitis with a true knee joint effusion. However, in the former the patella will not be palpable directly under the skin. It is important to distinguish between these two entities, since the examiner may be faced with a tensely swollen knee with significant superficial cellulitis. If the entity is an infected peripatellar bursitis and the knee joint is mistakenly aspirated, infection may be introduced into the joint.

Pain

Palpation of the location where the patient complains of pain should generally be performed after testing for ligamentous stability. If the examiner increases the patient's pain, the patient is more than likely to go into quadriceps and hamstring spasms that will significantly limit the subsequent examination for ligamentous stability.

Ligamentous examination

Since hamstring spasm can limit the examination, the least stressful tests should be performed first. It is my opinion that the sequence should be the Lachman test; the anterior-posterior drawer test; the varus-valgus tests at 30 and 0 degrees; the pivot-shift test; jerk test or Slocum test; and finally, the reverse pivot-shift test as described by Jakob.[5]

The *Lachman test* is the least stressful of all the ligamentous stability tests and is the most reliable test for anterior cruciate insufficiency.[2,6] It is an anterior drawer test performed with knee held in 10 to 20 degrees of flexion.[5] The examiner must palpate the hamstring tendons at the time of testing, since minimal hamstring spasm can negate this test. Any significant straight anterior translation of the tibia is pathognomonic of an anterior cruciate ligament tear. Care must be taken in evaluating a positive test, since a third-degree medial collateral ligament tear with extension of the tear into the posterior medial capsule will allow slight forward and mild to moderate external rotation of the tibia that may be confused with a true Lachman test. This has been called a pseudo-Lachman test.

The second test performed is an *anterior-posterior drawer test*, since this test is frequently not too painful to the patient. The knee is flexed to 90 degrees, and both knees are viewed from the side to see if there is any posterior tibial sag. The medial and lateral femoral condyles are then palpated with both thumbs. Both thumbs palpate down the condyles and a normal 8 to 10 mm step off of the anterior medial and anterior lateral tibial plateaus should be noted. If the thumbs come flush with the anterior tibia surface, then a posterior cruciate ligament injury should be suspected.[1]

An anterior drawer test is then performed. In the case of an acute anterior cruciate ligament injury, this test is often negative partly because of the wedging effect of the posterior horn of the medial meniscus. If it is significantly positive, there is frequently more ligamentous injury than just to the anterior cruciate ligament. The examiner must also be sure that a positive anterior drawer test is not the reduction of a posterior subluxed tibia resulting from a posterior cruciate ligament injury.

Varus-valgus testing is performed after the previous tests, particularly if there is any indication that either collateral ligament may have been injured. The knee is held in 30 degrees of flexion, and varus-valgus stress is applied. In this position the collateral ligaments are relatively isolated for testing. The knee is then fully extended, and again, varus-valgus testing is performed. The opposite knee should be examined first so the examiner can have a control for comparison. If there is significant laxity at full extension, then not only has the collateral ligament been injured, but one or both cruciate ligaments have also been injured.

The *pivot-shift test* as described by Galway and MacIntosh[3] is then performed. The knee is held in full extension by holding the heel in one hand. The other hand at the level of the fibula head applies an upward and inward (valgus) force, and the knee is slowly flexed. If there is a complete tear of the anterior cruciate ligament and sufficient laxity, the anterior tibia is initially subluxed forward and is held sub-luxed with the valgus force. At approximately 30 to 40 degrees of flexion, there is a sudden forceful and painful reduction as a result mainly of the pull of the iliotibial band.

A significant pivot-shift test has a high correlation with the development of func-tional instability. The Lachman test is only a test for anterior cruciate integrity and does not correlate with the likelihood of developing functional instability, whereas the pivot-shift test, when significant, has a high correlation in my experience.

The *jerk test* described by Hughston[4] is another test for anterior cruciate stability. The examiner starts with the patient's knee in flexion, and an upward and inward force is applied to the proximal tibia while the knee is extended. At approximately 30 degrees of flexion, a painful forward anterior tibial subluxation occurs. Unfortu-nately, those with a normal knee and excessive knee hyperextension may produce a similar type of anterior tibial translation at approximately 10 degrees of flexion, and this could be confused with a positive jerk test.

The *reverse pivot-shift test* has recently been described by Jakob.[5] This is a test for significant posterolateral rotatory instability. The patient's knee is fully flexed and the tibia is maximally externally rotated. The knee is then slowly extended while applying a valgus force to the proximal tibia and maintaining the tibia in external rotation. At approximately 40 degrees of knee flexion, there is a sudden visible and audible reduction of the tibia, which should not be confused with a forward sublux-ation of the tibia—a sign of anterior cruciate instability and therefore a positive jerk test.

When performing a reverse pivot-shift test in those patients with severe postero-lateral rotatory instability and accompanying anterior cruciate instability, the ex-aminer will hear two close but separate clunks. The first is the reduction of the tibia at 40 degrees (the reverse pivot) and the second, which occurs at approximately 30 to 20 degrees of flexion, is a forward subluxation of the tibia (a positive jerk test).

Severe posterolateral rotatory instability has been described to occur as an isolated entity, but it is more frequently associated with posterior cruciate ligament injury and to a lesser extent with anterior cruciate ligament injuries. Those patients with mild posterolateral laxity will often not have a reverse pivot-shift test. Noyes[7] recommends that to test for this mild laxity the examiner flexes the patient's knee and hip to 90 degrees. The tibia is completely rotated externally and internally while palpating the fibular head. The amount of external rotation is compared to the opposite knee. While rotating the tibia, the examiner should observe where the center of the axis of rotation lies.[7] It should be determined whether the center of rotation appears to be located about the medial femoral condyle or whether it appears to be located about the intercondylar notch. If it appears to be the former, then the examiner should suspect that there is some posterolateral component.

The McMurray and Apley tests for meniscal injury are sometimes used. If there has been any collateral ligament injury, then either of these tests will produce pain, since any twisting maneuver will load the injured ligament. The Apley test tries to differentiate between a meniscal lesion and a collateral ligament injury, but it does involve twisting the tibia and will probably be an unreliable test.

Extensor mechanism testing may also be performed. Significant subluxation, which is painful, or the presence of marked guarding to attempted lateral patellar displacement are strong indications of a patellar dislocation. Additionally, there should be significant pain on palpation at the insertion of the vastus medialis to the intermuscular septum just above the adductor tubercle.

RADIOGRAPHIC EVALUATION

Radiographs should be taken for all acute knee injuries. If there are signs of medial or lateral collateral ligament injury in a patient with open epiphyses, then stress radiographs should be obtained. If there has been a patellar dislocation and there are no signs of a loose body, then no further studies are indicated. If there has been a collateral ligament injury in which an adequate examination could be performed and there is no sign of an anterior or posterior cruciate ligament injury, there is no need for arthrography or arthroscopy.

ARTHROGRAPHY

An arthrogram is recommended for patients who have a suspected anterior cruciate ligament injury, because the accuracy of delineating a tear of the posterior horn of the medial meniscus is over 95%. Not only can a tear be defined, but quite frequently its location (peripheral or midsubstance) and whether there is a horizontal component can be demonstrated. This area of the meniscus is the most difficult to visualize by arthroscopy, and it is often close to impossible to determine whether there is a horizontal component to a peripheral tear. Anterior cruciate tears have a high association with peripheral meniscus tears, but the mechanism of injury is such that some of these peripheral tears will have a horizontal cleavage tear that will render them unrepairable.

An acute anterior cruciate tear with an absent or minimal pivot-shift test would not usually meet our criteria for surgical intervention. However, if there is a repairable meniscus lesion, then surgical repair of the meniscus, as well as a ligament repair and patellar tendon grafting, would be recommended. Thus performing an arthrogram would be helpful in recommending the various options to the patient.

EVALUATION UNDER ANESTHESIA AND ARTHROSCOPY

Evaluation under anesthesia should be recommended for any acute knee injury that appears to be significant and when adequate testing cannot be accomplished. An arthrogram should first be obtained, and then evaluation under anesthesia should follow.

If the examination indicates only a collateral ligament injury, there is no need to perform an arthroscopy. If the examiner is not sure whether there is a positive Lachman or a pseudo-Lachman test and the pivot-shift test is negative, then an arthroscopy should be performed to determine the status of the anterior cruciate ligament. If the Lachman test is positive, but there is an absent or minimal pivot-shift test, then an arthroscopy should be performed.

SUMMARY

Those patients who do not have any previous history of a knee injury and have a large tense effusion have probably sustained a serious knee injury. The most common injuries are a tear of the anterior cruciate ligament or a patellar dislocation.

Acute anterior cruciate ligament injury may be the result of a contact or noncontact injury. The noncontact injury is frequently the result of either a sudden deceleration, a hyperextension injury, or external rotation of the femur on a fixed tibia. A large tense effusion will usually develop by 24 hours. The Lachman test is almost always positive in a relaxed knee, whereas a significant pivot-shift test may not always be present.

Isolated posterior cruciate ligament injuries in sports are usually the result of a fall on a flexed knee with the foot in plantar flexion. A large tense effusion is usually not present with this injury. A mild posterior tibial sag and loss of the normal anterior tibial plateau step off is noted with the knee held in 90 degrees of flexion. A positive posterior drawer test may be misinterpreted as a positive anterior drawer test.

A patellar dislocation will usually have a large tense effusion, but will have a negative Lachman test. There will be medial parapatellar pain and additional pain to palpation of the distal insertion of the vastus medialis into the intermuscular septum just proximal to the adductor tubercle.

Isolated tears of the medial or lateral collateral ligament usually do not develop a large tense effusion. There may be significant laxity to stress testing at 30 degrees of knee flexion, but no laxity to stress testing at full extension. If there is significant laxity at full extension, then an additional cruciate injury should be suspected.

A thorough history and complete physical examination should lead to the appropriate diagnosis. An examination under anesthesia may be necessary to complete an adequate examination. Arthrography and arthroscopy are extremely important aids in confirming the suspected diagnosis.

REFERENCES

1. Clancy, W.G., Jr., and others: Treatment of knee joint instability secondary to rupture of the posterior cruciate ligament, J. Bone Joint Surg. **65A:**310, 1983.
2. DeHaven, K.E.: Diagnosis of acute knee injuries with hemarthrosis, Am. J. Sports Med. **8:**9, 1980.
3. Galway, R.D., Beaupré, A., and MacIntosh, D.L.: Pivot shift: a clinical sign of asymptomatic anterior cruciate insufficiency, J. Bone Joint Surg. **54B:**763, 1972.
4. Hughston, J.C., and others: Classification of knee ligament instabilities. I. The medial compartment and cruciate ligaments, J. Bone Joint Surg. **58A:**159, 1976.
5. Jakob, R.P.: Observations on rotatory instability of the lateral compartment of the knee, Acta Orthop. Scand. Suppl. **52:**191, 1981.
6. Noyes, F.R., and others: Arthroscopy in acute traumatic hemarthrosis of the knee, J. Bone Joint Surg. **62A:**687, 1980.
7. Noyes, F.R.: Lateral structures of the knee: clinical biomechanics, Paper read at the instructional course on the athlete's knee, Cincinnati, Ohio, June 11, 1983.
8. Torg, J.S., Conrad, W., and Katen, V.: Clinical diagnosis of acute anterior cruciate ligament instability in the athlete, Am. J. Sports Med. **4:**84, 1976.

15. Conservative treatment of acute knee ligamentous injuries

William G. Clancy, Jr.

Historically, conservative treatment has been synonymous with nonoperative treatment. Therefore when dealing with acute ligamentous knee injuries does conservative treatment mean that nonoperative treatment results will be less than ideal, particularly if there were a higher probability of better results if operative treatment were used? Since the immediate and long-term sequalae of both nonoperative and operative treatment should be assessed, conservative treatment should mean that the treatment selected has the highest probability of a successful end result and the least potential for morbidity.

To make a decision as to which is the best mode of treatment, certain questions must be answered. First, is there sufficient consistent data based on the patient's clinical examination to accurately predict the likelihood of achieving knee stability with either mode of treatment? Second, what is the likelihood of developing secondary problems, such as meniscal tears, late instability, or early traumatic arthritis with either form of treatment? Third, which mode of treatment will restore not only clinical stability but also biomechanical stability? Fourth, which mode of treatment has the higher probability of returning the patient to recreational or competitive sports or manual labor?

The patient's age, life-style, job demands, and willingness to follow a prolonged postsurgical rehabilitation program must be assessed. It must be remembered that it is the patient who is to select the treatment. It is the physician's responsibility to present the current scientific facts, possibilities, and probabilities of the treatments to the patient, so that the patient can make a decision as to what is best for himself.

The term *conservative treatment* will be used in this chapter for nonoperative functional rehabilitation of an acute ligament injury, which is believed to be the best treatment for the injury based on the clinical findings, a prolonged time interval between the injury and time of diagnosis, other extenuating circumstances, or the patient's desire for this form of treatment.

ACUTE ISOLATED MEDIAL AND LATERAL COLLATERAL LIGAMENT INJURY

O'Donoghue[21,22] believed that because of the significant associated injuries the best mode of treatment for collateral ligament injuries was surgical. In his series of medial collateral ligament injuries, the anterior cruciate ligament was also injured in 75% of the cases. However, with improvement in our clinical evaluation and use of the arthroscope, it is possible to separate those patients with isolated collateral ligament injury from those with accompanying cruciate ligament injury.

It is important to emphasize that a nonoperative functional rehabilitation program is indicated only in those patients with an isolated collateral ligament injury. There must be no signs of anterior or posterior cruciate ligament injury. The Lachman test and the pivot-shift test must be negative in the relaxed patient. An examination under anesthesia and arthroscopy should be used when there is any question about cruciate ligament integrity. Nonoperative treatment should not be used for a combined second- or third-degree collateral ligament and cruciate ligament injury. These injuries have too high a potential for significant long-term sequala to be treated nonoperatively except under the most unusual circumstances.

TREATMENT PROTOCOL FOR ISOLATED COLLATERAL LIGAMENT INJURIES

REHABILITATION OF FIRST-, SECOND-, AND THIRD-DEGREE ISOLATED MEDIAL AND LATERAL COLLATERAL LIGAMENT INJURIES

Day 1 to day 3:
1. Crutches with partial weight bearing
2. Compression dressing—loosen if ankle becomes swollen
3. Ice 3 to 4 times a day for 10 minutes
4. Quad sets—3 sets of 20 repetitions, 3 times per day
5. Straight leg lifts—3 sets of 20 repetitions, 3 times per day
6. Wear knee immobilizer at night

Day 3 to approximately day 7:
1. Whirlpool for range of motion (biking motion), cold water for first 3 to 4 days, then warm water
2. May use swimming pool instead, 30 to 45 minutes straight ahead flutter kick trying to bend knee
3. Straight leg raises with maximum weight that can be done 12 times; do 3 sets of 12 repetitions:
   a. Hip extension
   b. Hip flexion
   c. Hip abduction
      1. Knee kept straight
      2. No hip adduction

Continued.

TREATMENT PROTOCOL FOR ISOLATED COLLATERAL LIGAMENT INJURIES—cont'd

REHABILITATION OF FIRST-, SECOND-, AND THIRD-DEGREE ISOLATED MEDIAL AND LATERAL COLLATERAL LIGAMENT INJURIES—cont'd

Day 3 to approximately day 7:—cont'd
4. Continue with crutches and knee immobilizer and can bear weight as tolerated
5. Continue quad set exercises
6. Can discard knee immobilizer after seventh day

Day 7 to day 14 (if 90 degrees of knee flexion present):
1. Whirlpool or swimming for range of motion
2. Exercise bike for 15 minutes, if Fitron 60 rpm
3. Quad sets continued
4. Orthotron, speed 5—3 sets of 10 repetitions or Universal or Nautilus weight program
   a. Quadriceps—3 sets of 12 repetitions with maximum weight tolerated
   b. Hamstrings—3 sets of 12 repetitions with maximum weight tolerated
5. Crutches to be continued until patient can walk without a limp

Day 14 to completion (if full range of flexion and extension):
1. Whirlpool
2. Bike 15 minutes
3. Orthotron—3 sets of 10 repetitions at speed 3; 3 sets of 10 repetitions at speed 5 when equal to opposite side; then 3 sets of 10 repetitions at speed 7 Nautilus or Universal, 3 sets of 12 repetitions of maximum weights for quadriceps and hamstrings
4. Start running program—
   Jog 1 mile then:
   6 × 80 yards at ½ speed
   6 × 80 yards at ¾ speed
   6 × 80 yards at full speed
   6 × 80 yards at ½ speed cutting
   6 × 80 yards at full speed cutting
   Stop at any point when there is pain or a limp. Each day patient must start the entire running program over until it can be completed in 1 day.

To return to practice patient:
1. Must have full range of motion
2. Must have no pain
3. Must have quadriceps and hamstring strength within 90% of the normal leg
4. Must be able to complete the entire running program
5. Athlete should be rechecked by a physician when he completes the entire program if there has been a second- or third-degree ligament injury.

Excellent clinical results of nonoperative treatment of isolated collateral ligament injuries have been presented by Ellsasser[8] and Bergfeld and others.[3] Indelicato[15] used the arthroscope to report that there were no associated lesions in his patients with complete tears of the medial collateral ligament and also had excellent results with nonoperative treatment. Recently Andrews and others[1] recommended early functional rehabilitation of isolated third-degree medial collateral ligament injuries. The biomechanical studies of Häggmark and Eriksson[12] and Costill[6] demonstrate the significant deleterious changes that occur in the lower leg musculature with cast immobilization and the distinct advantage of early functional rehabilitation.

The functional rehabilitation programs for nonoperative treatment vary from researcher to researcher, with Andrews and others[1] recommending cast-bracing for a period of 3 to 6 weeks. The program in our clinic is more progressive, since immobilization ends after 1 week. The following protocol is used in our clinic for the treatment of first-, second-, and third-degree isolated collateral ligament injuries.

ACUTE ANTERIOR CRUCIATE LIGAMENT INJURIES

Unfortunately, there is still significant controversy over the long-term effect of insufficiency of the anterior cruciate ligament on the knee joint. Hughston,[14] McDaniel,[18] and Balkfors[2] believe that a high percentage of those patients with deficiencies of the anterior cruciate ligament but intact menisci will do well. In contrast to these studies, Clancy,[4] Feagin,[9] Fetto,[10] Jacobsen,[16] Marshall,[17] and Noyes[20] have documented the significant potential for those patients with functional deficiencies of the anterior cruciate ligament in the knee to tear at least one meniscus (50% to 78%) or both (38%), to develop significant early traumatic arthritic changes (54% noted at the time of surgery), or to have radiographic osteoarthritic changes noted on long-term follow-up (44%).

Obviously there must be some truth to both sides of the picture. There must be some patients with anterior cruciate deficiencies of the knee who can participate in all activities without functional instability and who do not develop meniscal tears or early traumatic arthritis. On the other extreme there are many well-documented series of patients with chronic anterior cruciate deficiencies of the knee who have developed functional instability, meniscal tears, and severe early traumatic arthritis.

The literature has not yet delineated a scientific means to differentiate those patients with potentially stable anterior cruciate deficiencies of the knee from those who will develop functional instability, meniscal lesions, and traumatic arthritis.

Although the Lachman test described by Torg,[23] and the flexion rotation test described by Noyes[19] are excellent clinical tests for determining anterior cruciate ligament integrity, these tests have little to do with predicting functional instability. However, when the pivot-shift test described by Galway and MacIntosh[11] and the jerk test described by Hughston,[13] are significant in patients with acute anterior cruciate ligament injuries, there appears to be a high probability of developing functional anterior cruciate instability. Clinically it has been noted that those patients with a negative or minimal pivot-shift test and chronic anterior cruciate deficiency

FUNCTIONAL REHABILITATION OF ACUTE ANTERIOR CRUCIATE LIGAMENT INJURIES

First and second week:
1. Crutches and partial weight bearing until the patient can walk without a limp. No form of knee immobilization is used.
2. Isometric leg raises with knee held in 30 degrees of flexion, 3 sets of 20 repetitions, 3 times a day.

Third through sixth week:
1. Range of motion with weights through a limited arc of 30 to 90 degrees, 3 sets of 12 repetitions with 50% of maximum tolerated weight.
2. Exercise bike, 15 to 30 minutes daily.

Seventh week on:
1. Progressive weight program through a full range of motion, 3 sets of 12 repetitions with maximum weight tolerated.
2. Start the running program as outlined in isolated collateral ligament injuries.

Return to sports activities or manual labor:
1. When quadriceps and hamstrings are within 90% strength of opposite knee.
2. When patient has completed the full running program.
3. When there is no effusion or pain.

Preventive measures:
1. Fit for a derotational brace to be used when engaging in recreational activities.
2. Teach patient how to cut only off the ball of the foot of the injured leg to decrease the valgus thrust.
3. Teach to land from a jump with the knee flexed to 30 to 40 degrees.

of the knee have a low incidence of functional instability. Based on these findings, it has been our protocol to treat those patients who, when examined under anesthesia, have an absent or minimal pivot-shift test and no repairable meniscal lesions with a nonoperative functional rehabilitation program.

If there is a significant pivot-shift test present with the acute injury, we believe that it will not disappear with time nor with a rehabilitation program, and therefore surgery is recommended because of the high probability of developing functional instability and its sequelae. If there is a negative or minimal pivot-shift test, but a repairable meniscal lesion, then repair of the meniscal lesion is recommended with an anterior cruciate ligament repair and patellar tendon augmentation. DeHaven's[7] high incidence of repeat tears of meniscal repairs (30%) in patients with anterior cruciate ligament deficiencies of the knee indicates that anterior cruciate ligament stabilization is necessary in these patients.

One of the most important preventative factors for those patients with anterior cruciate deficiency of the knee is teaching the athlete how to modify his cut, that is, the sudden change in direction made while playing sports. Athletes with chronic functional anterior cruciate instability continually reveal that the single most common mechanism of giving way is a sudden cut or change in direction to the side opposite the unstable knee. Observation reveals that the athlete cuts away from the injured leg while that heel and foot are firmly fixed to the ground, creating a valgus thrust at the knee. It is this valgus thrust that produces the painful subluxation or reduction of the femur on the tibia. In essence, the patient has performed his own pivot-shift test. If the athlete cuts off with only the ball of his foot fixed to the ground, the valgus thrust is markedly diminished, which decreases the likelihood of subluxation or reduction of that knee. Clinically it is almost impossible to perform the pivot-shift test or jerk test without applying a significant valgus stress. By eliminating or decreasing this valgus load on cutting by not allowing the heel to come into contact with the ground, the patient can decrease the potential for episodes of functional instability.

ACUTE ISOLATED POSTERIOR CRUCIATE LIGAMENT INJURIES

If there has been an avulsion of the posterior cruciate ligament with a piece of bony attachment, there is rarely any indication for nonoperative treatment. Only in extreme circumstances would a patient desire nonoperative treatment. Such circumstances would include multiple injuries, advanced age, the presence of a superficial wound infection, or a significant loss of skin about the involved area.

If surgical intervention is undertaken, it should be remembered that there may have been some significant interstitial failure of the ligament with a resulting increase in length. Therefore the fragment should either be countersunk in its anatomic site or should be distally advanced.

Those patients with acute isolated posterior cruciate ligament tears should have surgical repair and patellar tendon augmentation or augmentation with some other biologic substitute. The success of primary repair of interstitial posterior cruciate ligament has not been consistently successful, whereas repair and patellar tendon augmentation have yielded a high success rate.[5]

The nonoperative functional rehabilitation program for isolated posterior cruciate ligament injuries is the same used for the treatment of acute anterior cruciate ligament injuries.

Combined acute ligamentous injuries

I believe that there is no role for conservative treatment of significant combined acute ligamentous injuries. This would include (1) second- or third-degree medial or lateral collateral ligament injury and third-degree anterior or posterior cruciate ligament injury and (2) third-degree anterior or posterior cruciate ligament injury and third-degree posterolateral complex tears.

If any of the previous complex ligament injuries must be treated nonoperatively because of extenuating circumstances, then rigid immobilization for 6 weeks must be used so that the secondary restraints will heal as tight as possible.

•   •   •

In summary there is a definite place for conservative treatment of patients with acute isolated collateral ligament injuries and for patients with a deficient, yet stable, acute anterior cruciate ligament of the knee in which there are no repairable meniscal lesions. There is little, if any, role for nonoperative treatment of combined or complex ligamentous injuries. It also is my opinion that almost all acute posterior cruciate ligament injuries should be repaired and augmented.

REFERENCES

1. Andrews, J.R.: Treatment of complete tears of the medial collateral ligament, Paper presented at the annual meeting of the American Orthopaedic Society for Sports Medicine, Lake of the Ozarks, Mo., July 15, 1982.
2. Balkfors, B.: The course of knee ligament injuries, Acta Orthop. Scand. **53**(Suppl. 198):7, 1982.
3. Bergfeld, J.A., O'Connor, G.A., and Cox, J.S.: Functional rehabilitation of isolated medial collateral ligament sprains, Am. J. Sports Med. **7**:206, 1979.
4. Clancy, W.G., Jr., and others: Anterior cruciate ligament reconstruction using one-third of the patellar ligament augmented by extraarticular tendon transfers, J. Bone Joint Surg. **64A**:352, 1982.
5. Clancy, W.G., Jr., and others: Treatment of knee joint instability secondary to rupture of the posterior cruciate ligament, J. Bone Joint Surg. **65A**:310, 1983.
6. Costill, D.L., Fink, W.J., and Habansky, J.A.: Muscle rehabilitation after knee surgery, Physician Sports Med. **5**:71, 1977.
7. DeHaven, K.E.: Peripheral meniscus repair: 3 to 7 year results, Paper presented at the third congress of the International Society of the Knee, Gleneagles, Scotland, April 28, 1983.
8. Ellsasser, J.C., Reynolds, F.C., and Omohundro, J.R.: The nonoperative treatment of collateral ligament injuries of the knee in professional football players, J. Bone Joint Surg. **56A**:1185, 1974.
9. Feagin, J.A., Jr.: The syndrome of the torn anterior cruciate ligament, Orthop. Cli. North Am. **10**:81, 1979.
10. Fetto, J.F., and Marshal, J.L.: The natural history and diagnosis of anterior cruciate ligament insufficiency, Clin. Orthop. **147**:29, 1980.
11. Galway, H.R., and MacIntosh, D.L.: The lateral pivot shift: a symptom and sign of anterior cruciate ligament insufficiency, Clin. Orthop. **147**:45, 1980.
12. Häggmark, T., and Eriksson, E.: Cylinder or mobile cast brace after knee ligament injury, Am. J. Sports Med. **7**:48, 1979.
13. Hughston, J.C., and others: Classification of knee ligament instabilities. I. The medial compartment and cruciate ligaments, J. Bone Joint Surg. **58A**:159, 1976.
14. Hughston, J.C., and Barrett, G.R.: Acute anteromedial rotatory instability, J Bone Joint Surg. **65A**:145, 1983.
15. Indelicato, P.A: Nonoperative treatment of complete tears of the medial collateral ligament of the knee, J. Bone Joint Surg. **65A**:323, 1983.
16. Jacobsen, K.: Osteoarthrosis following insufficiency of the cruciate ligaments in man, Acta Orthop. Scand. **48**:520, 1977.
17. Marshall, J.L., and others: The anterior cruciate ligament: the diagnosis and treatment of its injuries and their serious prognostic implications, Orthop. Rev. **7**:35, 1978.
18. McDaniel, W.J., and Dameron, T.B., Jr.: Untreated ruptures of the anterior cruciate ligament: a follow-up study, J. Bone Joint Surg. **62A**:696, 1980.
19. Noyes, F.R., and others: Arthroscopy in acute traumatic hemarthrosis of the knee: incidence of anterior cruciate ligament tears and other injuries, J. Bone Joint Surg. **62A**:687, 1980.
20. Noyes, F.R., and others: The symptomatic anterior cruciate deficient knee, J. Bone Joint Surg. **65A**:154, 1983.
21. O'Donoghue, D.H.: Surgical treatment of fresh injuries to the major ligaments of the knee, J. Bone Joint Surg. **32A**:721, 1950.
22. O'Donoghue, D.H.: An analysis of end results of surgical treatment of major injuries to the ligaments of the knee, J. Bone Joint Surg. **37A**:1, 1955.
23. Torg, J.S., Conrad, W., and Kalen, V.: Clinical diagnosis of anterior cruciate ligament instability in the athlete, Am. J. Sports Med. **4**:84, 1976.

16. Treatment of anteromedial rotatory instability of the knee

Robert L. Larson

ANATOMIC AND BIOMECHANICAL CONSIDERATIONS

First I would like to review some of the physiologic anatomy of the medial side of the knee as it relates to providing stability. The support to the medial side of the knee is provided by three structural layers. These are from within out: the capsular layer, the ligamentous layer, and the muscular layer (Fig. 16-1). There are both dynamic and static elements that play a part in controlling knee stability. The activity of the dynamic layer is provided by the ligamentomuscular reflex (described in 1938 by Palmer[10]) through myelin-free fibers that are located in the ligaments. Tension in the ligaments produces a reflex contraction of the surrounding muscles that provides compression of the joint and aids in stabilizing the joint. Although this ligament reflex is too slow to provide protection in sudden injury, it does provide protection in those activities where the individual is consciously cutting, pivoting, or twisting.

Working with the ligaments are elements of the joint contour that allow the ligaments to tighten and relax.[3] Function of the leg requires balance in walking, running, kicking, and jumping. The ligaments must function together to provide a wide range of support from stance to speed, to provide propulsion and restraining mechanisms, to provide a stable pedal power for body movements, and to adapt to sudden changes of forces from the ground or body movement, which allow rapid change in direction, acceleration, or deceleration.[8]

The conical shape of the intercondylar eminence helps control rotation as long as the ligaments are intact (Fig. 16-1, *C*). With rotation the femur rides up on the eminence, minimizing the load on ligaments as rotation occurs. The femoral condyles are eccentrically shaped with a disparity in length. This provides a cam action that allows the fan-shaped ligaments to provide some degree of tautness in all degrees of flexion and extension. The oval shape of the femoral insertion of the medial collateral ligament provides that portions of this ligament will tighten as flexion-extension occurs (Fig. 16-1, *A*).

Although ligaments are considered to be static elements, they are dynamic, physiologic, and exactly placed tissues that respond to the laws of physics, mathe-

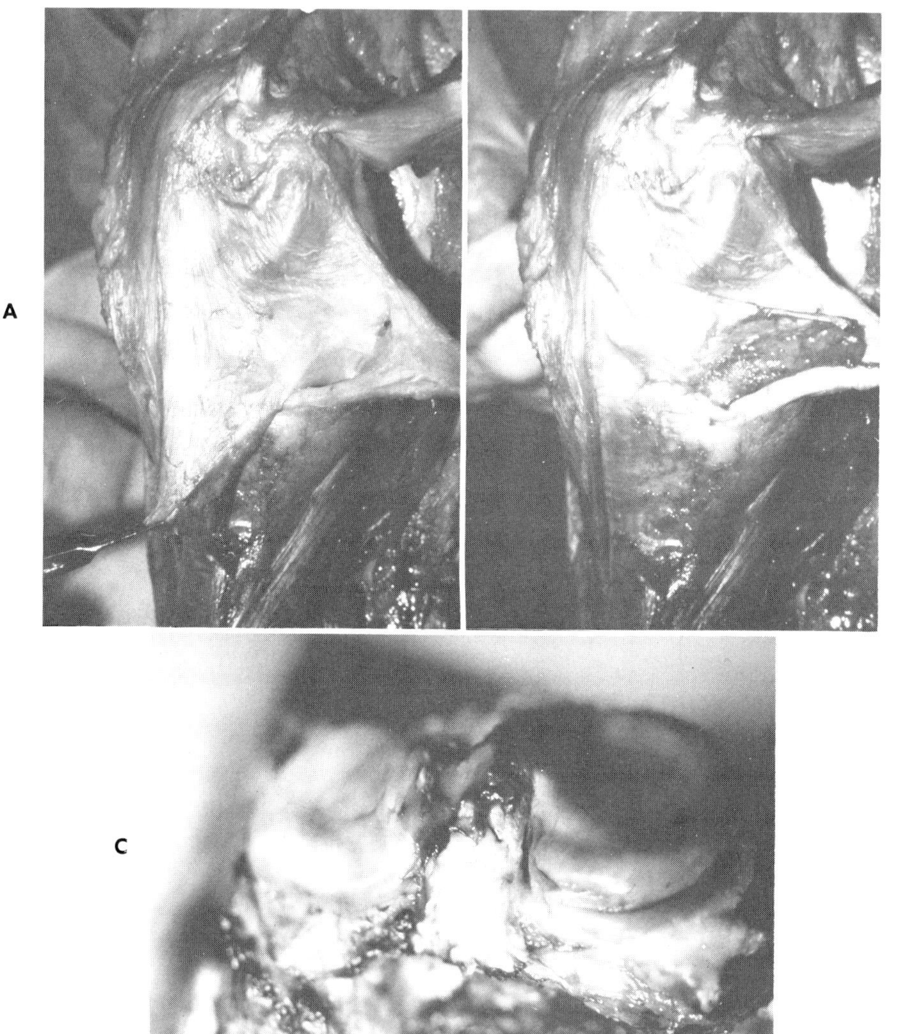

Fig. 16-1. A, Ligamentous layer of the medial side of knee. Distal (tibial) attachment of medial collateral ligament has been detached and is being held with clamp. Note firm longitudinal fibers of medial collateral ligament and relatively small oval-shaped proximal attachment of these fibers to medial femoral epicondyle. Posterior to these fibers are more dynamic fibers of this ligament. **B,** Medial collateral ligament has been lifted proximally, and capsular ligament can be seen tented up by instrument pushing from within joint. Capsular ligament attaches to meniscus forming meniscofemoral portion above meniscus and meniscotibial portion below meniscus. **C,** Intercondylar eminence controls rotation of femoral condyles as well as allowing condyles to move upward with flexion, which helps tighten ligamentous structures.

matics, and biomechanics. Müller[7] described the *dynamized ligament*. Portions of ligament have firm, bony attachments that have only a slight stretching potential. These fibers must be isometrically placed to conform to the mathematical principle of the Burmester curve. These bony attachments cannot be broad enough to allow all fibers to attach in the confines of the Burmester curve. There are therefore fibrous extensions of the vastus medialis, quadriceps anteriorly, and semimembranous posteriorly that act as dynamized fibers and are kept taut by the dynamic action of the muscles. These ligaments also act together with the physical construction of the knee that includes the elements previously mentioned. The configuration of the tibial plateau also aids in tightening the ligaments. The lateral tibial plateau is convex in its sagittal plane, which provides a lift of the femoral condyle and a tightening of these ligaments. The disparity of length of the femoral condyles allows the helicoid motion that is guided by the cruciate ligaments as the knee flexes and extends. There is a rolling action of the knee in the first 20 degrees of flexion, which is the degree of motion necessary for walking. A gliding or sliding action occurs past 20 degrees, with the ligaments, especially the cruciate ligaments, acting to keep the femoral condyles centered over the tibial plateau.

Beneath the superficial dynamic layer is the capsular ligament, which medially is firmly attached to the meniscus (Fig. 16-1, *B*). The posteromedial area is called the posterior oblique complex and the medial meniscus is a vital part. Hughston[2] has compared tears of the meniscofemoral portions to tears of the meniscotibial portion of this capsular ligament. Disruption of the meniscofemoral capsular ligament produces only a mild positive anterior drawer sign, whereas tears of the meniscotibial capsular ligament allow the meniscus to slide off the tibia posteriorly and produce a moderate to marked anterior drawer. The drawer is increased if the anterior cruciate ligament is torn in combination with a tear of the meniscotibial capsular ligament. Restoration of this area, particularly in acute knees with a preserved meniscus, returns the axis of rotation to its normal position, and the meniscus maintains its action and helps to stabilize the medial side of the knee. With chronic laxity allowing increased anterior and medial instability, the meniscus may fail because of the excess stress and shear produced by the excess rotation. If there is an associated deficiency of the anterior cruciate ligament with a marked anterior drawer, enhanced deterioration may occur. However, not every knee with a deficiency of the anterior cruciate ligament will deteriorate. Since joint conformity may be such that the knee can tolerate its loss, the medial meniscus may hold up through its increased demands, or the activity level may be such that this sequence may not occur.

The anterior cruciate ligament does play an important part in knee function (Fig. 16-2, *A*). It not only acts as a guiding mechanism and an anterior stabilizer to prevent anterior displacement of the tibia on the femur, it is also a secondary stabilizer against excess rotational movements of the knee.[9] When there has been tearing or stretching of the medial structures, increased demands are placed on the anterior cruciate ligament (Fig. 16-2, *B*). If it, too, fails, then a more complex type of instability occurs.

When dealing with a chronic medial instability, it is necessary to be aware of the

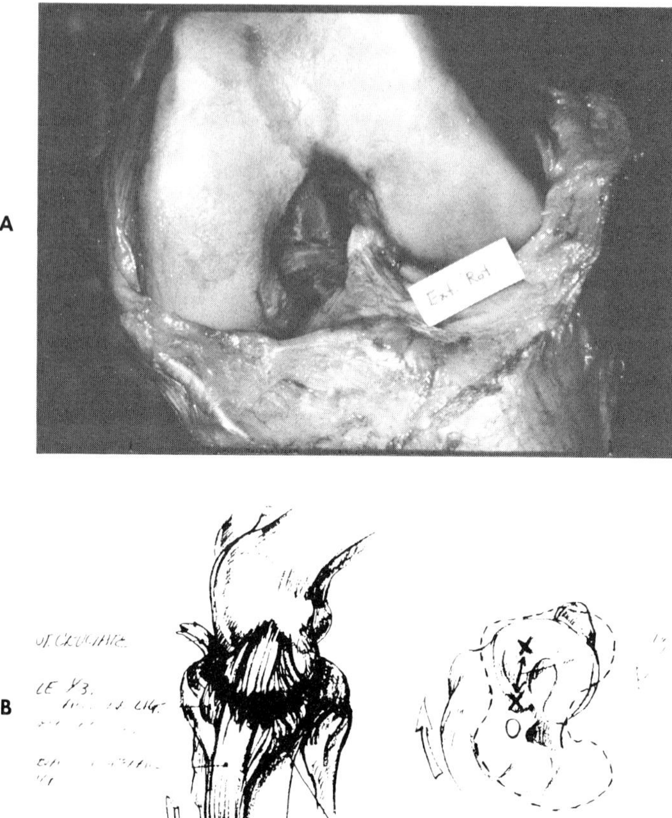

Fig. 16-2. **A,** Intercondylar area of knee showing anterior cruciate and its tibial attachment (just above card) and posterior cruciate ligament and its femoral attachment in left (medial) portion of notch. **B,** With tearing of medial structures as illustrated here, normal axis of rotation shifts from its more central position laterally. This allows excessive (unphysiologic) external rotation of tibial condyle beneath femur.

status of the anterior cruciate ligament. When attempting to control ligamentous instability that has an associated deficiency of the anterior cruciate ligament, the limitations of extraarticular repairs must be recognized. This leaves the deficient anterior cruciate ligament. It is difficult to control primary anterior displacement of the tibia forward from the rim only. Increased stress to other structures may lead to stretching of the extraarticular repair. If extraarticular repairs are used in the presence of a deficiency of the anterior cruciate ligament, a modification of activity level to protect this repair from stretching may be required. It may also require muscle strengthening and a maintenance program with possible bracing for recreational activities to protect the repair. Reconstruction of the medial aspect of the knee may require restoration of any or all of the medial side complex, which includes the posterior oblique ligament, the medial meniscus, the medial capsular ligament, the medial collateral ligament, and the overlying muscular complex that includes the semimembranous posteriorly, the pes anserinus group, and vastus medialis obliquus anteriorly.

HYPOTHESIS OF KNEE LIGAMENT SURGERY

Certain hypotheses can be developed relating to knee ligament surgery.[6]

1. Surgical repair of acute ligament disruption gives better results than later reconstruction.
2. Ligament stretching (interstitial tears) with elongation occurs before actual disruption.
3. The anterior cruciate ligament is the primary stabilizer for anterior movements of the tibia on the femur and a secondary stabilizer for excess rotary motions.
4. The anterior cruciate ligament defects do not fill in, although the blood supply is adequate.
5. Deficiency of one stabilizing structure produces additional stresses on other stabilizers of the knee.
6. The menisci contribute toward stability and functional demands of the knee.
7. Ligament healing requires 9 to 12 months.

Certain considerations should therefore be made before embarking on the surgical restoration for knee instability. These considerations are the degree of instability that is present, functional demands the patient requires, the disability that is produced, and the status of the joint wear. Surgical criteria are also necessary before recommending repairs for chronic instability. These include (1) a functional instability, either in running or walking activities; (2) episodes of swelling that indicate joint irritation; (3) signs of internal derangement, such as meniscal tearing; and (4) signs of extensor mechanism problems.

SURGICAL PROCEDURES FOR MEDIAL REPAIR

Several procedures are used to restore static and dynamic stabilization of the medial side of the knee. These procedures are pes anserine transfer, reefing of the posterior oblique ligament, semimembranous advancement, posterior capsule tightening, sartorial advancement, gracilis transfer, and vastus medialis advancement. These procedures are used alone or in combination, depending on the degree of the instability and the type of instability that requires correction.

Pes anserinus transfer was described by Slocum and Larson in 1968[11] when it was recognized that excessive external rotation of the tibia on an extremity that was planted and cutting in the opposite direction provided a functional disability, particularly in the athletically active individual. This procedure was described as providing a dynamic enhancement of the internal rotation power of the pes anserine group, as well as a sling beneath the flare of the medial tibial condyle that provides increased valgus support. The biomechanics of the pes anserine transfer is to move the semitendinous, which is the most powerful of the pes anserine group, proximally so that it increases its lever arm and enhances its internal rotation power (Fig. 16-3). If there is an associated anterolateral rotatory instability manifested as a pivot shift, the pes anserine transfer will not control this problem. It is therefore necessary to provide an additional anterolateral procedure to provide support to the proximal tibia from both the medial and the lateral sides.

Reefing of the posterior oblique ligament removes the elongation that has been produced by tearing or stretching this ligament.[12] Such elongation allows an increased external rotation of the tibia and provides increased stress to the posterior horn of the meniscus. In association with the tearing of the posterior oblique ligaments, there may be a tear of either the capsular attachment of the medial meniscus or the medial meniscus itself. One area of the posterior medial corner, which is important for this type of surgical repair, is the soft spot that is directly behind the trailing edge of the medial collateral ligament and just anterior to the posterior capsular ligament. This area is opened in an oblique direction beginning at the medial femoral epicondyle and obliquely proceeds posteriorly to the posterior medial edge of the tibia, using the anteromedial limb of the semimenbranous tendon as its stopping point (Fig. 16-4). This area is then double-breasted by bringing the anterior edge of this incision posteriorly and distally and the posterior edge anteriorly and supe-riorly. The anchoring stitch for the posterior advancement takes the suture through the distal portion of the anterior edge; through the posterior capsule and direct head of the semimembranous tendon, which attaches at the posterior tibial tubercle, then back through the posterior capsular area; and then through the anterior edge. This provides a mattress-type suture. These sutures are continued proximally until the anterior edge has been pulled posteriorly and distally. Care must be taken in doing this suturing, since overtightening this area will prevent normal knee extension. After this edge has been satisfactorily closed, the posterior edge is then brought over and attached to the medial capsular ligament.

Semimembranous advancement gives additional support to this posteromedial corner, as well as the dynamic action, and can be enhanced by bringing the conjoined tendon of the semimembranous tendon anteriorly and linking into the underlying posterior oblique ligament repair (Fig. 16-5). Again care must be taken to check the knee for full motion and extension and not to tighten this too tightly and prevent normal knee motion. Should normal knee motion be interfered with, the repair will stretch out, and since the physiologic action of the joint requires motion to occur, a permanent limitation of motion would be produced. After the conjoined tendon of the semimembranous tendon has been advanced, there is often a kinking of the anteromedial limb, which goes along the anteromedial edge of the tibia beneath the medial collateral ligament. This tendon can be detached from the tibia and exte-riorized, reattaching it superficially to the medial collateral ligament in the same alignment as the transferred conjoined tendon of the semimembranous tendon. Such advancement provides a dynamic enhancement of the tightening action of the semi-membranous tendon to the posterior medial corner of the knee.[4]

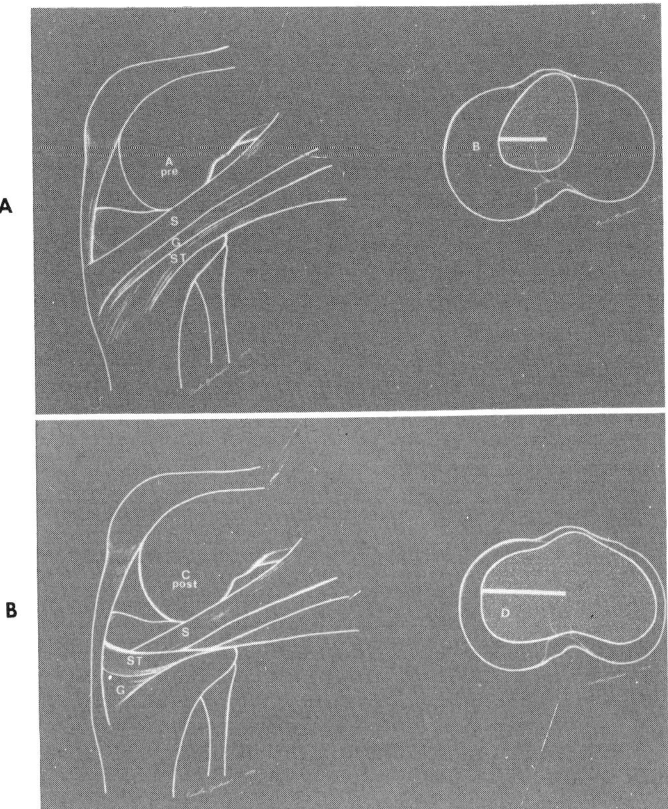

Fig. 16-3. **A,** Normal attachment of pes anserine group of muscles provides short moment arm for action as internal rotator of tibia. Strongest action is as knee flexor. **B,** Transplanting distal portion of pes anserine attachment proximally beneath flare of tibial condyle provides larger moment arm and enhances strength of these muscles to act as internal rotator of tibia. (From James, S.L.: Clin. Orthop. **146:**90, 1980.)

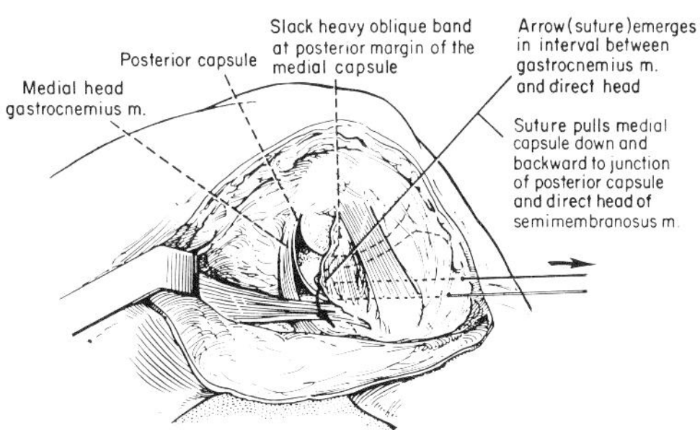

Fig. 16-4. Area just posterior to trailing edge of medial collateral ligament has been incised. Its anterior edge is brought posteriorly and distally. Initial fixation suture should be directed toward attachment of direct head to semimembranous tendon that attaches to posterior tibial tubercle. After advancement of anterior edge, posterior edge is brought anteriorly and superiorly to provide double layer and tightening of this layer. (From Slocum, D.B., Larson, R.L., and James, S.L.: Clin. Orthop. **100:**23, 1974.)

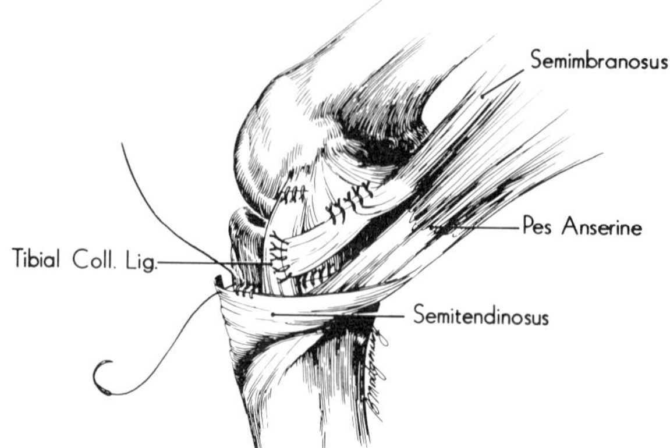

Fig. 16-5. Advancement of conjoined tendon of semimembranous and exteriorizing antero-medial limb of semimembranous. Pes anserine transfer has also been done. Additional sutures shown in figure are from repair of femoral attachment of medial collateral ligament and repair of meniscotibial portion of capsular ligament. (From Larson, R.L.: Dislocations and ligamentous injuries to the knee. In Rockwood, C.A., Jr., and Green, D.P., editors: Fractures, vol. 2, Philadelphia, 1975, J.B. Lippincott Co.)

If there is a posterior capsular laxity, this should be corrected before the posterior oblique ligament reefing is done. *Posterior capsule tightening* can be accomplished by detaching it from its tibial attachment and advancing it distally. It is necessary to extend the knee and determine the point of attachment that will not interfere with normal motion in extension and provide an isometric tension.

Sartorial advancement can be provided when there has been a deficiency produced over the medial collateral ligament[4] (Fig. 16-6). The sartorius is left attached at its anterior attachment on the proximal tibia and mobilized proximally. It is moved anteriorly and superiorly and attached to the medial aspect of the knee in line with the normal medial collateral ligament. The first anchoring stitch in this advancement is through the tendinous portion of the sartorius, which at this height often lies beneath the muscle belly, and this is attached to the tendinous portion of the vastus medialis obliquus. Sutures are then carried distally along the anterior edge of the sartorius tendon to provide fixation in the normal alignment of the collateral ligament. Such an advancement can also be used in an acute situation to provide scaffolding for markedly disrupted medial collateral ligament tissue.

When there has been an associated stretching of the anterior cruciate ligament and it is not felt that anterior cruciate ligament reconstruction repair is necessary, enhancement of its function can be provided by *gracilis transfer* (Fig. 16-7). In this situation the gracilis is detached distally at its tibial attachment.[5] It is then mobilized proximally. It is delivered through the posterior capsule beneath the oblique popliteal ligament to the notch area. A drill hole is placed in the proximal tibia beginning just medial to the tibial tubercle and extending into the notch, exiting just posterior to the anteromedial attachment of the anterior cruciate ligament. The gracilis is then delivered through this tibial drill hole to the anterior aspect of the tibia where it is affixed with sutures or stapling.

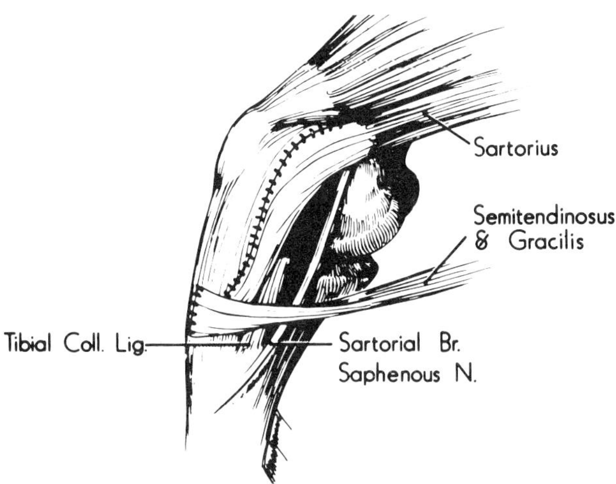

Fig. 16-6. Sartorial advancement produced by mobilizing its tendinous portion and leaving distal attachment intact. It is then sutured along line of deficient medial collateral ligament. (From Larson, R.L.: Dislocations and ligamentous injuries to the knee. In Rockwood, C.A., Jr., and Green, D.P., editors: Fractures, vol. 2, Philadelphia, 1975, J.B. Lippincott Co.)

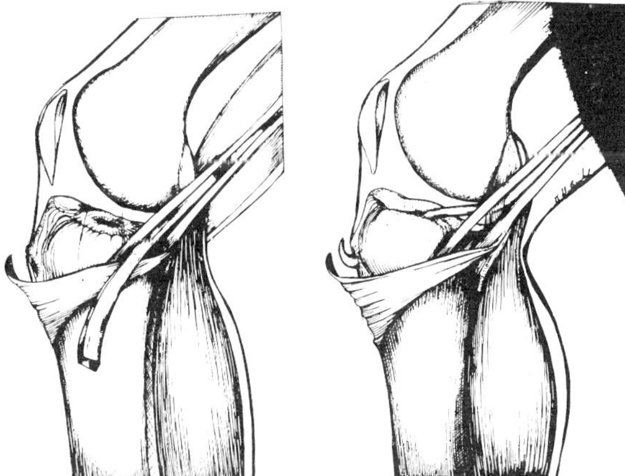

Fig. 16-7. The gracilis is detached distally and mobilized proximally. It is brought through midportion of posterior capsule beneath oblique popliteal ligament. It is then taken through drill hole in anterior tibia and fixed anteriorly. (From Larson, R.L.: Combined instabilities: combinations of surgical procedures. In American Academy of Orthopaedic Surgeons: Symposium on reconstructive surgery of the knee, St. Louis, 1978, The C.V. Mosby Co.)

Vastus medialis advancement is used when it is necessary to provide some dynamic support to a stretched-out medial ligament complex. The vastus medialis obliquus muscle is mobilized, leaving a small cuff of tendinous portion distally, bringing this distally, and reattaching it to the medial collateral ligament. When there has been marked stretching of the medial collateral ligament, fibrous nonelastic tissue results. A proximal or distal advancement of the entire medial collateral ligament attachment may be used to retighten this medial complex. Studies by Bartel and others[1] suggest that the distal advancement taken anteriorly and distally provides a more physiologic action of the joint than does the proximal advancement.

SUMMARY

Some of the problems that we face in providing a physiologic joint include (1) providing continuity and meniscal support by repair of the capsule because of ligament thinness in certain areas, (2) providing anatomic placement that produces a type of isometric tension and a biomechanical efficiency of the reconstructions of ligamentous tissue, and (3) definitely predicting the efficiency of the action of dynamic muscle transfers in reconstructive procedures. Because of these inadequacies, the decision to improve knee joint stability by surgery depends on our abilities to restore physiologic kinematics in a manner that the physiologic action of the joint will not provide a stretching out of repaired tissue, yet will still allow the normal arc of motion in flexion, extension, and rotation.

There is also a problem in assessing the various results after different types of reconstructive knee surgery. These variables include the constitutional factors of individuals, the ability of tissues to heal, the multiple surgical procedures that are performed in various combinations, the variation in immobility and length of the immobility provided, the differences in rehabilitation programs and the importance of various factors in rehabilitation, and the activity level to which the patient returns after the reconstruction procedure.

Certain externally regulated stimuli, such as joint motion, protect the articular cartilage from degenerative changes while certain amounts of physiologic stress provide an improved healing response and improved tensile strength of healing tissues.

Balanced against this is the adverse effect produced by the jeopardy of repair if too much tension is applied or the inflammatory response that may be produced if too much motion is allowed before muscle strength and joint recovery have been attained.

•　　•　　•

The restoration of stability of the knee requires an understanding of joint kinematics and an appreciation of the anatomic construction that allows physiologic motion. Reconstructive procedures that attempt to restore the harmony of normal knee motion with the stability necessary for vigorous use is a difficult task. Failures often relate to the placement of static tissue in a location that either limits motion or stretches with use. Stabilizing a joint as complex as the knee requires the application of principles of biomechanics, engineering, and mathematics, as well as surgical skills, for a successful result.

REFERENCES

1. Bartel, D.L., and others: Surgical repositioning of the medial collateral ligament, J. Bone Joint Surg. **59A:**107, 1977.
2. Hughston, J.C., and Barrett, G.R.: Acute anteromedial rotatory instability: long-term results of surgical repair. J. Bone Joint Surg. **65A:**145, 1983.
3. Kapandji, I.A.: The physiology of the joints, ed. 2, vol. 2, Edinburgh, 1970, Churchill-Livingstone Co.
4. Larson, R.L.: Dislocations and ligamentous injuries to the knee. In Rockwood, C.A., and Green, D.P., editors: Fractures, Philadelphia, 1975, J.B. Lippincott Co.
5. Larson, R.L.: Combined instabilities: combinations of surgical procedures. In American Academy of Orthopaedic Surgeons: Symposium on reconstructive surgery of the knee, St. Louis, 1978, The C.V. Mosby Co.
6. Larson, R.L.: Acute disruptions around the knee. In Straub, L.R., and Wilson, P.D., editors: Clinical trends in orthopaedics, New York, 1982, Thieme-Stratton, Inc.
7. Muller, W.: The knee: form, function, and ligament reconstruction, New York, 1983, Springer-Verlag, New York, Inc.
8. Nicholas, J.A.: Glossary of sports maneuvers in which the knee is immediately involved, Paper presented at the American Academy of Orthopaedic Surgeon's postgraduate course, Eugene, Ore., July 23-25, 1973.
9. Noyes, F.R., and others: Clinical biomechanics of the knee: ligament restraints and functional stability. In American Academy of Orthopaedic Surgeons: Symposium on the athlete's knee: surgical repair and reconstruction, St. Louis, 1980, The C.V. Mosby Co.
10. Palmer, I.: On the injuries to the ligaments of the knee joint. ACTA Chir. Scand. **81**(suppl 53):3, 1938.
11. Slocum, D.B., and Larson, R.L.: Pes anserinus transplant: a simple surgical procedure for control of rotatory instability of the knee, J. Bone Joint Surg. **50A:**226, 1968.
12. Slocum, D.B., Larson, R.L., and James, S.L.: Late reconstruction of ligamentous injuries of the medial compartment of the knee, Clin. Orthop. **100:**23, 1974.

17. Initial evaluation and management of acute anterior cruciate ligament ruptures

Russell F. Warren

Over the past 15 years much of the confusion regarding the function of the anterior cruciate ligament (ACL) and its major role in preventing the symptoms of giving way has been elucidated. In contrast, considerable debate continues to exist regarding the correct methods of managing this injury both acutely and chronically.

Some physicians still maintain that most patients do quite well without their ACL and advocate nonoperative treatment,[8] while others maintain that the results of nonoperative treatment are so poor and unpredictable that repair is not warranted, thus advocating either reconstruction or a "wait and see" approach with a late reconstruction when indicated.

PATIENT EVALUATION

Our experience has demonstrated several factors that will enable the physician to make a reasonable judgment in selecting the best course for a patient. The natural history following injury is variable, depending on the patient's activities and life-style. Overall, it appears that about 20% of the patients do quite well following ACL injury. Generally they are not loose-jointed and have no loss of secondary restraints. About 40% of the patients in our clinic have significant problems, but through bracing, exercise, and avoidance of specific activities they are able to tolerate their condition. Another 40% have major disabilities that require discontinuing an active life-style or having an ACL reconstruction. These percentages will undoubtedly vary from physician to physician, depending on the patient's activity level. Fortunately, only a few will have problems with daily activities in the first decade following injury. Symptoms are produced mainly in sports or work activities that require jumping, rapid deceleration, and cutting.

Other important factors to consider are the patient's ligamentous laxity and the status of the secondary restraints. Individuals who are loose-jointed with knee recurvatum, varus and marked tibial torsion, or a physiologic pivot shift appear to be at a greater risk for developing symptoms following isolated ACL injury. In addition, these same patients appear to do poorly following reconstruction, since they have stretched the secondary restraints over time. Thus we feel that the best way to handle these patients is with a primary repair of the ACL combined with semitendinous augmentation.

The role of secondary restraints is obvious to anyone who has seen a clinically stable knee of a patient with an absent ACL develop marked symptoms of instability following a complete medial meniscectomy. The role of the secondary restraints has become more important over time as the knees progressively fail. These patients may then require a medial meniscectomy and subsequently a lateral meniscectomy. We have previously found in a selective cutting study that the medial meniscus in the ACL-insufficient knee helps to prevent further anterior tibial translation on the femur (Fig. 17-1). In the ACL-insufficient knee, if a medial meniscectomy is performed there will be an 18% increase in tibial translation at 0 degrees of flexion increasing to 58% at 90 degrees of flexion. In contrast, it appears that the lateral meniscus plays only a minor role in increasing tibial translation following meniscectomy.[3]

Additional injury to the collateral ligaments is important, particularly the medial collateral ligament (MCL). We have found that the deep capsule and oblique component of the medial ligament at the posterior medial corner of the knee has no effect on anterior tibial translation.[11] In contrast, if the superficial MCL is incised, increased anterior tibial translation is seen if the ACL is absent. Thus in patients with known MCL or meniscal injury an increased probability of developing symptoms of giving way would be anticipated.

The age of the patient is an additional factor that we feel is of concern, since the young are most likely to participate in activities that will result in symptoms of

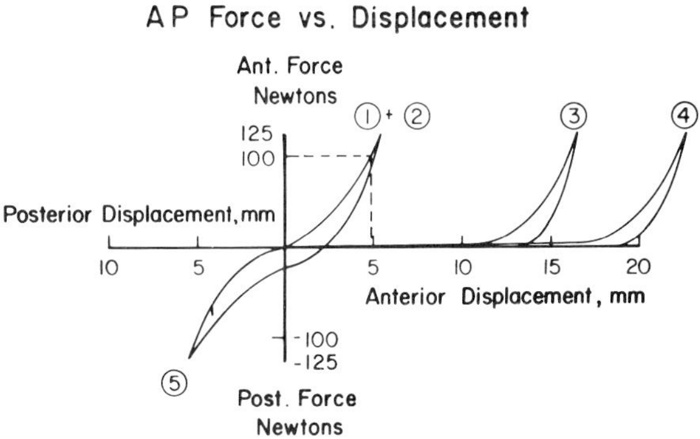

Fig. 17-1. Graph representing mean induced anterior tibial translation in intact knee *(1)*, following medial meniscectomy *(2)*, representing anterior tibial translation following ACL resection *(3)*, and *(4)* after medial meniscus was excised (marked increase was seen averaging 58% at 90 degrees of flexion vs 18% at 0 degrees of flexion). (From Levy, I.M., Torzilli, P.A. and Warren, R.F.: J. Bone Joint Surg. **64A:**885, 1982.)

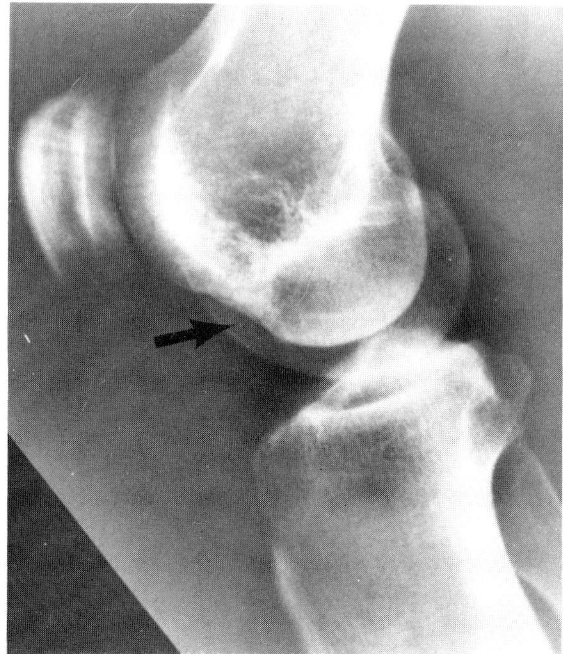

Fig. 17-2. Notch seen in lateral femoral condyle of patient with 3-year history of ACL rupture. Occasionally seen in acute ACL injury, but more common in chronic ACL injury.

instability and are also the group that will have to contend with the injury for 50 to 60 years. While we do not presently advocate primary repair as avoiding subsequent degenerative arthritis, it has been our observation in a retrospective study of 130 patients with chronic ACL injuries that degenerative changes frequently occur.[10] Generally these changes consist of periarticular osteophytes around the periphery of the joint, as well as superior and inferior spurs on the patella and peaking of tibial spines.

These changes are routinely seen after 5 years of ACL insufficiency. The degenerative changes consisting of joint-narrowing, sclerosis, and cyst formation occur toward the end of the first decade and are often marked by 20 years, irrespective of a previous meniscectomy. In addition, we have noted (Fig. 17-2) that a lateral notch will form on the lateral femoral condyle in some patients with chronic ACL injury.[4] With these criteria in mind, primary repair of the ACL is advocated for those patients felt to be "at risk." While it may represent overtreatment for some patients, it is appropriate for most. In addition, by using these selective criteria our conservative treatment and operative treatment will be improved.

ACL INJURY RECOGNITION

Previously the anterior drawer sign was felt to be the best test for noting the ACL injury. Unfortunately, many patients are unable to flex to 90 degrees, and, in

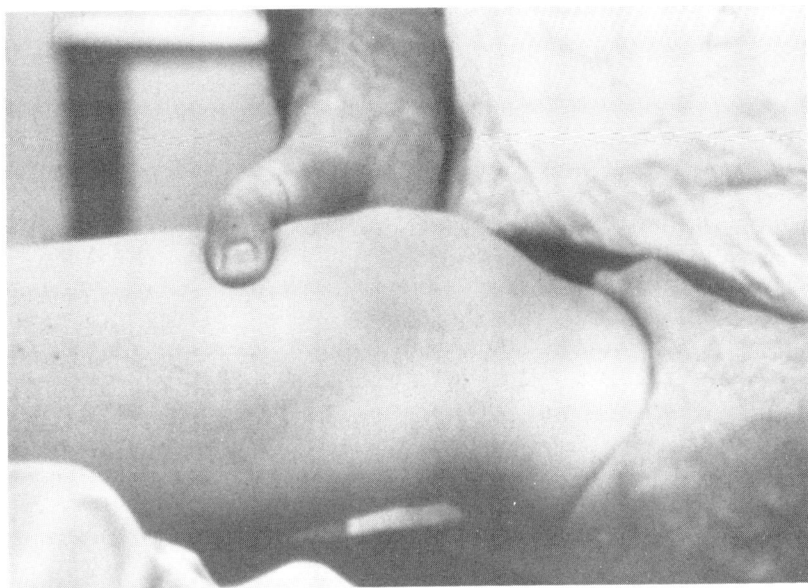

Fig. 17-3. Lachman test performed in 20 to 30 degrees of knee flexion.

addition, the increased excursion at 90 degrees following ACL disruption may be minimal. The Lachman test (Fig. 17-3) performed at 30 degrees has become the standard for recognizing acute ACL injury. The improved results with this test occur because the anterior tibial translation following ACL injury is maximum at 30 degrees, dropping off dramatically at 0 and 90 degrees.[2] In contrast, the posterior excursion secondary to posterior cruciate ligament (PCL) injury is maximum for 70 to 90 degrees of flexion. In performing the Lachman test, not only is increased tibial excursion noted, but more important, there is the loss of end point. End point is the jar that the examiner and frequently the patient will note on performing the Lachman test as the stiffness in the ACL increases and abruptly stops the tibial motion.

If this jar is absent, an injury to the ACL should be diagnosed. Rarely a displaced bucket-handle tear of the meniscus will alter the end point, but otherwise this test is accurate in the office in 99% of our patients. We have not found the pivot-shift test to be particularly helpful in the office, being positive in only 38%, but under anesthesia it will be positive in nearly 100% of the patients. The anterior drawer sign is more reliable if tested under anesthesia, but was still positive in only 54% of isolated ACL injuries. The positive percentage increased dramatically as the secondary restraints were lost. With combined ACL/MCL injury 89% were positive, and nearly 100% were positive if both menisci were torn.[1]

We have not found arthroscopy to be frequently required to evaluate these patients. In fact, we feel that arthroscopy is often overused, and a more thorough clinical examination would decrease the use of arthroscopy for diagnostic purposes. There are, however, certain indications for arthrography and arthroscopy.

We have found arthrography to be useful when the presence or absence of meniscus injuries will influence the subsequent treatment. Overall, approximately 25% of our ACL repairs have had a significant meniscus lesion requiring excision or reattachment. A well-performed arthrogram will demonstrate the presence and type of meniscus injury and suggest that primary reattachment may be possible. In addition, we have found a 96% accuracy rate in predicting the presence of a torn or normal ACL.[9]

Arthroscopy is reserved for those situations when the clinical tests are equivocal or the pivot-shift test under anesthesia is negative. In this situation there may be a partial ACL injury. While it is true that a much higher percentage of meniscal tears in association with acute ACL tears (70%) will be noted by arthroscopy, these are often insignificant partial vertical tears requiring no treatment.

Arthroscopy is also used to aid in making a decision about treatment in those patients whose damaged meniscus may determine the type of treatment. Thus a patient with a nonrepairable meniscus will be treated by meniscectomy, but meniscus reattachment is performed when possible and combined with ACL repair. An additional indication for arthroscopy is in those patients being considered for primary repair, but more than 2 weeks have passed since their injury.

SURGERY

Over the past 10 years we have advocated primary repair with augmentation for those patients who have poor quality ACL tissues.[7] Initially the iliotibial band was used, but over the past 3 years we have switched to the semitendinous, since it has better biomechanical characteristics. Overall, we will reinforce about 30% of our primary repairs, but, if in doubt, augmentation is preferred.

In addition, we have added a lateral sling procedure to our primary repairs over the past 3 years to act as a restraint against tibial translation and to decrease the pivot shift. This combined approach had a definite effect on our patients with chronic ACL insufficiency that lowered the pivot shift rate to 9% following quadriceps tendon substitution. Whether this has been beneficial in our primary repair group will be determined in our 5-year follow-up study.

TECHNIQUE OF REPAIR

Having decided on a primary repair, we use a long anterior lateral incision (or medial and lateral incisions if there is MCL damage) (Fig. 17-4). After exploring the joint and assessing the status of the menisci, reattachment of the meniscus is performed when possible. We have become aggressive in performing meniscus reattachment, particularly medially where we will attempt to repair tears that include the midportion of the meniscus (Fig. 17-5). To accomplish this repair, vascular access channels may be created to allow the ingrowth of vessels into the meniscal defect. In creating these channels, care must be taken to avoid further destabilization of the meniscus. Repair is then done using 3-0 Dexon sutures. After completing the meniscal repair the knee is flexed to 100 degrees, and the ACL stumps are dissected out.

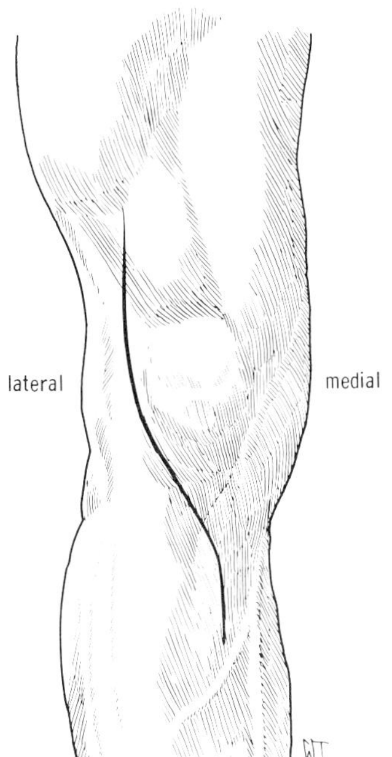

Fig. 17-4. Lateral approach for ACL repair is generally used. (From Warren, R.F.: Acute ligamentous injuries. In Insall, J., editor: Surgery of the knee, Edinburgh, 1984, Churchill-Livingstone.)

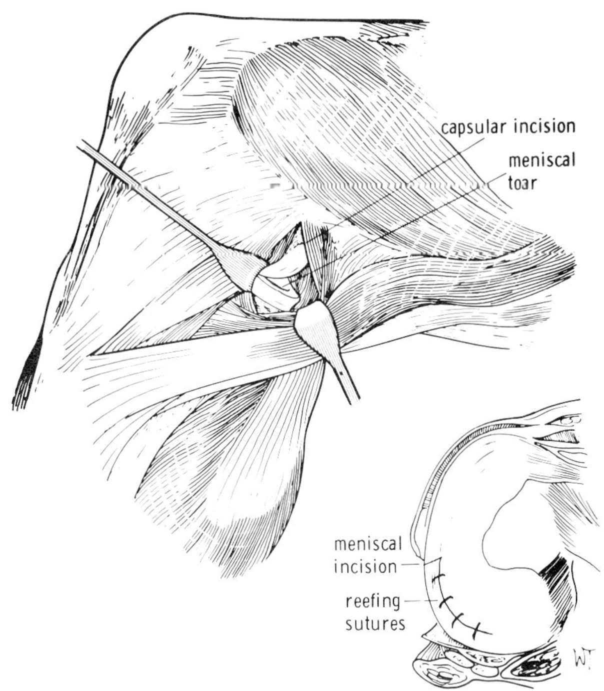

Fig. 17-5. Incision behind medial ligament will expose posterior horn of the meniscus allowing meniscus repair. (From Warren, R.F.: Acute ligamentous injuries. In Insall, J., editor: Surgery of the knee, Edinburgh, 1984, Churchill-Livingstone.)

Generally the tear is spiral, running from anterior proximal to posterior distal in the ACL. In over 80% of the patients the tear is essentially the midportion of this type, while in about 15% it is essentially an avulsion proximally. While performing the repair, the multiple loop suture technique is used to dissipate the stresses throughout the ligament (Fig. 17-6). The sutures are placed at varying depths down to the fibrocartilaginous insertion on the femur and tibia. Drill holes are then placed in the tibia and femur. The placement is critical, particularly on the femur where it must be posteriorly well positioned. If the ligament is advanced anteriorly, it will either limit flexion or stretch out. Generally only one hole is placed in the femoral condyle and the second set of sutures is placed over the top of the lateral femoral condyle (Fig. 17-7).

The lateral sling is then constructed by taking a strip of iliotibial band running from Gerdy's tubercle proximally for 6 inches. It is about 1.5 cm wide, and after tubing it is passed deep to the lateral collateral ligament (LCL) at its femoral attachment site (Fig. 17-8).

If it is felt that the suture repair of the ACL was inadequate or if there is collateral ligament damage, then an augmentation using the semitendinous tendon is performed (Fig. 17-9). The tendon is dissected proximally and detached at the muscle tendon junction. The tendon is passed through the tibia and over the top of the lateral femoral condyle where it is stapled in place. Before suturing the ACL the lateral sling is stapled in place with the knee at 90 degrees of flexion. Then the sutures are tied in place.

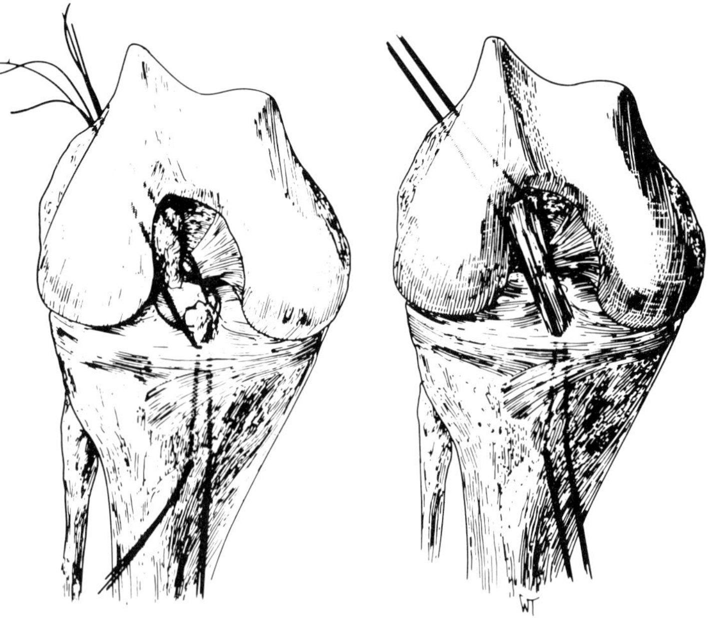

Fig. 17-6. Marshall multiple loop suture technique for primary repair of ACL ruptures. (From Marshall, J.L., and others: Clin. Orthop. **143**:99, 1979.)

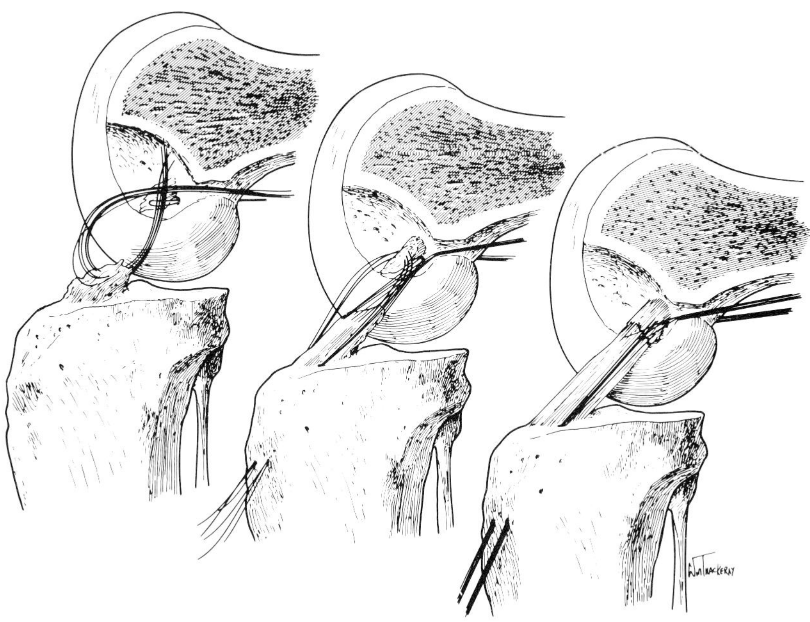

Fig. 17-7. Lateral view of Marshall multiple loop suture technique for primary ACL repair. (From Marshall, J.L., and others: Clin. Orthop. **143**:99, 1979.)

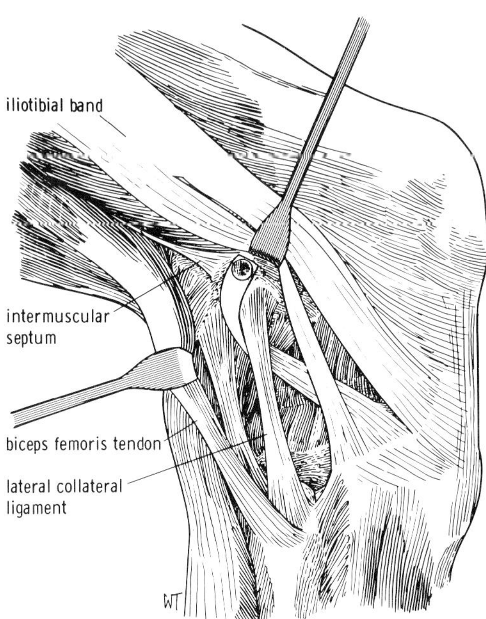

Fig. 17-8. Lateral sling procedure used in primary ACL repair. Graft passes from Gerdy's tubercle beneath femoral attachment of lateral collateral ligament.

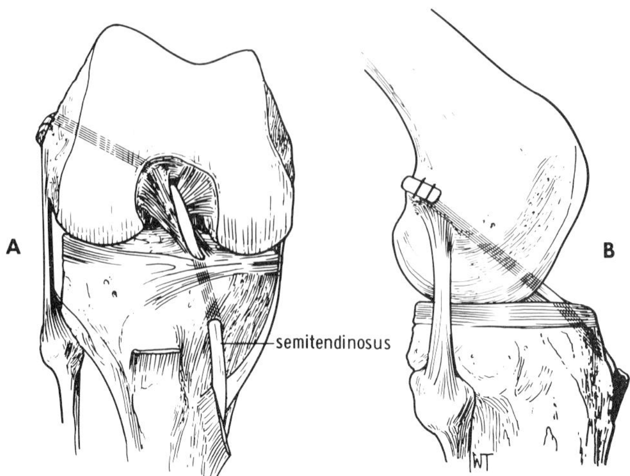

Fig. 17-9. A, Anterior view of semitendinous augmentation of primary ACL repair. **B,** Lateral view of semitendinous augmentation of primary ACL repair. (From Warren, R.F.: Acute ligamentous injuries. In Insall, J., editor: Surgery of the knee, Edinburgh, 1984, Churchill-Livingstone.)

The tourniquet is then released, and drains are placed. A plaster splint is applied over a Jones dressing with the knee flexed 30 degrees. On the fourth to fifth postoperative day a fiberglass cast is applied and then worn for 5 additional weeks. At that time a limited motion brace is applied with motion from 30 to 60 degrees. During this period physical therapy will work only on flexion. Subsequently, the brace is adjusted to −10 degrees of extension and a derotation strap is used. At 3 months the hamstrings are exercised, and at 4 months limited-arc quadriceps exercises are begun, avoiding the terminal 30 degrees of extension.

Bracing is continued full time for 5 months, and running is begun about the sixth month. Sports are initiated after 7 to 8 months initially using the brace, but subsequently discarding it if the follow-up examination is satisfactory.

FOLLOW-UP

We have carried out two follow-up studies on our initial patients. The initial study reported by Marshall and others[7] consisted of 70 patients with an average follow-up of 29 months. Sixty-one patients had ACL repair alone, and nine had augmentation with the fascia lata. Patients were evaluated on the HSS 50-point knee scoring system with an average score of 42.7. No patients had developed giving way or symptoms of instability. In addition, no patient required subsequent meniscectomy, a frequently noted occurrence in ACL-insufficient knees. Overall 93% of the patients were active in sports.

This past year we have completed a long-term follow-up of 52 of the initial patients at a minimum of 5 years with an average of 82 months. At follow-up each patient was scored on our 50-point system with an average of 41.8. Eighty-nine percent of the patients were active in some sport, 63% had no restrictions, and 26% had some limitations. Five patients (9.6%) were considered to be failures. These patients complained of giving way and unpredictable instability. Each of these patients had a 2 + or 3 + pivot shift. Overall, 15 patients had a positive pivot shift, but 10 of these were a minimal grind that many would not consider as a positive shift. These patients were not symptomatic and had no giving way. In addition, we tested 28 patients with the KT-1000 machine designed by Malcolm. When tested at 30 degrees and 20 pounds of force, there was an average difference of 2.5 mm from the surgical knee to noninjured knee in the asymptomatic patients. There was a marked increase in the five clinically unstable patients, with a difference of 6.6 mm found in the injured knee.

Overall, we have not been impressed by any significant deterioration over time following primary ACL repair despite continued sports activity in 89% of our patients. This is supported by the lack of significant meniscal deterioration requiring meniscectomy in these patients. Of the five patients complaining of giving way at 82 months, three patients had a 2 + or 3 + pivot shift at the 29-month follow-up and were regarded as failures. Thus our failure rate of 9.6% in our active population must be compared to untreated populations like those reported by McDaniel and Dameron.[8] In their study of 52 patients with untreated ACL injuries, 83% had a positive pivot shift and 79% complained of giving way despite only 47% participating in unrestricted sports.

It is our opinion that in the carefully selected patient primary repair offers a distinct advantage. If the tissue is deemed inadequate, then semitendinous augmentation should be added to the repair. In addition, we recommend combining this with an extraarticular lateral sling to aid in decreasing the incidence of pivot shift.

REFERENCES

1. Donaldson, W., and Warren, R.F.: A comparison of acute cruciate ligament examinations initial vs examination under anesthesia, Paper presented at the meeting of the American Orthopedic Society for Sports Medicine, Williamsburg, Va., July, 1983.
2. Fukuybashi, T., and others: An in vitro biomechanical evaluation of anterior-posterior motion of the knee, J. Bone Joint Surg. **64A:**258, 1982.
3. Gould, J.D., and others: The effect of lateral meniscectomy on anterior posterior motion of the knee, Trans. Orthop. Res. Soc. Atlanta **5:** 1984.
4. Kaplan, N., and Warren, R.F.: The lateral notch: a case review, In preparation, 1984.
5. Kaplan, N., Warren, R.F., and Wickiewicz, T.L.: Long-term follow-up of primary surgical treatment of anterior cruciate ligament ruptures, In preparation, 1983.
6. Levy, I.M., Torzilli, P.A., and Warren, R.F.: The effect of medial meniscectomy on anterior-posterior motion of the knee, J. Bone Joint Surg. **64A:**883, 1982.
7. Marshall, J.L., Warren, R.F., and Wickiewicz, T.L.: Primary surgical treatment of anterior cruciate ligament lesions, Am. J. Sports Med. **10:**2, 1982.
8. McDaniel, W.J., and Dameron, T.B.: Untreated ruptures of the anterior cruciate ligament, J. Bone Joint Surg. **62A:**696, 1980.
9. Pavlov, H., and others: The accuracy of double contrast arthrographic evaluation of the anterior cruciate ligament, J. Bone Joint Surg. **65A:**175, 1983.
10. Sherman, M., and others: A clinical and radiographical analysis of 127 anterior cruciate insufficient knees, Paper presented at the Hospital for Special Surgery, New York, 1980.
11. Sullivan, D., and others: Medial restraints to anterior-posterior knee motion, J. Bone Joint Surg., 1984. (In press.)

18. Advances in biologic substitution for cruciate deficiency

William G. Clancy, Jr.

The fact that anterior cruciate ligament insufficiency can lead to functional instability, meniscal tears, and degenerative arthritis has been demonstrated in dogs by McDevitt[22] and Marshall,[20] and in humans by Jacobsen,[15] Clancy,[10] and Bergfeld.[4] That posterior cruciate ligament (PCL) insufficiency can lead to early traumatic arthritis has been reported by Kennedy[16] and more recently by Clancy.[11] It would appear therefore that in some if not most of those patients with anterior or posterior cruciate ligament insufficiency stabilization may be of significant benefit. To date there have been a number of procedures proposed and used to correct anterior cruciate ligament insufficiency. These procedures consist of an intraarticular substitution, an extraarticular tenodesis, or a combination of both.

Logic would dictate that intraarticular substitution should be the procedure of choice. A number of procedures have been proposed and performed using an intraarticular biologic substitute. The various substitutes have consisted of patellar tendon,[10,12] semitendinosus,[7,18] gracilis,[23] and fascia lata,[25] or combinations of these. Until recently there were few reports of long-term follow-up of these procedures. More importantly there has been little research on the revascularization, histologic change, and biomechanical properties of these substitutes.

There are a number of factors that must be considered in evaluating and selecting a biologic substitute. The biologic substitute must initially be of sufficient tensile strength to withstand the loads that occur in the knee joint. The substitute, if avascular, must readily revascularize. The substitute must also regain sufficient tensile strength to tolerate the demands placed on it. In addition, the substitute should readily achieve bone-to-bone or tendon-to-bone union. Finally the substitute must be placed so that it is as isometric as possible through the full range of motion.

Thus the substitute must have a high tensile strength, must readily revascularize, and must regain reasonably high tensile strength. The graft placement must be such that it is isometric and will not stretch out with motion.

POTENTIAL BIOLOGIC SUBSTITUTES

Noyes[24] has studied the tensile strength of the anterior cruciate ligament and compared it to the tensile strengths of the various potential biologic substitutes. He found that the tensile strength of the semitendinosus tendon was 75%, the gracilis tendon was 49%, the distal iliotibial tract was 53%, and the patellar tendon, patellar retinaculum, and quadriceps tendon were 15% to 21%. This quadriceps, patellar tendon, and patellar tendon retinaculum is different from the one-third patellar tendon with its bony attachments. The patellar tendon inserts into the lower one third of the patella, and the quadriceps tendon inserts into the proximal portion of the patella. The two structures are connected by only a thin superficial layer of aponeurotic fibers, and it is this structure that is the significant weak link in the quadriceps patellar tendon graft (QPTG) with a tensile strength of only 15% to 21%. The one-third patellar tendon with its bony attachments has been shown by Noyes[24] to be 163% to 175% the strength of the anterior cruciate ligament. Kennedy's tensile testing[17] found that the posterior cruciate ligament was almost twice the strength of the anterior cruciate ligament. Thus the one-third patellar tendon with its bony attachments would be initially 90% of the strength of the posterior cruciate ligament.

From these studies it would appear that the one-third patellar tendon with its bony attachment has the highest initial tensile strength. The semitendinosus and gracilis tendons when used together or the combination of semitendinosus tendon and iliotibial tract would appear to be reasonable secondary procedures for anterior cruciate ligament substitution.

GRAFT PLACEMENT

The various procedures reported for intraarticular substitution have not recognized the importance of graft placement and graft length. To prevent the stretching out of the substitute the graft must be placed as isometrically as possible. Since none of the potential grafts can reduplicate the broad insertion pattern of the normal anterior cruciate ligament, the substitute should be placed so that it lies in the anatomic center of the insertional sites on the tibia and the femur.

Girgis and Marshall[14] have extensively studied the insertional area of the anterior cruciate ligament. From their studies it become apparent that any tunnel placed in the tibia must be placed eccentrically so that the posterolateral circumference of the tibial tunnel will coincide with the anatomic center of the anterior cruciate ligament insertion. Since the substitutes are relatively flat structures and since their direction of pull is posterior and lateral toward the lateral femoral condyle, the graft must lie along the posterolateral circumference of the tibial tunnel. Girgis and Marshall's study demonstrates that the anterior cruciate insertion on the tibial eminence is medially eccentric. Therefore the K wire must be eccentrically anteromedial so that when it is overdrilled the posterolateral circumference will lie at the anatomic center of the original anterior cruciate ligament.

For the same rationale, the K wire must be placed eccentrically posterior and superior to the anatomic center of the anterior cruciate ligament insertion on the lateral femoral condyle. When the K wire is overdrilled the anterior and inferior circumference of the tunnel will lie at the anatomic center, and, since the substitute is directed anteriorly and medially to the tibia, this is where the graft will lie.

Both McIntosh[19] and Marshall[21] have advocated placement of the substitute around the lateral femoral condyle with fixation on the lateral side of the femur. It was their conjecture that the graft would lie along the entire insertion of the anterior cruciate on the lateral femoral condyle. However, our observations on cadaver knees reveal that the graft lies along the insertion site from full extension to approximately 45 degrees of flexion at which time the graft loosens up. It appears that the graft loosens up because of the *cam* shape of the lateral femoral condyle and because the substitute is not fixed to the lateral femoral condyle. This laxity allows for increased anterior tibial translation. If this type of lateral femoral condyle placement is desired, then a trough must be made in the insertional area of the lateral femoral condyle. The graft should be fixed to this point so that the substitution will become united to the femur in the trough.

Adequate tendon length is necessary so that it can be placed in the appropriate location on the tibia and the lateral femoral condyle. Wirth[29] has demonstrated that one third of the patellar tendon, when left attached to the tibia, was not long enough in 87 of 100 cadaver knees to reach the anatomic center on the lateral femoral condyle. Thus osteotomy of the tibial attachment should allow the graft to slide proximally in the tibial tunnel. Vascular studies by Scapinelli[27] have shown that there is no osseous vascular contribution to the patellar tendon from its bony attachment site, so it is a free graft whether or not it is left attached to the tibia.

HISTOLOGIC, MICROANGIOGRAPHIC, AND BIOMECHANICAL ANALYSES OF CRUCIATE SUBSTITUTION

In 1974 Alm[1] was the first to report detailed histologic and microangiographic analyses of patellar tendon substitution for the anterior cruciate ligament. This study was performed in 29 dogs. Ten dogs were not immobilized after surgery, nine were immobilized for 1 week, and ten were immobilized for 2 weeks. Histologic and microangiographic analyses were performed over a 5-month period. When sacrificed, only 12 of the 29 dogs (41%) had an intact substitute; however, those rigidly immobilized for 2 weeks had a much higher success rate (80%).

Microangiographic studies during the first 8 weeks in those with intact substitutes revealed that the distal portion of the substitute that laid in the tibial groove vascularized rapidly, while the midportions and proximal portions in which the sutures were placed did not revascularize until approximately 8 weeks. Revascularization was noted to come from contributions of the posterior cruciate synovium, the fat pad that was sutured to the graft, and the tunnel or cavity created in the lateral femoral condyle.

Histologically it was noted that by the fourth day vessels from the fat pad sutured to the graft were noted to anastomose with the endoligamentous vessels in the midpart of the transplant.

In the first week the fibrocytes in the substitute were noted to lose their ability to stain. There was also increased disintegration and fragmentation of the collagen in the substitute. By 8 weeks the substitute had become revascularized. By the twentieth week the patellar tendon substitute resembled a normal ligament. An 80% success rate (8 of 10 dogs) was found in the group that was rigidly immobilized for 2 weeks. Unfortunately, no tensile testing was performed on these substitutes. There was only a 40% success rate in those not immobilized (4 of 10 dogs) and complete failure (9 of 9 dogs) in those immobilized for only 1 week.

Chiroff[6] performed histologic analysis on patellar tendon substitutions for the anterior cruciate ligament in eight knees of four dogs. The substitute was placed over the tibia and into a femoral tunnel. The leg was immobilized for 4 weeks. He found that the substitute initially underwent necrosis followed at 8 weeks by syn-ovialization with concurrent ingrowth of fibroblasts. At 4 weeks the patellar bone was incorporated at its margin to the femoral tunnel and was completely incorporated at 1 year. At 1 year there were still some areas of necrosis present as well as continued fibroblastic activity. All joints were found to be stable at the time of sacrifice.

Arnoczky and others[2] studied the vascular response in a partial injury to the anterior cruciate ligament and noted that the repair reaction including the vascular response was mainly from the fat pad and synovial membrane surrounding the lig-ament. When the fat pad and the synovium were resected, they noted a decrease in the vascular and repair response. It was their opinion that this study justified the recommendation of O'Donoghue[25] that the fat pad be sutured to repaired anterior cruciate ligament or substitution. These authors also noted, as Scapinelli[27] had in humans, that there was no vascular communication between the tibial tubercle and the patellar tendon attachment. Thus the patellar tendon graft, when used as a cruciate substitute, was a free graft even if left attached to the tibial tubercle.

Microangiographic, histologic, and biomechanical analyses of the medial third of a patellar tendon with its tibial and patellar bony attachments used as both an anterior and a posterior cruciate substitute was studied by Clancy and others.[9] Their studies revealed that synovialization was complete at 8 weeks and that the graft was signif-icantly revascularized. The revascularization appeared to be derived from the pos-terior synovial fold and the fat pad and endosteal vessels from the tibial and femoral tunnels. Subsequent studies at 3 months revealed complete revascularization. At 6, 9, and 12 months there was no significant change in the vascular pattern in and about the substitute.

Histologic evaluation at 8 weeks revealed that a significant portion of the graft contained viable cells. In a later study Arnoczky[3] noted a similar histologic picture. These findings tend to substantiate the theory of synovial fluid nutrition.[13] There were numerous areas where cellular invasion of the graft occurred. The leading cells in these areas appeared to be histocytes or tissue macrophages, and behind those there were abundant fibroblasts. Serial sections suggested that these macrophages were digesting the areas of necrotic graft and the fibroblasts were laying down new collagen. Histologic evaluations at 3, 6, 9, and 12 months confirmed this creeping substitution–remodeling reaction. These findings were also noted by Arnoczky.[3] At 1 year the graft used for both anterior and posterior cruciate substitution had been completely remodeled and histologically resembled a normal ligament.

Biomechanical analysis of anterior cruciate ligament substitution was performed on three rhesus monkeys at each interval of 3, 6, and 9 months and five rhesus monkeys at 12 months. Evaluation of posterior cruciate ligament substitution was performed on one rhesus monkey at 2, 3, 6, 9, and 12 months.

The control medial one-third patellar tendons with their bony attachments were 300 ± 58 N, the control anterior cruciate ligaments were 600 ± 132 N, and the control posterior cruciate ligaments were 450 ± 12 N. All failures at the time of testing were interstitial. The results of patellar tendon substitution for the anterior cruciate ligament, when compared to the control one-third patellar tendon, revealed that it was 53% at 3 months, 52% at 6 months, 81% at 9 months, and 81% at 12 months. When compared to the opposite control anterior cruciate ligaments, it was 26% at 3 months, 43% at 6 months, 38% at 9 months, and 52% at 12 months.

The posterior cruciate patellar tendon substitute, when compared to the control one-third patellar tendon, was 43% at 2 months, 75% at 3 months, 89% at 6 months, 119% at 9 months, and 71% at 12 months. When compared to the opposite control posterior cruciate ligament, it was 31% at 2 months, 51% at 3 months, 68% at 6 months, 93% at 9 months, and 47% at 12 months. Only one monkey was studied at each time interval.

It is important to note that there are certain differences in the normal strengths of the rhesus monkey's patellar tendon and anterior and posterior cruciate ligament strengths when compared to those of the human. Noyes' study[24] revealed that in humans the one-third patellar tendon with its bony attachments was approximately 175% the strength of the normal anterior cruciate ligament. In our study of rhesus monkeys, the one-third patellar tendon was only 50% the strength of the anterior cruciate ligament. Our tensile testing results for the control anterior cruciate ligament in rhesus monkeys was essentially the same as reported by Cabaud.[5] Our studies of the strength of the posterior cruciate ligament in rhesus monkeys revealed it to be only 75% the strength of the anterior cruciate ligament and the patellar tendon to be 67% the strength of the posterior cruciate ligament. Kennedy[17] found that in humans the posterior cruciate ligament was approximately 200% the strength of the anterior cruciate ligament.

In evaluating these reports and the results of our tensile testing, we can state that in rhesus monkeys the patellar tendon substitution after revascularization and recollagenization at 9 months and at 1 year regains approximately 80% of its initial strength. If this same remodeling repair would occur in the human knee, then the one-third patellar tendon substitution theoretically would achieve 150% of the strength of the anterior cruciate ligament and approximately 70% of the strength of the posterior cruciate ligament. Unfortunately, this is only a supposition that needs far more laboratory and clinical investigation.

These results would suggest that the one-third patellar tendon is more than adequate for anterior cruciate ligament substitution in humans and that its substitution for the posterior cruciate ligament may be adequate, but an additional tendon substitution may be beneficial.

The reported clinical results of the use of patellar tendon, semitendinosus and gracilis tendons, or semitendinosus tendons in humans have been most encouraging as to functional stability. The long-term reports of the patellar tendon, patellar aponeurosis, and quadriceps tendon over the top procedure have yielded reasonably good functional results, but somewhat less satisfactory static stability.[28] However, the patellar tendon with its bony attachments placed in the appropriate tibial and femoral tunnels has yielded a higher static stability result.[10] Neither of these procedures or other intraarticular biologic substitute procedures have consistently eliminated all traces of anterior tibial translation at long-term follow-up.

There are several reasons for this. First, in the majority of the patients with chronic anterior cruciate ligament instability, the secondary restraints have become lax. In addition, one or both menisci may have been removed, eliminating their stabilizing effect. The biologic substitute being avascular also develops a marked decrease in tensile strength during the first 4 to 6 months. Motion and weight bearing probably lead to some stretching out of the substitute, particularly when the secondary restraints are lax.

VASCULARIZED PATELLAR TENDON GRAFT

To combat the stretching out of the graft during the period of low tensile strength, Paulos and Noyes[26] developed the concept of trying to maintain a vascular supply to the graft with the hope of minimizing the amount of necrosis in the graft and thus maintaining a high tensile strength graft. In their procedure they try to preserve the middle superior and the middle inferior geniculate blood supply to the medial one third of the patellar tendon. A review of Scapinelli's microangiography of the human knee[27] suggests that an adequate blood supply to the patellar tendon could also be achieved by maintaining the fat pad attachment to the medial third of the patellar tendon. His study indicated that the lateral inferior geniculate blood supply coursed through the fat pad to the proximal one third of the patellar tendon. An additional contribution from the anterior tibial recurrent vessels was also noted. Thus we have for the past 2 years left the fat pad attached to the proximal one third of the patellar tendon substitute.[8] Because this fat pad pedicle is usually not of sufficient length to allow the patellar bone to be placed into the lateral femoral condyle, the graft is flipped 180 degrees so that the tibial bone is placed in the lateral femoral condyle, and the patellar bone is placed in the tibial tunnel.

A preliminary microangiographic study was performed in dogs to see if the contributions from the lateral inferior geniculate and anterior tibial recurrent vessels were sufficient, and, if so, whether or not at 10 days after substitution there was still adequate vascularity of the graft. In two dogs the medial one third of the patellar tendon with its bony attachments and fat pad pedicle was developed, but not placed in the appropriate tunnels. The femoral artery was cannulated and injected with micropaque. In two more dogs the vascularized patellar tendon graft was developed and then turned 180 degrees. The graft was placed and fixed in the appropriate tunnels, and then the femoral artery was cannulated and injected with micropaque. In two more dogs the vascularized graft was developed, turned 180 degrees, and fixed in the appropriate tunnels. The wounds were closed and the knees immobilized. At 10 days the femoral artery was cannulated and injected with micropaque. The microangiographic studies revealed that at least one dog in each study group had maintained its normal vascular pattern. These studies, as well as those of Paulos,[26] strongly suggest that a vascularized patellar tendon graft is feasible and may lead to better static stability. Long-term follow-up with accurate measurement of not only anterior-posterior tibial translation, but measurements of all planes of motion, will be necessary before one can be satisfied that substitution with a biologic substitute has achieved its desired result. To date the clinical results are most encouraging.

REFERENCES

1. Alm, A., and Strömberg, B.: Transposed medial third of patellar ligament in reconstruction of the anterior cruciate ligament: a surgical and morphologic study in dogs, Acta Chir. Scand. (suppl) **445**:37, 1974.
2. Arnoczky, S.P., Rubin, R.M., and Marshall, J.L.: The microvasculature of the cruciate ligaments and its response to injury: an experimental study in dogs, J. Bone Joint Surg. **61A**:1221, 1979.
3. Arnoczky, S.P., Tarvin, G.B., and Marshall, J.L.: Anterior cruciate ligament replacement using patellar tendon: an evaluation of graft revascularization, J. Bone Joint Surg. **64A**:217, 1982.
4. Bergfeld, J.A., and others: Two to five year evaluation of anterior cruciate reconstruction using patellar tendon and Ellison iliotibial band transfer, Paper presented at the annual meeting of the American Academy of Orthopaedic Surgeons, Anaheim, Calif., March, 1983.
5. Cabaud, H.E., Rodkey, W.G., and Feagin, J.A.: Experimental studies of acute anterior cruciate ligament injury and repair, Am. J. Sports Med. **7**:18, 1979.
6. Chiroff, R.T.: Experimental replacement of the anterior cruciate ligament: a histological and micro-radiographic study, J. Bone Joint Surg. **57A**:1124, 1975.
7. Cho, K.O.: Reconstruction of the anterior cruciate ligament by semitendinosus tenodesis, J. Bone Joint Surg. **57A**:608, 1975.
8. Clancy, W.G., Jr.: Anterior cruciate ligament functional instability: a static intraarticular and dynamic extraarticular procedure, Clin. Orthop. **172**:102, 1983.
9. Clancy, W.G., Jr., and others: Anterior and posterior cruciate ligament reconstruction in rhesus monkeys: a histological, microangiographic, and biomechanical analysis, J. Bone Joint Surg. **63A**:1270, 1981.
10. Clancy, W.G., Jr., and others: Anterior cruciate ligament reconstruction using one third of the patellar ligament augmented by extraarticular tendon transfers, J. Bone Joint Surg. **64A**:352, 1982.
11. Clancy, W.G., Jr., and others: Treatment of knee joint instability secondary to rupture of the posterior cruciate ligament, J. Bone Joint Surg. **65A**:310, 1983.
12. Ericksson, E.: Sports injuries of the knee ligaments: their diagnosis, treatment, rehabilitation, and prevention, Med. Sci. Sports **8**:133, 1976.
13. Ginsburg, J.H., Whiteside, L.A., and Piper, T.L.: Nutrient pathways in transferred patellar tendon used for anterior cruciate ligament reconstruction, Am. J. Sports Med. **8**:15, 1980.
14. Girgis, F.G., Marshall, T.L., and Al Monajem, A.R.S.: The cruciate ligaments of the knee joint: anatomical, functional, and experimental analysis, Clin. Orthop. **106**:216, 1975.
15. Jacobsen, K.: Osteoarthritis following insufficiency of the cruciate ligaments in man: a clinical study, Acta Orthop. Scand. **48**:520, 1977.
16. Kennedy, J.C., and Grainger, R.W.: The posterior cruciate ligament, J. Trauma **7**:367, 1967.
17. Kennedy, J.C., and others: Tension studies of human knee ligaments: yield point, ultimate failure, and disruption of the cruciate and tibial collateral ligaments, J. Bone Joint Surg. **58A**:350, 1976.

18. Lipscomb, A.B., and others: Secondary reconstruction of anterior cruciate ligament in athletes by using the semitendinosus tendon: preliminary report of 78 cases, Am. J. Sports Med. **7**:81, 1979.

19. MacIntosh, D.: Anterior cruciate deficient knee: natural history management of acute and chronic problems, Paper presented at the American Academy of Orthopaedic Surgeons instructional course on the athlete's knee and arthroscopy, Palm Beach, Fla., June, 1981.

20. Marshall, J.L., and Olsson, S.-E.: Instability of the knee: a long term experimental study in dogs, J. Bone Joint Surg. **53A**:1561, 1971.

21. Marshall, J.L., and others: The anterior cruciate ligament: a technique of repair and reconstruction, Clin. Orthop. **143**:97, 1979.

22. McDevitt, C.A., and Muir, H.: Biochemical changes in the cartilage of the knee in experimental and natural osteoarthritis in the dog, J. Bone Joint Surg. **58B**(1):94, 1976.

23. McMaster, J.H., Weinert, C.R., Jr., and Scranton, P., Jr.: Diagnosis and management of isolated anterior cruciate ligament tears: a preliminary report of a new procedure. Clin. Orthop. **118**:30, 1976.

24. Noyes, F.R., and others: Intraarticular cruciate ligament reconstruction, Clin. Orthop. **172**:71, 1983.

25. O'Donoghue, D.H.: A method for replacement of the anterior cruciate ligament of the knee: report of twenty cases, J. Bone Joint Surg. **45A**:905, 1963.

26. Paulos, L.E., and others: Intraarticular cruciate reconstruction. II. Replacement with vascularized patellar tendon, Clin. Orthop. **172**:78, 1983.

27. Scapinelli, R.: Studies on the vasculature of the human knee joint, Acta Anat. **70**:305, 1968.

28. Warren, R.F., and Kornblatt, I.B.: Long-term follow-up of anterior cruciate ligament reconstruction using quadriceps tendon substitution for anterior cruciate insufficiency, Paper presented at the annual meeting of the American Academy of Orthopaedic Surgeons, Anaheim, Calif., March, 1983.

29. Wirth, C.J., and Artmann, M.: Ist die Länge der Patellarsehne für die vordere Kruzbandplastik ausreichend? Arch. Orthop. Trauma Surg. **79**:149, 1974.

19. Prosthetic anterior cruciate ligament repairs: current status

H. Edward Cabaud
William G. Rodkey
John A. Feagin

Debate, research, and controversy continue over the management of the injured anterior cruciate ligament. Instability, pain, degenerative changes, disability, and even multiple surgeries may result in the patient with anterior cruciate ligament insufficiency. In an effort to resolve the problem of the acutely injured anterior cruciate ligament, we have conducted a series of experimental studies.[4-6]

Our initial studies[6] involved simple primary repairs of surgically transected anterior cruciate ligaments in dogs and monkeys. The anterior cruciate ligaments were repaired with a single size O-Dexon suture, and the limbs were immobilized for 6 weeks in long-leg casts. The animals were evaluated 4 months postoperatively, and the anterior cruciate ligaments were healed grossly in all of the monkeys and 7 of the 10 dogs. All animals, however, had degenerative joint changes, as well as functional and clinical instability. Maximum strength of the repaired anterior cruciate ligaments in the dogs was less than 10% of the normal anterior cruciate ligament.

In 1976 Feagin and Curl[10] had published the results of their 5-year follow-up study of isolated anterior cruciate ligament repairs in West Point cadets. Follow-up in 32 of the 64 patients in the operated group revealed that 12 were functionally impaired, 24 felt they were athletically handicapped, and 8 were dissatisfied with the results.

Based on evidence from the experimental and clinical studies, we reasoned that simple primary repair was not an appropriate method, and that further studies testing procedures to augment or reconstruct the injured ligament should be conducted. When an injury occurs, the anterior cruciate ligament may stretch 30% to 40% by

□ The opinions or assertions contained in this chapter are the private view of the authors and are not to be construed as official or as reflecting the views of the Department of the Army or the Department of Defense. In conducting the research described in this chapter the authors adhered to the *Guide for Laboratory Animal Facilities and Care* as promulgated by the Committee on the Guide for Laboratory Animal Resources, National Academy of Sciences, National Research Council.

the time it fails. There is a tenuous blood supply, which is markedly disrupted by an injury. Inadequate immobilization and stress following repair also may be contributing factors to an unsatisfactory result. In an effort to preclude the problems associated with primary repair, a surgical technique using the medial one third of the patellar tendon was developed to augment or reconstruct the repaired anterior cruciate ligament.[4] The purpose of this approach was to provide an additional blood supply, have the transferred patellar tendon act as an internal splint for the healing anterior cruciate ligament, and perhaps provide additional strength to the repaired complex.

Eleven dogs were used in the agumentation study. All anterior cruciate ligaments were transected at the femoral origin of the anterior cruciate ligament, since this location most commonly is associated with clinical injuries. The anterior cruciate ligament was repaired with O-Dexon sutures, and the medial one third of the patellar tendon was then transferred and placed in the intercondylar notch in the manner of Eriksson.[9] Thus the transferred patellar tendon lay adjacent to the repaired anterior cruciate ligament and supported it.

All repaired and augmented anterior cruciate ligaments healed.[4] All dogs had clinical and functional stability in the extremity. There were minimal or no degenerate changes in the joints, and a thick synovial envelope surrounded the repaired complexes. Six of the dogs were sacrificed at 4 months, and five of the dogs were sacrificed at 8 months. The load deformation curves of the failure testing are shown in Fig. 19-1. By 8 months bony ingrowth had occurred at the repair site and during mechanical testing interstitial failure occurred. In fact, one of the repaired complexes was stronger than its control anterior cruciate ligament.

As a result of this augmentation study,[4] we believe that primary repair with reconstruction or augmentation has become an accepted principle for acute ligament injuries. Although long-term studies are not yet available, augmentation has the potential to produce the best clinical result in acute anterior cruciate ligament injuries.

In the next phase of our studies, we sought to develop a biodegradable intraarticular ligament that would function as the intraarticular splint.[5] By using a biodegradable ligament, autogenous tissue grafts, such as a portion of the patella tendon, would be avoided. Potentially the need for postoperative immobilization would be precluded, and the anterior cruciate ligament could be expected to heal while the joint was allowed some protected motion.

Braided polyglycolic acid (PGA) was selected as the material of choice from which to construct the ligament. This material is strong, easy to handle, readily absorbed over 4 to 6 weeks, well-tolerated intraarticularly, and produces little tissue reaction. Several hand-braided patterns were evaluated until a Y-shaped design was selected that had physical properties that approximately matched those of the normal canine anterior cruciate ligament. Fig. 19-2 shows the comparison between a normal anterior cruciate ligament and a polyglycolic acid ligament that was used in this study.[5] The prosthetic ligament was approximately 80% as strong as a normal anterior cruciate

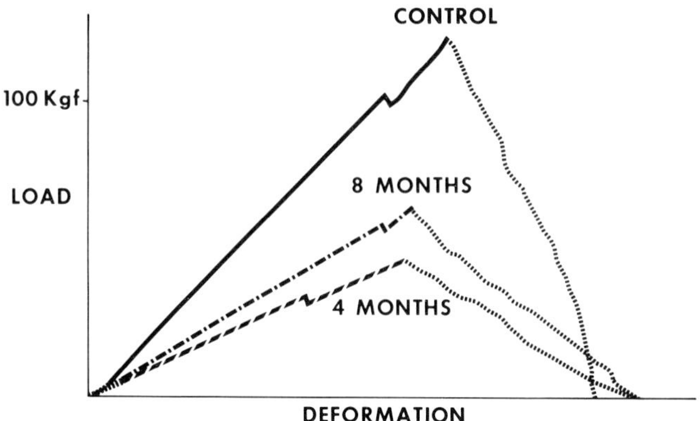

Fig. 19-1. Schematic load deformation curves of normal control dog anterior cruciate ligament compared to repaired anterior cruciate ligaments augmented with patellar tendon at 4 months and at 8 months postoperatively.

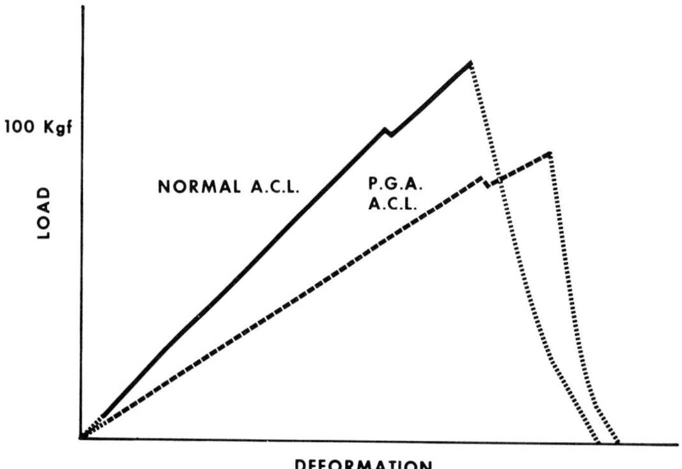

Fig. 19-2. Schematic load deformation curves of normal dog anterior cruciate ligament compared to polyglycolic acid prosthetic ligament. (From Cabaud, H. E., Feagin, J. A., and Rodkey, W. G.: Am. J. Sports Med. **10:**295, 1982.)

ligament, but it was slightly more compliant. The strains and energy absorbed to failure were similar between the normal and the prosthetic ligaments, but the prosthetic ligament had higher ultimate stress and modulus of elasticity as a result of its smaller diameter.

We evaluated the biodegradable intraarticular ligament in canine stifle joints. Following transection of the anterior cruciate ligament at the femoral condyle and repair with an O-Dexon suture, we reinforced the repair with the polyglycolic acid ligament. The tails of the Y-shaped ligament were passed through parallel drill holes in the femoral condyle. Then the bulk of the ligament was passed through a vertical hole in the tibia and two transverse holes in the tibial tubercle. The biodegradable prosthesis was placed with slightly greater tension than the O-Dexon sutures used to repair the anterior cruciate ligament.

The dogs were killed humanely, the legs were amputated, and the knee joints were evaluated. One dog was evaluated at 2 weeks postoperatively, one dog at 5 weeks, and the remaining ten dogs at 4 months, including one dog that had not been immobilized. In the dog evaluated at 2 weeks, the ligament constructed of PGA was intact with no evidence of degenerative changes, with no synovitis, and with mild residual hemorrhage from the arthrotomy. The repaired complex required over 40 kg of force (kg_f) to rupture. In the dog evaluated at 5 weeks, the majority of the prosthetic ligament had been resorbed. The remaining extraarticular portions of the ligament were still intact and showed little change from the time of their insertion. Intraarticularly there was no synovitis or degenerative changes, but a thick vascular synovial envelope had developed around the complex. Failure testing required 16 kg_f to disrupt the healing anterior cruciate ligament, which failed partially interstitially and partially from its repair site on the femoral condyle.

The remaining dogs were all evaluated 4 months postoperatively. All repaired and reinforced anterior cruciate ligaments had healed, including the one in the nonimmobilized knee. As in the augmentation study,[4] there were minimal or no degenerative changes, and a thick residual synovial envelope was present around the repaired anterior cruciate ligament. Clinical evaluation revealed that the length of the anterior cruciate ligament at 4 months was 20.4 mm, compared to a normal anterior cruciate ligament in the dog of 19.2 mm. Anterior drawer testing normally is 1 mm or less in the dog, and at 4 months five of the dogs had normal drawer tests and five measured between 2 and 3 mm. Fig. 19-3 shows load deformation tests comparing the normal canine anterior cruciate ligament with the augmented patellar tendon and the polyglycolic acid ligament reinforced curves at 4 months. In addition, several of the repaired and control anterior cruciate ligaments were incubated in tissue culture with sulfur-35 to determine proteoglycan production. This technique is an evaluation of cellular viability, and the repaired anterior cruciate ligament showed 142% more activity than the control ligaments 4 months postoperatively.

We felt that, as a result of these studies with the biodegradable polyglycolic acid ligament, it was safe, strong, well-tolerated, and had satisfactorily provided the splinting function desired to provide clinical and functional stability in the dogs. However, the material had resorbed by 5 weeks, and a ligament intended for human clinical use must provide support over a longer period of time.

This brings us to the question of a permanent prosthesis for anterior cruciate ligament reconstruction and the current status of this problem. Any permanent prosthesis must meet the functional, physiologic, and biomechanical characteristics of a normal anterior cruciate ligament.[24,26] Such a prosthesis must be biocompatible and durable, show comparable mechanical properties, and be surgically implanted with relative ease, yet allow for tissue incorporation or replacement over an appropriate period of time.

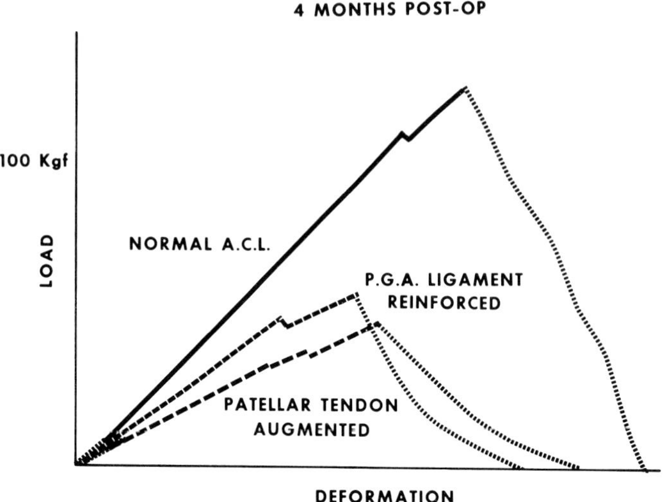

Fig. 19-3. Schematic load deformation curves of normal dog anterior cruciate ligament compared to repaired anterior cruciate ligaments either reinforced with polyglycolic acid ligament or augmented with patellar tendon at 4 months postoperatively. (From Cabaud, H. E., Feagin, J. A., and Rodkey, W. G.: Am. J. Sports Med. **10**:295, 1982.)

The anterior cruciate ligament biomechanically provides stability to the knee joint, guides joint motion, and prevents excessive motion. As surgeons we find ourselves attempting to restore biomechanic stability of the knee joint with repairs (with or without reconstruction) following acute ligament injury or with autogenous tissue reconstruction for knees with chronic instability. Currently, surgeons are considering replacing the anterior cruciate ligament with a permanent prosthesis.

Biologically a prosthetic anterior cruciate ligament could be biodegradable, biodegradable and replaced, partially biodegradable, or permanent. A variety of materials* have been evaluated, but the only truly biodegradable substance evaluated is polyglycolic acid.[5] Partially biodegradable or biodegradable and replaced materials include carbon-fiber ligamens and a PGA-Dacron material, which we are currently evaluating. Permanent materials that have been evaluated have included Dacron, Marlex, polyethylene, polypropylene, Proplast, Silastic, stainless steel, and Teflon (Table 19-1).

Our current approach is to develop a partially biodegradable ligament that undergoes controlled degradation and appropriate replacement by fibrous tissue. We have attempted to match the physical characteristics more exactly by varying weave patterns and composition, yet allow for a design in which fibrous tissue ingrowth can occur over a reasonable period of time. We believe that such a material can not only potentially be used for prosthetic repairs, either for acute injuries or chronic instability, but also for prosthetic reconstruction. The major problem in prosthetic

---

*References 2, 3, 5, 7, 8, 11-23, 25-28.

Table 19-1. Evaluation of permanent materials for prosthetic anterior cruciate ligament.

Material	Physical properties*		
	Stress	Strength	Elongation
Braided Dacron-silicon[13]	—	—	—
Braided wire[25]	—	123.75 kg$_f$†	—
Carbon fibers			
PLA coated[1]	1.5-2.76 GP$_a$	—	0.4%-3.0%
Plain[17,18]	—	—	—
Dacron (polyethylene tereph- thalate)			
Heat set[14]	40-50 psi	—	50%-80%
Knitted/Teflon coated[25]	—	29.25-40.50 kg$_f$†	—
Velour[23]	—	34.2 kg$_f$†	—
Woven[23]	—	34.2 kg$_f$†	—
Ethilon[25]	—	36.0 kg$_f$†	—
Nomex-Teflon-Proplast-carbon[16]	—	68 kg$_f$‡	2.4%†
		158 kg$_f$†	23.6%†
Polyethylene[12] (ultrahigh mo- lecular weight)	—	420 N†	10%
Polypropylene			
Braid[22]	—	1506 ± 12 N†	50 ± 1 mm§
Monofilament twisted[23]	—	9.3 kg$_f$†	—
Silastic-Dacron[26]	Variable, depending on construction		
Teflon[8]	—	115 lb†	—
Tevdek[26]	—	56.25 kg$_f$†	—

*Reported by authors or patents.
†Value at ultimate failure.
‡Value at yield point.
§Based on initial length of 250 mm.

management of anterior cruciate ligament injury or insufficiency is the intraarticular environment. There is rapid tissue breakdown, and the blood supply to the inter-condylar notch structures is limited. There is rapid absorption of degradable materials and delayed fibrous ingrowth that remains disorganized over a prolonged period of time. There are also extreme torsional and tensile stresses in the knee joint. We are exploring the literature to find methods in which we can alter the synovial fluid environment to enhance its tissue nutrition and minimize the adverse effects of the degradative enzymes.

A variety of permanent prosthetic ligaments have been evaluated. One of the initial models was a Proplast stent, which consisted of a core containing Teflon and a textile fiber coated by Proplast that contained carbon fiber to stimulate fibrosis and attachment.[16] The ligament had adequate strength and extensibility and was readily fixed with a metallic staple. The ligament was initially designed as an internal splint to ensure stability in a cast, maintain a normal path of motion in the joint, and allow sound healing of repaired and reconstructed ligaments and tendons. It was anticipated that eventual breakage would occur. The results of a clinical study using Proplast stents (19 patients) was published by Woods and others.[28] All patients had extensive extraarticular reconstruction, but at follow-up eight patients had broken stents and 50% had lost stability. Several patients required removal of the Proplast stents. They considered anterior cruciate ligament reconstruction with a Proplast stent a salvage procedure and expected this prosthetic ligament would fail.[28] The Proplast stents therefore showed more promise as ligament augmentation devices, and thus provided additional length or better fixation with patellar tendon-anterior cruciate ligament reconstructions.[28]

Dacron has been evaluated for anterior cruciate ligament reconstruction.[11,14] It is somewhat more compliant than the Proplast, shows good bony ingrowth through bony canals, and some fibrous ingrowth occurs into the interstices of the ligament. It is well-tolerated intraarticularly, but has been unsuccessful in dogs as an isolated replacement.

Arnoczky[2] has demonstrated excellent vascular ingrowth by microangiography techniques into Dacron velour grafts with associated fibrous tissue ingrowth. The fibrous tissue has remained disorganized. To date Arnoczky has not evaluated the strength of this Dacron velour reconstruction.

We are still searching for a prosthetic ligament with sufficient strength and appropriate compliance and adequate porosity to allow fibrous ingrowth. A ligament that has a scaffold principle is one possibility. Our preliminary studies with a woven PGA-Dacron combination *scaffold* has the potential of allowing fibrous tissue ingrowth as the PGA is resorbed and the Dacron fibers remain to provide the porous matrix for fibrous ingrowth. The weave pattern that we have evaluated is not satisfactory; as the PGA is resorbed the weave pattern becomes more open and allows a markedly increased compliance of the prosthetic ligament.

Studies of carbon fibers and carbon fibers coated with polylactic acid as ligament replacements have been conducted both in animals and in humans.[1,3,17,18] Although the carbon fibers stimulate extensive fibrosis and collagen formation as they break up and degrade, as anterior cruciate ligament replacements these materials have not been successful. The carbon fiber is extremely brittle and has insufficient elasticity to meet the demands of the anterior cruciate ligament. To protect the carbon fibers in the intraarticular environment, it appears that an autogenous tissue graft, such as the semitendinosus or patellar tendon, is required.

The question remains: is a composite graft needed to meet both the mechanical demands and fibrous tissue ingrowth requirements? A composite permanent prosthesis developed in Canada constructed of a compressible Silastic core covered by high tensile Dacron fibers woven over the Silastic has appropriate mechanical properties, yet the complexity of this design would not withstand the test of time in the knee joint nor would it allow fibrous tissue ingrowth.[26]

Collagenous tissues undergo plastic deformation before failure. The anterior cruciate ligament is no exception. It has an elastic phase in its physical properties that allows 20% to 30% deformation before reaching the plastic phase.[6] Loading of ligaments in this phase would allow collagenous tissues to remodel under mechanical demands, and we believe the loading would convert unorganized weak fibrous tissue into organized stronger tissue that can withstand the stresses of a normal cruciate ligament. Once satisfactory bony fixation is achieved with a prosthetic ligament, gradual transition of the loads from the prosthetic ligament to the regrown or ingrown fibrous tissue should allow a permanent prosthesis to function over a prolonged period of time. We believe that a synthetic substitute is needed. Limited success with ligament augmentation devices has already been apparent. Polypropylene stents as augmentation devices have been used in goats and in humans with encouraging results.[20]

The clinical and investigational goals are momentous, but achievements in newly formulated materials, both biodegradable and permanent, as well as improvement in surgical technique with a better understanding of the anatomy and mechanics will facilitate development of prosthetic ligaments. The goals that we must strive for include the development of a prosthesis that is biologically compatible, has adequate strength and compliance, is easy to insert surgically or potentially arthroscopically, mechanically functions as a normal anterior cruciate ligament, and yet provides a satisfactory scaffold for fibrous tissue ingrowth.

REFERENCES

1. Alexander, H., and others: Bioabsorbable composite tissue scaffold, U.S. Patent 4,329,743, May 18, 1982.
2. Arnoczky, S.P.: Personal communication, Feb. 1, 1982.
3. Butler, H.C.: Teflon as a prosthetic ligament in repair of ruptured anterior cruciate ligaments, Am. J. Vet. Res. **25**:55, 1964.
4. Cabaud, H.E., Feagin, J.A., and Rodkey, W.G.: Acute anterior cruciate ligament injury and augmented repair, Am. J. Sports Med. **8**:395, 1980.
5. Cabaud, H.E., Feagin, J.A., and Rodkey, W.G.: Acute anterior cruciate ligament injury and repair reinforced with a biodegradable intraarticular ligament: experimental studies, Am. J. Sports Med. **10**:259, 1982.
6. Cabaud, H.E., Rodkey, W.G., and Feagin, J.A.: Experimental studies of acute anterior cruciate ligament injury and repair, Am. J. Sports Med. **7**:18, 1979.
7. Denny, H.R., and Goodship, A.E.: Replacement of the anterior cruciate ligament with carbon fibre in the dog, J. Small Anim. Pract. **21**:279, 1980.
8. Emery, M.A., and Rostrup, O.: Repair of the anterior cruciate ligament with 8 mm tube Teflon in dogs, Can. J. Surg. **4**:111, 1960.
9. Eriksson, E.: Sports injuries of the knee ligaments: their diagnosis, treatment, rehabilitation, and prevention, Med. Sci. Sports **8**:133, 1976.
10. Feagin, J.A., and Curl, W.W.: Isolated tear of the anterior cruciate ligament: 5-year follow-up study, Am. J. Sports Med. **4**:95, 1976.
11. Gerdes, M.H., Haynes, D.W., and Nelson, C.L.: The failure of Dacron as an anterior cruciate ligament, Trans. Orthop. Res. Soc. New Orleans **7**:257, 1982.
12. Grood, E.S., and Noyes, F.R.: Cruciate ligament prosthesis: strength, creep, and fatigue properties, J. Bone Joint Surg. **58A**:1083, 1976.
13. Gupta, B.N., and Brinker, W.D.: Anterior cruciate ligament prosthesis in the dog, J. Am. Vet. Med. Assoc. **154**:1057, 1969.
14. Hoffman, H.L.: Ligament and tendon prosthesis of polyethylene terephthalate and method of preparing same, U.S. Patent 4,209,859, July 1, 1980.

15. Hinko, P.J.: The use of a prosthetic ligament in repair of the torn anterior cruciate ligament in the dog, J. Am. Anim. Hosp. Assoc. **17**:563, 1981.
16. James, S.L., Woods, G.W., and Hornst, C.A.: Cruciate ligament stents in reconstruction of the unstable knee: A preliminary report, Clin. Orthop. **143**:90, 1979.
17. Jenkins, D.H.R.: The repair of cruciate ligaments with flexible carbon fibre: a longer term study of the induction of new ligaments and of the fate of the implanted carbon, J. Bone Joint Surg. **60B**:520, 1978.
18. Jenkins, D.H.R.: The role of flexible carbon-fibre implants as tendon and ligament substitutes in clinical practice, J. Bone Joint Surg. **62B**:497, 1980.
19. Johnson, F.L.: Use of braided nylon as a prosthetic anterior cruciate ligament of the dog, J. Am. Vet. Med. Assoc. **137**:646, 1960.
20. Kennedy, J.C.: Intraarticular replacement in an anterior cruciate ligament-deficient knee, Am. J. Sports Med. **8**:1, 1980.
21. Leighton, R.L., and Brightman, A.H.: Experimental and clinical evaluation of a new prosthetic anterior cruciate ligament in the dog, J. Am. Anim. Hosp. Assoc. **12**:735, 1976.
22. McPherson, G.K., Mendenhall, H.V., and Sanford, T.B.: Mechanical properties of polypropylene braid: an augmentation device for anterior cruciate ligament repair, Proceedings of the seventh annual meeting of the Society for Biomaterials, Troy, New York, May 28-31, 1981.
23. Meyers, J.F., Grana, W.A., and Lasker, P.A.: Reconstruction of the anterior cruciate ligament in the dog, Am. J. Sports Med. **7**:85, 1979.
24. Noyes, F.R., and others: Comparative mechanical properties of prosthetic primate and human cruciate ligaments, Trans. Orthop. Res. Soc. New Orleans **1**:15, 1976.
25. Saidi, K., Beauchamp, P., and Laurin, C.A.: Prosthetic replacement of the anterior cruciate ligament in dogs, Can. J. Surg. **19**:547, 1976.
26. Tremblay, G.R., Laurin, C.A., and Drovin, G.: The challenge of prosthetic ligament replacements, Clin. Orthop. **147**:88, 1980.
27. Vaughan, L.C.: A study of the replacement of the anterior cruciate ligament in the dog by fascia, skin, and nylon, Vet. Res. **75**:537, 1963.
28. Woods, G.W., Hornsy, D., and Prewith, J.: Proplast leader for use in cruciate ligament reconstruction, Am. J. Sports Med. **7**:314, 1979.

Index